W9-CLY-798

OUTSMARTING
Alzheimer's
What *You* Can Do to Reduce Your Risk

- Understand the six keys to protecting brain health
- Personalize your 3-week plan based on the latest science
- Make fun and easy lifestyle changes

Kenneth S. Kosik, MD
with Alisa Bowman

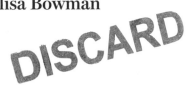
DISCARD

Reader's
digest

The Reader's Digest Association, Inc.
New York, NY • Montreal

A READER'S DIGEST BOOK

Copyright © 2015 Trusted Media Brands, Inc. (fka The Reader's Digest
Association, Inc.)
All rights reserved. Unauthorized reproduction, in any manner, is prohibited.
Reader's Digest is a registered trademark of Trusted Media Brands, Inc.

Fitness illustrations by Alison Muñoz.

Library of Congress Cataloging-in-Publication Data
Kosik, K. S. (Kenneth S.), 1950-
  Outsmarting alzheimer's : what you can do to reduce your risk / Kenneth S. Kosik,
MD, with Alisa Bowman.
      pages cm
  Includes bibliographical references and index.
  ISBN 978-1-62145-244-7 (hardback) -- ISBN 978-1-62145-348-2 (paperback) --
ISBN 978-1-62145-245-4 (epub) 1. Alzheimer's disease--Prevention. 2. Self-care,
Health. I. Title.
  RC523.K68 2015
  616.8'31--dc23
                    2015025509

We are committed to both the quality of our products and the service we provide
to our customers. We value your comments, so please feel free to contact us.
          Reader's Digest Adult Trade Publishing
          44 South Broadway
          White Plains, NY 10601

For more Reader's Digest products and information, visit our website:
          www.rd.com (in the United States)
          www.readersdigest.ca (in Canada)

Printed in China

10 9 8 7 6 5 4 3 2 (HC)
10 9 8 7 6 5 4 3 2 1 (PB)

NOTE TO OUR READERS
The information in this book should not be substituted for, or used to alter,
medical therapy without your doctor's advice. For a specific health problem,
consult your physician for guidance.

Mention of specific companies, organizations, or authorities in this book
does not imply endorsement by the author or publisher, nor does mention of
specific companies, organizations, or authorities imply that they endorse
this book, its author, or the publisher. The brand-name products mentioned
in this book are trademarks or registered trademarks of their respective
companies. Internet addresses and telephone numbers given in this book
were accurate at the time it went to press.

R0448910447

Contents

Introduction

If you picked up a book like this one 20 years ago, you'd find little hope between its covers. Back then, many scientists believed that dementia (a noticeable loss of mental functioning caused by Alzheimer's or any number of other brain diseases) was a natural and inevitable consequence of aging.

In your 40s or 50s, so it was thought, you'd start to experience mild "senior moments," such as occasionally losing your reading glasses or car keys. Into your 60s and 70s, you'd increasingly find that you'd walked into a room but had forgotten why. Maybe, during conversations, you'd lose your train of thought. New tasks, such as learning how to program the television, would make your head hurt. If you were fortunate enough to live into your 80s and 90s, your mind would continue to unravel. Your family members would seem like strangers. Eventually you'd no longer remember basic self-care and personal hygiene. Ultimately you'd die from infections like pneumonia or bed sores.

The only thing that would stop you from eventually dying of complications from dementia: dying of heart disease, cancer, or some other disease first.

Well, I'm happy to report that all of this has dramatically changed for the better. More than 73,000 research papers about causes and treatments for dementia have been published in the past 20 years. That's an average of 10 papers a day.[1] In recent years, thanks to the development of functional magnetic resonance imaging (fMRI for short), we've been able to peer inside of the human brain while people are still alive, studying brain activity in real time. This new tool has led to several exciting, scientific developments that have changed our understanding of the aging brain and also of Alzheimer's disease, the most common cause of dementia. We now know that:

Our brains are remarkably resilient. They're not stuck in time. Rather, they're capable of maintaining and repairing themselves, a phenomenon we refer to as *plasticity*. This is why some stroke victims eventually recover and regain the ability to talk and move. Their brains build new connections, relearning how to form words and how to move affected muscles. This is particularly true if we provide our brains with what they need to complete these important maintenance tasks. Just as a state-of-the-art highway system needs maintenance work-ers, new asphalt, and the occasional construction crew to change continually for the better, our brains need a rich environment with social, cognitive, and physical stimulation. *Outsmarting Alzheimer's* will show you how to create the optimum environment for continual brain maintenance. The Brain Smarts prescriptions in Part Two will teach you what you need to do to remodel your brain for the better.

Old brains can grow new cells. The size of your brain is, in part, determined by the number of brain cells (also called *neurons*) it contains. If new brain cells are created at the same pace that older cells die off, your brain volume remains constant. If cells die off faster than cells are created, the brain shrinks, and cog-nitive health declines. What does it take to stop the brain from shrinking as we age? Exercise, a healthy diet, a rich social life, good sleep habits, and a combina-tion of other Brain Smarts suggested in *Outsmarting Alzheimer's*. These strate-gies can protect your brain even if you are genetically predisposed to developing Alzheimer's disease. When researchers from the Cleveland Clinic in Ohio used fMRI machines to scan the brains of 100 men and women who had a family history of Alzheimer's disease, they found that the hippocampal brain regions of people who exercised remained the same size over an 18-month period, a time period that would normally be associated with a small amount of brain shrink-age.[2] Other research finds that a healthy lifestyle, similar to what we suggest in *Outsmarting Alzheimer's*, can even *increase* the volume of the hippocampus by 1 to 2 percent over one year.[3] This is important because the hippocampus is the region of the brain most affected by Alzheimer's disease.

When we change our lifestyles for the better, our brains change for the better, too. I've spent the past 25 years researching Alzheimer's disease, first at Harvard Medical School and later at University of California, Santa Barbara. As a neurologist, I've treated patients who either have already been diagnosed with Alzheimer's disease or who are at risk for developing it. During this time, I've watched as fascinating research trends have unfolded. On the one hand, studies have dashed our hopes over and over again when it comes to finding a prescrip-tion medicine or technological treatment for Alzheimer's disease. On the other hand, a vast and growing body of research shows that lifestyle habits—what you eat, whether you exercise, how you sleep, the quality of your social connections, what you do to buffer stress, whether you challenge your mind—can dramatically reduce your risk for developing this disease.

Risk is a statistical term that describes your chances of getting a disease. We all have some risk for developing Alzheimer's disease, but some of us—because of our genes, a history of concussions, and high blood pressure, among many other factors—are at a greater risk than others, just as people who live in Seattle are at a greater risk of experiencing a rainy day than people who live in San Diego. No matter your current level of risk, however, you can reduce the chances of suffering the symptoms of Alzheimer's disease, just as people who live in Seattle reduce their risk of getting wet by carrying umbrellas wherever they go.

Scientists and researchers have never been more optimistic about our ability to help you tackle this disease. A recent statistical review concluded that modifiable risk factors—things like diabetes, inactivity, smoking, high blood pressure, depression, lack of education, and so on—contributed to a third or more cases of Alzheimer's disease.[4] Other research estimates that lifestyle changes may prevent as many as half of all Alzheimer's cases.[5]

Yes, healthy living has always been a good idea. This, in itself, is not news. Depending on how closely you follow breaking health news, the strategies that will help you reduce your risk for Alzheimer's disease may or may not seem familiar. You've heard that you should exercise and eat more vegetables, for example, to reduce your risk for heart disease, diabetes, cancer, and many other diseases. But, until recently, the incredible impact of healthy living on the brain wasn't clear.

Alzheimer's disease, perhaps the most frightening disease we know, does not have to loom in your later years as some inevitable fate. It's not an inevitable consequence of aging, a condition for which we have no cure, but a disease that every single one of us can combat with clear and effective steps.

Many years of scientific evidence have revealed the risk factors for Alzheimer's disease as well as the strategies to reduce many of those risks. So why not embrace these strategies? Just as you save for retirement, why not put good-health bucks in your cognitive account? Why not rack up some cognitive savings by adopting the brain-healthy habits so you are less likely to incur the problems that are shockingly common among seniors? Why not provide yourself with the best chance for enjoying the happiest time of your life? Yes, the happiest time! Among all age groups, seniors are the happiest, with one exception: those in poor health.

The suggestions here don't require testing and treatment from a tertiary care center. In fact, much of what is in this book does not require a doctor at all. That's because, in *Outsmarting Alzheimer's*, we are focusing on health whereas, unfortunately, the medical system is preoccupied with disease. Few doctors will take the time to fully explain the lifestyle habits that affect your health and keep your brain in top shape. In contrast, we have packed this book with 80 suggestions that will help you live out your senior years with happiness, good health, and a sharp mind.

Not long ago, a team of Finnish and Swedish researchers revealed the encouraging results of a large study that followed more than a thousand people aged 66 to 77 who were considered to be at high risk for developing Alzheimer's disease. It was called the Finnish Geriatric Intervention Study to Prevent

Cognitive Impairment and Disability (FINGER), and the initial results were just published in the spring of 2015.[6] After several years, study participants who overhauled their lifestyles to include nutritious eating, regular exercise, and intellectual pursuits performed at least 25 percent better on tests of memory, thinking, and problem solving than did other study participants who didn't take steps to improve their lifestyles. On tests of executive function (the ability to organize and regulate thought processes), they scored 83 percent higher, and their processing speed (how quickly they responded to new information) was 150 percent higher. All told, this was enough to delay a dementia diagnosis by two years, and reduce the prevalence by 25 percent. Had the interventions been started earlier in life, there's good reason to suspect that the results would have been even more dramatic.[7]

A separate study by a team at Rush University Medical Center in Chicago found that people who consumed a diet rich in leafy greens, veggies, nuts, berries, beans, and other wholesome foods slashed their risk for Alzheimer's disease by up to 53 percent over nearly five years.[8]

Finally, based on results from nearly 2,000 people enrolled in the Mayo Clinic Study of Aging, we also know that intellectual hobbies like the ones suggested in Chapter 7 may delay Alzheimer's symptoms by up to 10 years.[9, 10] In other words, if, based on your genes and past lifestyle, you would have normally developed problems with memory and thinking around age 85, intellectual pursuits may postpone those symptoms until around age 95.

It was research results like the ones I just described that prompted me to start the Center for Cognitive Fitness and Innovative Therapies (CFIT) in Santa Barbara in 2009. CFIT was one of the first programs in the country dedicated to helping people reduce their risk for Alzheimer's disease. I wanted to help people adopt lifestyle habits that would help them avoid getting this disease altogether or, at the very least, put off its symptoms for as long as possible. When people came to CFIT, they were cared for by a comprehensive team of professionals that included nutritionists, exercise physiologists, stress-reduction experts, physical therapists, and cognitive psychologists. Rather than a medical center, it was more like a gym for the brain.

The recommendations in this book are based on the practical lessons I learned from CFIT as well as the extensive medical literature. The prescriptions you'll find within *Outsmarting Alzheimer's* pages represent the best thinking on how to reduce your risk of developing this terrible disease.

Now Is the Time to Outsmart Alzheimer's

It really is possible to live into your 60s, 70s, 80s, and beyond with sharp wits and excellent powers of recall. You can outsmart Alzheimer's disease, and enjoy old age with a healthy, vibrant mind. *Outsmarting Alzheimer's* will show you the way. Throughout the pages of *Outsmarting Alzheimer's,* you'll find scientifically sound strategies that have been shown to reduce your risk for poor brain health and cognitive deterioration such as memory loss. When incorporated into your life, these strategies can help to:

Reduce your risk of developing Alzheimer's disease. In the past few years there's been a shift in the thinking for many of us who study dementia. We've come to the conclusion that the best time to treat Alzheimer's disease is *before* the earliest symptoms surface.

This shift has been brought on by new technology that allows us to peer inside the human brain. In 2012 the US Food and Drug Administration approved the use of a substance (called a *tracer*) that could be injected into the bloodstream and allow specific substances in the brain to light up during a positron emission tomography (PET) scan. Thanks to this and other techniques, we now know that the Alzheimer's plaques begin to proliferate 10 or even 20 years before the first Alzheimer's symptoms become noticeable.[11]

This is not unlike other disease processes. Take heart disease. Long before the first hint of chest pain, fatty deposits are silently coating artery walls. By the time you first feel chest pain or suffer from shortness of breath, you're well on your way to having your first heart attack. It's the same with cancer. Tumors silently grow long before the first ache, bout of fatigue, or dizziness. In all of these diseases, it's during this silent phase that treatment is most effective.

Yet most people are diagnosed with Alzheimer's only after serious symptoms have already set in. By this time many brain cells have died or become irreparably damaged because they have filled up with rope like structure called *tangles* that strangle the cells. At the same time the space between the cells fills up with a hardened, sticky protein called *plaque*. Together the *plaques* and *tangles* make up the classic hallmarks of Alzheimer's disease. Treating Alzheimer's at this stage is a lot like treating cancer after it has already spread throughout the body or like treating heart disease after the first heart attack has already taken place. It's much more effective to treat these diseases during their earliest stages—and even more effective to prevent them from developing in the first place. Though we don't currently have a widely available diagnostic test that can definitively predict whether the Alzheimer's disease process is already silently spreading through your brain, there are a few clues that can give you a sense of your current level of risk, and you'll learn more about them in Chapter 2. No matter how many or how few risk factors you may have, however, now is the best time to incorporate the strategies from *Outsmarting Alzheimer's* into your life.

Delay the onset of Alzheimer's disease. Maybe you're reading this book because you're already experiencing frustrating episodes of forgetting. If so, you may be wondering, "Is it too late?" New research from Sweden's Karolinska

Institutet's FINGER trial mentioned earlier tells us that it's not. I mentioned this research just a few pages back. After following the health outcomes of more than 1,200 people over two years, the researchers found that even people already experiencing early symptoms of dementia benefited from a comprehensive program that included Brain Smart eating, exercise, intellectual pursuits, and medical care. They performed better on tests of memory, planning, judgment, and problem solving than did other study participants who didn't participate in the same program.[12] This was true of all of the study participants who took part in the program, even those in their late 70s. So I hope it's comforting to know that it may never be too late to take steps to improve your brain's health. No matter your age and no matter how many symptoms you have, a healthy lifestyle can help. In *Outsmarting Alzheimer's* you'll find dozens of simple strategies to slow the progression of the disease as much as possible, delaying the full onset of the disease by as many as 10 years.[13, 14]

Improve your well-being. *Outsmarting Alzheimer's* is for *everyone* affected by Alzheimer's disease. Whether you are trying to prevent Alzheimer's disease, already have it, or are caring for someone who does, you'll find advice to help you to reduce stress, live life to the fullest, and find peace of mind.

Who Benefits from *Outsmarting Alzheimer's*?

In short, just about everyone.

IF YOU ARE YOUNG AND/OR HEALTHY: *Outsmarting Alzheimer's* can help you remain mentally sharp for years to come. It's never too early to take steps to reduce your risk of Alzheimer's disease.

IF YOU WANT TO PERFORM AT YOUR BEST: The prescriptions in Part Two of this book can help you boost your brain power at any age and for many different lifestyle pursuits, including sporting activities and even demanding careers. This side benefit became clear to me years ago when, one day, a perfectly fit 45-year-old athlete showed up in our Cognitive Fitness Center. I asked him why he came and he said that for an athlete, the razor-thin edge between coming in first or second is totally a matter of mind, so he wanted to be sure his brain was optimized for top performance. His testing revealed a slightly elevated systolic blood pressure, which is a clear risk for cognitive decline later in life. His blood pressure was easily treatable, and we were able to drop his risk for developing Alzheimer's and help him protect his competitive edge, too.

IF ALZHEIMER'S DISEASE RUNS IN YOUR FAMILY: You are at a higher risk of developing this terrible disease than someone who doesn't have a family history of Alzheimer's, but an Alzheimer's diagnosis isn't necessarily inevitable. For one, there's a 50 percent chance that you didn't inherit the gene that has affected your other family members. Two, even if you did inherit the gene, the right foods, exercise, and other lifestyle changes may allow you to outsmart your genetic heritage.

IF YOU ARE EXPERIENCING THE EARLIEST SYMPTOMS OF ALZHEIMER'S: Lifestyle changes may allow you to slow the progression of the disease, putting off further mental decline for as long as possible.

IF YOU ARE CARING FOR SOMEONE WITH ALZHEIMER'S: You'll not only learn how to bolster the health of your loved one but also how to ease the stress of caregiving.

The Myths of Alzheimer's Disease

Why aren't more people taking steps to reduce their risk of Alzheimer's disease? The answer to that question is complex, but at least some of it stems from pervasive societal myths about who is at risk for this disease. Understanding these myths can help you to put them in their place, as well as find the motivation you need to get off the couch, stock the fridge with produce, and sign up for that yoga class. Let's take a look at some of the more common myths that may stand between you and your ability to outsmart Alzheimer's.

Myth #1: "If I live long enough, I will get Alzheimer's disease." Many people assume that forgetting and a lack of mental clarity are normal consequences of aging. They're not, and the best way to show this is with a story about a remarkable autopsy. Within hours after 115-year-old Hendrikje van Andel-Schipper died of cancer, scientists transported the Dutch woman's body to the University of Groningen in the Netherlands. As expected, during autopsy they found tumors in Andel-Schipper's stomach, liver, kidneys, and armpit. It's what they didn't find that stunned them. In her brain, they'd expected to see tangles of dead or damaged cells and clusters of plaque, both signs of Alzheimer's disease. To their amazement, however, they found no hardened plaque and very few tangles. Her blood vessels were equally free of disease. And when the scientists tediously counted the number of a specific type of brain cell in one part of Andel-Schipper's brain—and then counted again just to be sure—the tally reached higher than 16,000, roughly the number of cells they would have expected to find in a healthy 60-year-old in the equivalent region of the brain. They concluded, ". . . in contrast to general belief, the [age] limits of human cognitive function may extend far beyond the range that is currently enjoyed by most individuals. . . ."[15]

She's no anomaly. Though scientists didn't have the opportunity to dissect their brains, we can infer from their life accomplishments that many others lived into old age with vibrant cognitive health. The artist Pablo Picasso produced a torrent of etchings and paintings in the years just before his death at age 92. Actor George Burns won an Academy Award at the age of 79, starred in a film just two years before his death at age 100, and remained witty. When asked his secret of achieving old age, he famously said, "If you live past one hundred, you've got it made. Very few people die past that age." Jimmy Carter, Henry Kissinger, Betty White, and many others have remained sharp-witted well into their 90s.

And then there's Jeanne Calment, who lived to age 122. French neuropsychologist and epidemiologist Karen Ritchie examined Calment four years before her death. Ritchie found that the then 118-year-old Calment was incredibly sharp-witted. After meeting with Calment several different times over a period of many months, Ritchie concluded that Calment had "no evidence . . . of senile dementia."[16]

Can I promise that *Outsmarting Alzheimer's* will help you stay sharp and vibrant until your hundredth birthday and beyond? No, but I can promise you this: The solutions and personalized approach in this book will definitely *give you your best shot at doing so.*

Myth #2: "If Alzheimer's disease runs in my family, I'll eventually get it no matter what I do." The genes that we inherit from our parents do influence whether we will eventually develop Alzheimer's disease, among others. But we've learned that they don't predict our future with absolute certainty. Whether we carry an Alzheimer's gene or not, our risk for developing the disease doubles every five years after age 65, and it reaches nearly 50 percent after age 85. In other words, we all have close to a 50 percent chance of developing Alzheimer's disease after age 85.[17] For someone who has one copy of the *ApoE4* gene, however, risk reaches 50 percent a decade earlier, by age 75. Someone with two copies of this gene (inheriting one from each parent) has a 50 percent chance of developing Alzheimer's disease by age 65.

Those statistics, however, are not quite as dire as they may seem. First, while *ApoE4* raises risk, other genes may also be present that lower risk. Second, as research is showing, with Brain Smarts, you can outsmart the *ApoE4* gene and diminish the likelihood of future cognitive impairment.

For example, in one study, fit study participants who were carriers of the *ApoE4* gene had brain scans comparable to those of people at low risk for developing Alzheimer's disease, whereas sedentary study participants who were carriers of the same gene experienced a 3 percent shrinkage in this area of the brain over the same period of months.[18] In another study, participants who were carriers of the *ApoE4* gene were able to postpone the development of Alzheimer's disease by almost a decade if they spent their adult lives immersed in intellectually enriching activities.[19]

It's important to understand, however, that you can't outsmart all Alzheimer's genes. Several years ago, neurologist Francisco Lopera told me of 12 interrelated families in Antioquia, Colombia, whose members were experiencing Alzheimer's symptoms often around age 45. For most people, dementia symptoms don't set in until after age 65 or later. Intrigued, I agreed to help Lopera discover the gene mutation that might be at work. We soon learned that the extended family members with early-onset dementia numbered in the thousands, and they were passing on a segment of DNA from one generation to the next that contained a defective gene called *presenilin 1* (PSEN1).[20] If one parent has this particular gene mutation, there's a 50 percent chance that each of his or her children will have it, too. Those who inherit the mutant gene will develop early-onset Alzheimer's and, at the moment, there's nothing they can do to stop it.

I tell you the story of this large Colombian family because sometimes people confuse the *ApoE4* with this or other PSEN1 gene mutations that they may have heard or read about in news reports, mistakenly thinking that, based on their family history, an Alzheimer's diagnosis is inevitable when, in reality, it's not. If you have a strong family history of Alzheimer's disease, you can quickly get a sense of which gene your family members are likely passing down by considering two questions:

1. Have any of your family members developed Alzheimer's *before* age 60?

2. Did you develop Alzheimer's symptoms *before* age 60?

If you answered "no" to both questions, then you probably do not have one of the rare, very serious mutations such as the one in the presenilin gene. Yes, you may have one or two copies of *ApoE4*, but these are the genes you can challenge and possibly outsmart.

If you answered "yes" to either or both questions, remember that these gene mutations are exceedingly rare, so you may not have any detectable mutation. However, you may wish to undergo genetic testing. Genetic testing is expensive, and it is not usually reimbursed by insurance. It's also a serious undertaking, which not only affects you but also your children and your grandchildren. But it may help you to plan for the future.

Myth #3: "I don't need to worry about Alzheimer's disease because no one in my family has it." It may surprise you to know that you can develop Alzheimer's disease even if you can't think of one family member with this disease.[21] We're all at risk for Alzheimer's. Remember the statistics I mentioned earlier: We all have a 50 percent chance of developing Alzheimer's disease after age 85.[22] Most people diagnosed with late-onset Alzheimer's disease do not test positive as carriers for any of the known Alzheimer's genes.[23]

In addition to genetics, many other factors play a role in determining your risk for developing Alzheimer's. You may be at higher risk for Alzheimer's because of a past history of concussions, because of high blood pressure or another health problem, or because of your lifestyle.

No matter whether you can trace Alzheimer's disease through several generations of your family or not, it's still important to take steps to outsmart this disease. This disease is very common as we age, so everyone is at risk.

The Different Types of Alzheimer's Disease

Early-onset Alzheimer's disease: If you are diagnosed with Alzheimer's disease before age 60, then you're said to have the early-onset type. This type of Alzheimer's is rare, affecting less than 5 percent of the 5.3 million people living with Alzheimer's disease.[24] It's usually inherited and tends to progress more quickly than the late-onset type.

Late-onset Alzheimer's disease: The other 95 percent of people with Alzheimer's disease have the late-onset type. This form of Alzheimer's is diagnosed after age 60. Though genetics can increase your risk for developing late-onset Alzheimer's, your lifestyle can influence how those genes ultimately play out.

How You'll Outsmart Alzheimer's Disease

In the United States, about 5.3 million people have Alzheimer's disease. To put that in perspective, that's the same number of every single man, woman, and child currently living in Scotland. Worldwide, the numbers are even more staggering, reaching 36 million people.[25]

And those numbers are growing. By 2030, it's estimated that 66 million people will have Alzheimer's disease; by 2050, 115 million.[26]

Alzheimer's disease is one of the biggest worries that we have as we age, and yet it's hard to find viable medical solutions. To date, there is no surgery, procedure, or medicine that can cure Alzheimer's disease. The available Alzheimer's medications do not modify the disease course; they simply provide modest amelioration of symptoms for a short time, and they don't work for everyone.

Now for the good news: You may not need prescription Alzheimer's medication to outsmart this terrible disease. Within the pages of this book, you'll find everything necessary to create your best chances of beating it. The Brain Smart prescriptions in Part Two can all be found outside of a pharmacy. More important, they're fun, pleasurable, and easy to adopt.

And they may surprise you.

Did you know that within the produce section of your grocery store are countless ways to reduce your risk for Alzheimer's? Or that you're lowering your risk of Alzheimer's every time you plan a dinner party and puzzle over what to cook, who should sit next to whom, and how to ensure all your dishes are ready around the same time the guests arrive? Planning, which we call executive function, is an excellent brain excercise.

How fun would it be to know when you step out onto the dance floor you are taking a step away from Alzheimer's? How relaxing and soothing would it be to know that you're protecting your brain whenever you unroll your yoga mat, take a morning walk, or relax with a short, early afternoon power nap? Did you know that a morning cup of coffee may prevent this disease, but a late afternoon cup of joe might *increase* your risk? Or that one glass of wine with dinner offers delicious protection, but more glasses after dinner do not?

How motivating would it be to know that all of those hobbies and interests that you've been putting off—acting lessons, world travel, singing, even bingo— work to reduce your risk of getting Alzheimer's disease?

It's all true. These are just a few examples of the dozens of prescriptions you'll find throughout the pages of this book. They all add up to a well-rounded, comprehensive, and personalized plan that will help you to powerfully improve the health of your blood vessels, your heart, your cells, and, yes, your brain—for the better. In *Outsmarting Alzheimer's*, I'll share with you the six keys that have the most scientific evidence for protecting the health of your brain. These keys form the Brain Smart Plan:

S = Social Smarts. Slash your risk of cognitive decline by leaning on the support of your friends and family.[27]

M = Meal Smarts. Key diets from around the world have been shown to reduce disease, improve longevity, and protect the health of the brain. Rich in plant foods and low in highly processed foods, these eating patterns preserve brain function and overall health.[28, 29] Here's more: Brain Smart eating includes many of the foods and beverages you already have come to know and love: fruit, coffee, wine, and much more.

A = Aerobic Smarts. The more you move, the fewer brain cells you lose. Exercise may even boost the production of new brain cells.[30] Best of all: Brain Smarts are easier to fit into your schedule than you may think. You can take powerful steps to boost your physical fitness in just seven minutes a day. Learn more in Chapter 5.

R = Resilience Smarts. Long-term, unremitting stress is bad for your entire body, including your brain. So are depression, anxiety, and other chronic emotional problems, raising your risk of Alzheimer's by as much as 135 percent! On the other hand, meditation, deep breathing, massage, and other relaxing activities help to keep the brain resilient, so it more easily weathers daily stressors. Also, not all stress is bad for the brain. Some of it actually keeps your brain sharp. Learn the difference in Chapter 6.[31]

T = Train-Your-Brain Smarts. The more you challenge your brain—by learning new languages, playing musical instruments, contemplating brain teasers, and more—the better your brain's ability to fend off Alzheimer's. Based on results from nearly 2,000 people enrolled in the Mayo Clinic Study of Aging, we know that a college education, a mentally demanding profession, and intellectually engaging hobbies all have the ability to delay declines in brain functioning. Study participants who were carriers of one of the Alzheimer's genes were able to postpone the development of Alzheimer's disease by almost a decade if they spent their adult lives immersed in intellectually enriching activities. Study participants without the gene postponed the development of the disease even longer.[32]

S = Sleep Smarts. Men who reported poor sleep habits had a higher risk of developing Alzheimer's disease within the next 40 years compared to men who reported normal sleep.[33] But this doesn't necessarily mean you must force yourself to sleep seven to nine hours every night. Nor do we know yet whether improved sleep habits will reduce risk. Nevertheless, find out the best amount of sleep for your body—as well as several effective strategies to ensure the sleep you do get is more restorative—in Chapter 8.

In addition to the Brain Smart prescriptions in Part Two, be sure to know your numbers. By numbers, I'm talking about the test results for health conditions that can affect your cognitive health. Those include your blood pressure, cholesterol, and blood sugar levels. When these numbers fall outside the normal range, safe medications, treatments, and lifestyle changes are available to correct them, including some of the lifestyle suggestions in the pages of this book.

It's also important to keep the pounds off. Excess weight raises your likelihood for developing diabetes, high blood pressure, and elevated blood cholesterol, all of which raise your risk for Alzheimer's. People who are overweight are more likely to be diagnosed with dementia than people who remain slender.[34]

You'll learn more about the interplay between all of these medical conditions and Alzheimer's in Chapter 2.

The best approach to preventing and delaying Alzheimer's is a personalized one. The 3-week plan in Chapter 9 will help you to choose and organize the right strategies for you into a successful program that you can adopt and maintain for years to come. And, most important, you'll also find out how to make change possible. It's one thing to know what to eat or how much to exercise. It's quite another to do it. By personalizing an array of choices, you really can embrace your new healthy lifestyle. Within the pages of this book, you'll also find helpful advice on how to stay motivated as well as how to turn unfamiliar healthy behaviors into habits.

A Comprehensive Approach

Throughout the pages of *Outsmarting Alzheimer's*, you'll find sound medical advice that will help you guide your decisions about what to eat, how much to sleep, when and how to exercise, and much more. You'll also discover what you *don't* need to worry about. Do you need to buy and take an arsenal of supplements? To forego every trace of aluminum foil? To stop using antiperspirant? Probably not, and you'll find out why.

The onslaught of temptations waged against the brain is multipronged: menus with seductively photographed high-calorie desserts; full email inboxes and computer work that keep you sitting in your office chair for hours; mindless TV reruns that are on air at any time of the day or night; the constant feeling of being "on call" as your phone pings, dings, and buzzes late into the night.

Because the attacks on our brains are pervasive, the solution must be comprehensive, too. Nowhere in these pages will you find a single magic bullet. There is no expensive wonder food, no rare tea found only in the high mountains of a faraway place, no single yoga position, or breathing style, or crossword puzzle, and certainly no miracle supplement that is the secret to lifelong cognitive health. It would be naïve to think that one remedy can undo years of a sedentary lifestyle, fast food consumption, loneliness, stress, and boredom.

Instead, use this book to devise an entire package of risk-reducing measures. Pick what fits your lifestyle and health needs, but cover all bases. New research from the FINGER trial I mentioned earlier shows that this type of personalized, comprehensive approach offers the most promise for maintaining lifelong cognitive health. This two-year intervention did not study just one drug, one eating approach, one exercise plan, one way to connect with others, or one type of brain-training system. Rather, participants in the study learned and practiced a personalized combination of *all* of these strategies. Miia Kivipelto, MD, PhD, a professor at the Karolinska Institutet Center for Alzheimer's Research in Sweden, and her team followed the health outcomes of more than 1,200 people over two years, and they found that every measure of cognitive performance—including measures of memory, planning, and problem solving—improved.[35]

During the July 2014 Alzheimer's Association International Conference in Copenhagen, Denmark, Kivipelto presented the latest findings, commenting, "It's never too late to do something. It is possible."[36] By flexing your Brain Smarts, you really can outsmart Alzheimer's disease. It's never too early, and it's never too late. No matter your family history, age, or symptoms, now is the time to take steps to outsmart this terrible disease.

PART ONE

Why Everyone Needs to Outsmart Alzheimer's

Every person on this planet is at risk for developing Alzheimer's disease. This is true regardless of our age, family history, or current state of health.

That's the bad news. The good news is that nearly all of us are equally capable of dramatically reducing our risk and living well into our old age with vibrant health and sharp minds. In this part of the book, you'll learn what Alzheimer's is, how it affects our brains, and why right now is the best time to do something about it. It's never too early, and it's never too late to elevate your well-being and decrease your chances of devolving into dementia. You'll also take a quiz designed to give you an idea of your personal Alzheimer's risk score and how you might improve it.

CHAPTER 1

Your Brain on Alzheimer's

When physician Alois Alzheimer came to examine her, Auguste Deter was sitting on the hospital bed, a helpless expression on her face. Alzheimer asked, "What's your name?"

"Auguste," answered the 51-year-old patient at Frankfurt Hospital.

"Last name?"

"Auguste," she repeated.

"What's your husband's name?"

"Auguste," she said, sounding confused. "I think."

"Your husband?"

"Ah, my husband."

"Are you married?"

"To Auguste."

Later, while she was eating cauliflower and pork for lunch, Alzheimer asked, "What are you eating?"

"Spinach," Deter answered.

"What are you doing?" he asked.

"Potatoes."

Throughout the examination, Alzheimer took meticulous notes, jotting down the conversation word for word and commenting on Deter's impaired compre- hension and memory, disorientation, paranoia, anxiety, and auditory hallucina- tions. Deter, he wrote, didn't know what year it was, could not perform basic math, and was unable to write her name. Alzheimer found himself repeating every word so Deter could comprehend his basic questions and instructions.

At the time, in 1901, doctors had no term to describe Deter's condition. Her symptoms were much like the senility known to affect the oldest of the old. At the time, it was thought that the brain wore out over time much as joints did, leaving the elderly forgetful and confused. If that were true, though, how was it possible for a middle-aged woman to be suffering from "old age"? Alzheimer was fascinated. Even after leaving his post at Frankfurt Hospital, the German doctor continued to keep tabs on Deter.

In 1906 Deter died at age 55, and Alzheimer subsequently autopsied her brain. Just by holding it in his hands he could tell that it had shrunken. Her brain was roughly half the size of a normal one. Then, when he examined slices of her brain tissue under a microscope, he found the cause. Inside the neurons Alzheimer observed thick fibers that wrapped around the cell's interior, crushing its normal contents. These structures are called neurofibrillary tangles. He also observed clumps of a smooth plaquelike material that filled the space around the cells and distorted their shape. These structures are called senile plaques.[37]

When he published his findings, he referred to Deter's condition as "an unusual disease of the cerebral cortex" that caused memory loss and disorientation and eventually depression and hallucinations. Within the next five years, other physicians began diagnosing patients with the same disease and publishing their findings. A few years later, the disease was named after the physician who first described it, and we now know it as "Alzheimer's disease."[38]

The Most Common Cause of Dementia

The story of Auguste Deter is unsettling. In her case history, Alzheimer describes a condition that no one wants. Indeed, according to surveys, many of us fear an Alzheimer's diagnosis more than we fear any other disease, including cancer, stroke, or heart disease.[39]

It's the kind of disease that we wish had remained rare and obscure. We would like to read about Alzheimer's disease and be able to say, "That won't happen to me." Yet statistics tell us otherwise. Though the early-onset form of the disease that Deter had is relatively rare, the late-onset form is not. If we're not diagnosed with Alzheimer's ourselves, we'll know someone who is.

While reading about this disease may make us uncomfortable, knowledge is power. The more you understand about Alzheimer's, the better your chances of doing everything possible to prevent it or slow its progression.

What is Alzheimer's disease? It's a disease that affects the brain, leading to a decline in cognition: the mental process of acquiring, understanding, and using the information we gather through our senses. Its diagnostic feature is the presence of senile plaques and neurofibrillary tangles (discussed in detail on page 5). Though new diagnostic tests called beta-amyloid imaging allow us to peer into the brain and see these plaques, the imaging is expensive, not widely available, and is generally only offered to patients who already have persistent symptoms. For the majority of people, the disease is diagnosed based on its symptoms. It's not until after death and during an autopsy that these hallmark features are observed. One of the many brain regions that the disease attacks is called the hippocampus, where newly learned information is first processed. As a result, the memory problems suffered by Alzheimer patients often begin with impaired learning of new information.

When these symptoms become severe enough to interfere with everyday life—for example, making it difficult to drive without getting lost—we say you have "dementia." *Dementia* is an umbrella term that describes many different types of cognitive symptoms that can interfere with everyday tasks. Of the many different diseases that lead to dementia, Alzheimer's is the most common, accounting for somewhere between 60 and 80 percent of all dementia cases.[40]

Other types of dementia include:

Vascular dementia: In this type of dementia, hardened, blocked, and leaking blood vessels stop blood from flowing to affected parts of the brain, causing brain cells to die. When physicians use MRI or CT scanners to peer inside the brains of patients with vascular dementia, they often discover that these patients have had multiple small strokes. Often these strokes were silent, meaning the individual is unaware that a small volume of brain tissue has died. Symptoms of this form of dementia vary, depending on which parts of the brain are affected, and they often overlap with symptoms of Alzheimer's disease: confusion, trouble paying attention, difficulty with planning and decision making, restlessness, agitation, depression, and memory loss.

Dementia with Lewy bodies: Named after Frederick H. Lewy, MD, Lewy bodies are microscopic, abnormal clumps of protein that form throughout the cerebral cortex of the brain, causing nerve cells to degenerate. This form of dementia can be difficult to distinguish from Alzheimer's disease in living individuals. It tends to lead to problems with walking and balance, hallucinations, dizziness, and other nervous system issues, and sleep disturbances.

Parkinson's disease: Lewy bodies can also cause Parkinson's disease. In this case, they form deep in the brain, in an area called the *substantia nigra*, causing tremors and problems with movement.

Frontotemporal dementia: Affecting the front and side of the brain, this type of dementia leads to changes in personality and behavior. As the disease erodes the areas of the brain responsible for inhibiting behavior, patients with frontotemporal dementia can become impulsive, and some even show a disinhibited creativity, by taking up painting for example. Inappropriate and compulsive behaviors are common, as is a flagrant lack of empathy for others.

Normal pressure hydrocephalus: Derived from the Greek words *hydro* (water) and *cephalus* (head), this condition was once referred to as "water on the brain." Caused by the buildup of spinal fluid in the brain, it's called "normal pressure" because spinal fluid pressure remains normal when measured during a spinal tap. This rare form of dementia can bring on intense headaches and dizziness, changes in personality and behavior, trouble walking, and thinking and reasoning problems.

An early symptom in these patients that may occur even before memory loss is urinary incontinence. Patients with normal pressure hydrocephalus are unaware of the urge to urinate. This form of dementia can sometimes be corrected with the surgical installation of a shunt that drains the excess fluid from the brain to the abdomen.

What Causes Alzheimer's Disease?

Exactly what causes Alzheimer's disease is a mystery that we've yet to solve, but it's thought to involve at least two distinct processes:

Plaques: A dangerous protein fragment called *beta-amyloid* lurks in all our brains. For most of us, the brain clears away these fragments in the same way we wipe the dust off our furniture, and this regular brain dusting operates best while we sleep. But in some of us, these fragments build up over time. While diffusing through the fluid-filled spaces between cells, the fragments start to clump together into plaques, one of the villains of our story. As the beta-amyloid molecules accumulate, they damage and destroy brain cells and impair the communication between them. A type of immune cell called *microglia* then interpret the formation of plaques as an injury. As these immune cells rush in to repair the plaques (a process known as *inflammation*), they can further damage your brain cells.

Tangles: While the plaques penetrate the spaces between brain cells, another insidious process begins to cause damage inside the brain cells themselves. An otherwise normal protein called *tau* turns against the brain, and in partnership with other tau proteins, twists itself into a long, tangled thread that gradually strangles the neuron. The misfolded tau proteins cannot perform their usual functions. The normal function of tau is to keep cellular traffic flowing throughout the cell—all the proteins and other building blocks of the cell are busy all the time getting to work so the cell can function. However, just as a fender bender causes a major traffic jam on a highway, tau tangles can interfere with the transport of nutrients in and out of cells, causing brain cells to degenerate and die. If this damage affected only one brain cell, the effect would be inconsequential. But, the true malevolence of tau is its ability to damage tau in neighboring cells, spreading this tendency to *misfold* and consequently inducing these long threads widely throughout the cells of the brain.

We're not sure which of these processes—the accumulation of beta-amyloid plaque or of tau tangles—is primarily responsible for the disease. Does one of these processes play the starring role as the villain in the Alzheimer's saga, whereas the other serves merely as a sidekick? Are both equally involved? Does one cause the other? Or perhaps we've got the progression backward, and something else causes both of them.

We just don't know for sure. As a result, for many years, heated debates erupted at neurology meetings, with some scientists (known as the BAPtists) arguing that *beta-amyloid plaques* were the more important of the two processes, and others (known as the TAUists) saying that it was the *tau proteins* that were primarily responsible for causing the disease. Each group believed strongly that they were right.

Today, we don't see the issue as quite so black and white. My view is that science is about evidence. It's not about belief. Though we might hypothesize that one protein or the other is primarily responsible, the proof will come from the remedies that cure the disease. With enough study, we will learn the truth.

No matter the actual cause, though, the end result is the loss of brain cells. Among the regions most intensely affected are the *hippocampi* (the seahorse-shaped brain structures involved in memory formation and storage), the *amygdala* (an almond-shaped brain structure that plays an important role in emotions), and *raphe nuclei* (a part of the brain stem that is involved in sleep). As more and more brain signals are lost in the hippocampi, it's increasingly difficult to form new memories. Over time, it also becomes harder to pull older memories out of storage. The loss of neurons in the amygdala accounts for many of the emotional issues and personality changes observed in Alzheimer's. As more and more of the raphe nuclei is affected, sleep disturbances result.

The Symptoms of Alzheimer's Disease

Initially, Alzheimer's disease silently snakes its damage through the brain. Plaques and tangles may spread through the hippocampi as much as 10 to 20 years before symptoms set in. It's often not until the brain starts to shrink that memory loss and other symptoms become noticeable.

In the initial stages of the disease, many people are tempted to blame their symptoms on "getting older." They experience the kind of forgetting that middle-aged and older people like to joke about: *Where are my reading glasses? What is that woman's name? Did I feed the dog yet? Why can't I ever remember how to switch the TV over to Hulu or Netflix? What's my password again?*

Eventually those symptoms go beyond anything we might think of as normal aging. People with mild Alzheimer's disease might repeat themselves, telling the same story more than once. Or they might continually forget appointments, become confused when attempting to follow directions, become lost or disoriented when driving or when in unfamiliar places, or struggle to balance their checkbook or budget their finances. They may abandon a task when it's only partially finished.

At a different stage in the disease, people with Alzheimer's might not recognize people they once knew. They can see their daughter-in-law or grandchildren and only have a vague sense, "I should know who this person is." The same may happen with common objects. They don't just lose their car keys; they don't know what car keys look like or what they are supposed to use them for. They may pick up a Frisbee and say, "Is this someone's shoe?" Or, you might ask them to turn off the light, and they may stare blankly. They don't understand your instructions because they don't know what a "light" is.

As the disease erodes the hippocampi and spreads to other parts of the brain, people with Alzheimer's lose themselves bit by bit. When you lose your memories, you lose your ability to think about the future because thinking about the future is based upon your memories and experiences of the past. How can you know what you want to eat for dinner if you can no longer remember what foods you like and which ones you don't? Depending on which areas of the brain are affected, Alzheimer's disease may also bring on listlessness, depression, poor judgment, disorientation, confusion, behavior changes, and/or difficulty speaking, swallowing, and walking.

Memory enriches our thoughts. It provides the details that personalize our experience. It adds dimensions to how we ponder the future. Ask an Alzheimer patient about his or her plans for vacation, and the answer will contain little detail. Ask a child the same question, and you will be flooded with images of daring amusement park rides and sand castles and the top flavors of ice cream. From the perspective of the Alzheimer patient, this paucity of memory feels like emptiness. The saddest thing an Alzheimer patient ever said to me was in response to my inquiry about what concerned her most. This former high school language teacher said, "I have nothing to think about."

The Stages of Alzheimer's Disease

Alzheimer's disease progresses through several stages. Technically, when you are in Stage 1 or Stage 2, we don't say you have "Alzheimer's disease." It's not until you've reached Stage 3, and you have symptoms of cognitive problems (such as forgetting) coupled with evidence of plaque formation in the brain that you would get an "Alzheimer's disease" diagnosis.

Stage 1: A Symptom-Free Condition

The Alzheimer disease process begins long before any symptoms are apparent with amyloid deposits in the brain. At this stage, without any cognitive symptoms we cannot say that someone has Alzheimer's disease, although the risk of progressing to Alzheimer's disease is very high. Although at the very earliest stage most people do not experience symptoms, some people note a subjective sense of declining memory that is difficult to pinpoint. This stage of the disease can span many years, even a decade. All the while, plaques and tangles are forming, and the brain may be shrinking, but there are no noticeable problems with memory.

Brain imaging can pick up these early amyloid plaques, which can appear as long as ten years before patients experience any cognitive decline. The imaging procedure is generally only offered to people who are enrolled in an Alzheimer's study because these tests are expensive, involve radiation, and are not practical to administer to large numbers of people. Also, they do not show neurofibrillary tangles.

Stage 2: Mild Cognitive Impairment (MCI)

The changes people might notice at this stage are not severe enough to interfere with their independence. Though they might have trouble remembering what someone just said, have trouble judging how long various tasks might take or the sequence of steps needed to complete a complex project, they can still eat, bathe, and take care of other personal needs without assistance.

At this stage, it can be difficult to tell whether the memory lapses (such as increased difficulty retrieving names) experienced really stem from the proliferation of plaques and tangles. Because the symptoms of Alzheimer's disease overlap with the symptoms of a few other diseases, some people who have been diagnosed with MCI will not get Alzheimer's disease. They may be under stress, they may have an exaggerated sense of the very small amount of memory decline nearly all people incur with aging, they may have symptoms of menopause (discussed later) or have another disease that leads to symptoms of dementia (such as Parkinson's), or their symptoms may stem from a treatable condition such as thyroid disease. Sometimes, if the underlying disease is treated, the symptoms of memory loss resolve.

Only about half of people with MCI go on to develop dementia due to Alzheimer's. Some progress to Stage 3 quickly, while others live with MCI for 10 years or longer. We don't currently have the ability to determine how quickly any one person's Alzheimer's will progress. For some people, it progresses rapidly. For others, it's the opposite. If you are already at this stage, it's possible that you may be able to remain in Stage 2 for a long time.[41] Brain Smarts are important, both for putting off Stage 3 and also for improving your overall health, energy level, and mood. Embracing a healthy lifestyle and especially getting medical problems (such as high blood pressure) under control may slow the progression of the disease.

Stage 3: Dementia Due to Alzheimer's

This is when enough plaques and tangles have formed to cause the brain to start to shrink. Symptoms become clearly noticeable, with the patient having repeated trouble finding the right word, forgetting new names and faces, not being able to absorb new information, losing or misplacing objects, and feeling muddled when attempting to plan and organize. As memory continues to worsen, people with Alzheimer's disease may still recognize those close to them but not always remember their names. Sleep patterns become seriously disrupted. They have trouble controlling their bladder or bowels, and they tend to wander or become lost. In the most severe form, people with Alzheimer's lose the ability to talk and control their movements.

Meet Your Brain

Weighing roughly three pounds, your brain consists of folded masses of white and gray matter that are composed of billions of cells called *neurons*, and others called *glia*. Unlike the round shape of most other cells in your body, each of your nerve cells is equipped with several long, spidery legs called *axons* and *dendrites*. And these legs extend toward other nerve cells, creating a complex web.

These weblike connections allow each of your nerve cells to connect with thousands of others. All told, throughout your brain, there are hundreds of trillions of connections—as many as there are leaves in the Amazon rainforest. These connections between and among brain cells are often referred to as the brain's *wiring*.

So as the information from this book enters your brain, it is passed from one nerve cell to another in the form of electrical signals (or impulses). These signals travel along many spidery legs of a variety of neurons until they reach the end— the *toes* of this leg called a *synapse*. Within these toes are small packets filled with chemicals called *neurotransmitters*. When the electrical signal reaches these tiny packets the chemical contents get released into a gap between the end of one neuron and the beginning of the next. The neurotransmitters diffuse across the gap and stimulate a receptor on the opposite side of the synapse to renew the electrical signal. These receptors are proteins tailor-made for the neurotransmitter to fit within them and re-initiate the signal in the next neuron in the chain of neurons that make up a neuronal circuit.

Now, let's say you just read the above paragraph, and your eyes glazed over. Perhaps you've rarely seen words like *synapse* and *neurotransmitter*. In that case, your eyes glazed over for a good neurological reason—you don't yet have the cell-to-cell connections needed for the previous paragraph to sound familiar. But the more often you encounter a piece of information, the stronger the connections and the faster that information can get to its destination.

This is not unlike our transportation system. The first human traveler to go from point A to point B has to forge a rough dirt path. It's hard work that can require some bushwhacking, and the result often isn't terribly easy for other humans to follow. As more and more people walk the same path, however, the path becomes smoother and wider. As the path becomes more traveled, someone might lay down macadam or asphalt or replace a downed tree with a bridge, making it still easier to travel.

The same process takes place in your brain. The stronger the connections between neurons, the easier it is to absorb, retain, and recall new information. So even if words like *axon* and *neurotransmitter* might feel foreign to you right now, with repeated exposure, they can eventually roll in and out of your memory and on and off your tongue as easily as other words like *dog* and *belt buckle*.

How the Brain Works

Many of the first clues about what happens inside the brain we owe to a few unlucky humans whose brains suffered undue trauma. One of them was Phineas Gage, the foreman for a railroad construction gang in the mid-1800s. He was using a three-and-a-half-foot tamping iron to pack blasting powder into a rock when he accidentally triggered an explosion. The blast launched the tamping iron into his left cheek, through the left frontal cortex of his brain, and out the top of his head. The iron landed several yards behind him.[42]

Amazingly, Gage survived the accident and was even discharged from the hospital within 10 weeks, but he was forever changed. His physician noted that the once capable and efficient foreman was now impatient, irreverent, fitful, obstinate, and grossly profane. His friends remarked that he was "no longer Gage," and the railroad refused to employ him. Gage eventually joined the circus as a sideshow act.

The tale of his life is a sad one, but it's nonetheless one that has greatly advanced our understanding of the brain. Thanks to Phineas Gage, we now know that the frontal cortex is where much of our personalities is housed, and damage to this area of the brain can cause our personalities to change dramatically.[43]

We learned about the importance of another area of the brain, called the hippocampus, from a similarly unlucky person named Henry G. Molaison (known only as "H.M." until his death in 2008).

In 1953, at age 27, Molaison suffered from frequent and severe epileptic seizures that did not respond to anticonvulsant medications. His disease had disabled him, preventing him from working and forcing him to live with his parents. Out of desperation, he agreed to undergo an experimental treatment, during which portions of his medial temporal lobes—including most of his hippocampi—were removed.

Shortly after the surgery, Molaison's physician noticed that something was wrong. Though Molaison's seizures had abated, the young patient failed to recognize the staff who attended to him day after day. Molaison could carry on a conversation, but then, just minutes later, could not remember the conversation had occurred or even the person he'd spoken to.

For the rest of his life, Molaison kindly allowed neuroscientists such as Brenda Milner and later Suzanne Corkin to interview him over and over again. Though she met with him repeatedly over a 30-year span of time, "every time I walked into the room, it was like we'd never met," Milner told *The New York Times*.[44]

In one of those interviews, about four years after Molaison's surgery, Corkin asked, "I understand that you have a little bit of trouble remembering things?"

Molaison replied, "Yes, I do."

"How long have you had trouble remembering things?"

"That I don't know myself. I can't tell you, because I don't remember."

"Well do you think it's days, or weeks? Months, or years?"

"Well, see, I can't put it exactly on a day, week, or month, or year basis."[45]

His memory had been frozen in time. He did not remember what he'd eaten for breakfast or lunch on any given day. Nor did he remember anything that had taken place after his surgery. On the other hand, he *could* remember most of what had taken place in his life before the operation.

Molaison eventually would go on to donate his brain to science, allowing us to learn just how important the hippocampi are in making long-term memories out of short-term ones.[46]

The Brain's Filing Clerk

There are two hippocampi in the brain, one in each hemisphere. Named after the mythological seahorselike creature they resemble, these structures are among the brain's star players when it comes to memory. Information must pass through either hippocampus before it can be stored. In this way, the hippocampi serve as filing clerks that separate useless memories from useful ones and put like memories together.

To understand how this works, let's, for a moment, imagine that you are at a social gathering. Your friend Wendy introduces you to her date Jim. You reach out your hand and say, "Nice to meet you, Jim." In that moment, you know this man's name. But an hour or so later—when the two of you meet again, perhaps while ordering drinks at the bar—will he still be Jim? Or will he be "what's-his-name, Wendy's date"?

Or will you be confused when he says hello, causing you to wonder why he seems to know you, but you don't have any idea of how you know him?

The answers to those questions depend, in large part, on what happens inside your brain during the moment that Wendy introduces you.

For you to remember Jim's name hours later, that memory message must be transmitted across synapses, from neuron to neuron, as it travels through the hippocampus, which sorts the information, compares it to other memories, creates associations, and then sends it for storage.

Let's say, as Wendy was introducing you to Jim, you were distracted by something else. Maybe someone walked by with a tray of chocolate truffles. Or perhaps someone in your direct line of sight spilled a drink, causing your attention to drift away from the words Wendy was saying. Or maybe you were indulging in one of the largest weapons of mass distraction ever invented: a smartphone. End result: You went through the motions of saying hello to Jim, but you didn't really register his name at all. Will you still remember his name an hour or so later? No, because you never really learned his name in the first place. Perhaps the sound waves of *Jim* traveled to your ears, and a brief sensory memory of Jim began to form. But, because you were not paying attention, the memory quickly vanished, as did the memories of other useless information gathered through your senses that night: the sound of your car keys jingling as you reached into your pocket or purse; the brief hint of perfume as someone walked by; the muted color of the carpet you were standing on.

Now, let's say you were paying attention as you were introduced. It might have taken less than 5/100ths of a second for the message "Jim" to pass through hundreds of thousands of neurons, all working in synchronicity to deliver that message to the hippocampus. Once there, the hippocampus compared the information of Jim's name and linked it with the information of his face, which was compared to stored memories you may have had of Wendy, of the cologne Jim might have been wearing, of his facial hair that resembles your cousin's, of the sound of his voice, which may have reminded you of your brother, or of the ways he said the word "boat" which reminded you of a recent trip to Canada. All the while, various synapses needed to make new proteins to cement the memory in place.[47] The synapses enlarged, growing spiny protrusions that allowed them to fire more efficiently so you could recall the memory of Jim's name more readily.

Even if the information of Jim's name had been stored, however, you still may not have been able to recall it later, and here's why: After hearing Jim's name only once, your brain only had one narrow path to follow to retrieve that info. On the other hand, if, just after being introduced, you said Jim's name a few times ("It's so nice to meet you, Jim. You know, Jim, that's a nice tie. Where did you get it? Jim, Wendy is one of my dearest friends.") you were able to build several memory paths in your brain, beefing up the connections needed to bring those memories out of storage and to the front of your mind. Similarly, you might have associated his name with other memories, perhaps of another Jim you know. Now you'd created an even stronger connection. So an hour or so later, when you were face-to-face at the bar, these strong connections made it easier for you to say, "Hey, Jim, how's it going?"

Now, let's consider what happens after the social gathering. How long will you remember Jim? Every time you reactivate a memory, you strengthen it. So if, after this social engagement, you met Jim repeatedly, the connections got stronger and stronger, making his name easier and easier to recall. If, on the other hand, it was more than a decade before you saw Jim again, you might not have continued to remember him.

Why We Forget

You may have noticed that children learn and recall information much more easily and quickly than the rest of us. They can store cryptic computer passwords like, "3xT9LYz#?" in their heads, whereas adults usually must write such things down, sometimes only to forget where we've put the piece of paper on which we've written such information. It's our children and grandchildren who remember the names of everyone in the neighborhood, including the names of all the neighborhood pets. They learn new information—Spanish, algebra, the lyrics to the latest #1 hit—in a fraction of the time it takes us, if we are able to learn it at all.

Why do children have such an edge on us? As we accumulate experiences, much of our daily lives may seem less novel and therefore less memorable. But though we don't know for sure, there are likely some other things happening inside the brain as it ages. Some good guesses are:

Inflammation: Our immune systems respond to danger by sending out pro-inflammatory proteins that create heat, swelling, redness, and pain as they go about their germ-killing business. In the short term, inflammation helps us survive a case of the flu. But if inflammation becomes chronic, it can also kill healthy cells, including brain cells. While a certain amount of inflammation is normal, too much of it accelerates aging all over the body, including the brain. Though many questions remain, chronic inflammation is also thought to be involved in Alzheimer's disease.[48]

Oxidation: As cells use oxygen to create energy, they create toxic, "oxidized" by-products that, when left unchecked, can speed up aging throughout the body, including in the brain. Cells throughout our bodies and brains are capable of manufacturing antioxidant enzymes that have the ability to neutralize these oxidized molecules, but when the oxidized molecules outnumber our antioxidant enzymes, damage results.

Wear and tear: Over time synapses may wear out, slowing and hindering the connections between and among neurons. The stringlike fibers that conduct a cell's electrical impulses may also weaken. And we may lose nerve cells throughout the brain. Unlike some other areas of the body, the brain isn't able to replace many of its neurons once they are damaged. (The hippocampus is an exception with some ability to replicate neurons well into our 90s.) So as brain cells are lost, our brains begin to shrink about 0.2 to 0.5 percent a year after age 35.[49]

As this happens, we can still think, learn, remember, and solve problems, but these tasks tend to take longer.[50] When a child recalls a cryptic computer password, the information can often travel in a straightforward route. When we do the same, the password memory might have to travel through a more haphazard maze, bypassing and detouring around synaptic connections that don't perform as well as others.

As key synapses are affected, the ability to retrieve certain memories and connect past experiences with the present will decline.[51, 52] The formation of new memories can also become more vulnerable, making it easier to remember the name of a high school classmate but harder to remember the name of the person you met last night during that social event. ("It was Jim, right?") Finally, we may experience more and more difficulty with multitasking; for instance it may be harder to try to talk on the phone while scrolling through email.

But not all brain aging is bad. Some of it actually gives us an edge. It's not until our late 20s or early 30s that the nerve connections in the frontal lobe of the brain fully mature. Mature nerve connections are encased in a protective coating of fatty material called myelin, much as the electrical wiring in your home is encased in insulation. In addition to protecting the nerves, myelin allows impulses to travel from one nerve cell to another more quickly. The frontal lobe (the very front of your brain) is the last part of the brain to fully mature. This is the part of the brain that is involved in planning, reasoning, problem solving, and decision making. When it's fully mature, we're less impulsive and better able to fully weigh the pros and cons of our actions.[53, 54] This is why we often read news stories about 20-year-olds getting arrested or ending up in the emergency room after a night of partying but rarely read the same stories about 40-year-olds.

Older brains are also wiser, thanks to years and years of learning. Every moment allows us to gain experience, adding to the richness of our knowledge. The older you are, the more you know and the more wisdom you have to draw from.

It's partly because of the years and years of wisdom stored in our brains that our processing speed slows. Consider what happens to a computer when you load up the hard drive with as many files as its memory can handle. It completes each task more slowly, and running too many programs at once can bring everything to an abrupt halt. At the same time, it can do more than the same computer with fewer files. It simply takes more time for it to get it all done.

It's the same with the brain, according to German researchers who programmed computers to act like humans.[55] This may partly explain why you can't quite pull a piece of information off the tip of your tongue at the moment you need it. Then, hours later, the memory surfaces, "Jim! His name is Jim!"

With more data in the brain, there's also more opportunity to forget. Consider how easy it is for a 10-year-old child to remember the birthdays of all five of his friends. Consider how much more difficult it is for a 60-year-old to remember the birthdays of 250 Facebook friends. It's much harder but, thankfully, Facebook remembers them for us!

In addition to computerized reminders, we can also lean on tried and true memory aids. For example, if you struggle to remember a particular word (such as *neuron*), you can instead say a word or phrase that you can remember (such as *nerve cell*).[56] If you can't remember the phrase *cognitive health*, you can instead say *brain health*. You can also use strategies to retain and recall important information—such as repeating names over and over and associating them with other stored memories. If what's-his-name is on the tip of your tongue, you might recall thoughts of the sights, sounds, and scents of that night you met, thus stimulating the same area of the brain where the memory of what's-his-name is stored. You remember what a certain truffle tasted like, and then you think, *Oh, right, that's it. Jim!*

Don't Ignore These Symptoms

The earlier you implement prevention measures, the better. If you notice any of the following symptoms or signs of mild cognitive impairment, make an appointment with a health professional for a thorough health assessment.

FORGETTING NEW INFORMATION. It's normal to forget information if you never really learned it in the first place because you were distracted by your phone or your very full to-do list. If you don't know why you continually lose track of what others have told you, however, it's worth mentioning it to your doctor.

FORGETTING IMPORTANT APPOINTMENTS. At some point in life, nearly all of us will show up for a party on the wrong day or time, and it's normal to forget an appointment every once in a while. But doing so regularly is not. If you have difficulty keeping track of important events or planning for the future or if you sometimes forget where you are or how you got there, it's time to see a doctor.

TROUBLE RECALLING INFORMATION. It's normal not to recall a word occasionally or have an "it's on the tip of my tongue" sensation. If this happens regularly, however, or you sometimes feel lost in conversations or have a tendency to repeat yourself, it's time to get checked.

FEELING CHALLENGED WHEN PLANNING OR SOLVING PROBLEMS. This could show up as the inability to make change, balance a checkbook, keep track of the bills, or calculate a tip, especially if such activities once came easily for you. Or it might show up as trouble following a recipe or other types of step-by-step instructions, such as putting together furniture or assembling Lego creations.

DIFFICULTY COMPLETING FAMILIAR TASKS. Perhaps you start off on an errand but forget where you are going. Maybe you can't remember the rules of a game you once played a lot. Or something that once came easily to you at work now takes much longer. If this happens only occasionally, it might be normal. But if it happens repeatedly, it's a good idea to mention it to your doctor.

LOSING THINGS. It's normal to misplace our keys or reading glasses occasionally. It's not normal to misplace items regularly and especially concerning if you tend to find lost items in strange places, such as a wallet inside the medicine cabinet or the car keys inside the freezer.

In addition to considering whether you are experiencing any of those symptoms, ask yourself: *Do I think I'm losing my memory?* Most of us, as it turns out, are good judges of whether our memories are fading. Researchers at the University of Kentucky asked 531 older adults if they'd noticed any changes in their memories in the previous year. Then they tested the memories and thinking skills of these study participants once a year for 10 years. After death, the researchers examined the participants' brains for evidence of Alzheimer's disease. The researchers found that study participants who reported changes in their memories were three times more likely to eventually be diagnosed with *mild cognitive impairment (MCI)*. The study participants noticed the memory and thinking problems as many as 12 years before these issues became apparent on annual tests.[57]

The Forgetting That Isn't Alzheimer's

Quite often, when I tell people what I do for a living, they end up telling me about their memory troubles. And so it was during a recent flight. The woman seated next to me told me about recent issues she'd had with her short-term memory. She'd initially gone to her family doctor, telling him that her thinking was muddled. It was increasingly difficult for her to concentrate at work. She was fatigued, and she often forgot small details such as lunch dates. She felt as if she was losing her mind.

Her doctor referred her to a neurologist who referred her to a rheumatologist. Eventually she was referred to a major academic hospital. All told, over a year's time, she met with several doctors and underwent countless tests, including numerous blood tests, brain scans, and even a spinal tap. They ruled out Lyme disease, brain cancer, ALS, Alzheimer's disease, and multiple sclerosis.

They could find nothing wrong with her. Finally, she visited her OB-GYN, who told her: "You're not losing your mind. You just have perimenopause."

During the transition to menopause, levels of the female hormone estrogen fluctuate, rising and falling unevenly. This can bring on symptoms such as hot flashes and sleep problems, and it seems to also be responsible for what has now been documented as memory loss.

Researchers at the University of Rochester asked 75 highly educated women aged 40 to 60 to undergo a battery of tests to gauge their ability to learn and retain new information, to mentally manipulate new information, and to sustain their attention. The researchers found that many of the women with perimenopausal symptoms such as hot flashes did poorly on tests that measured working memory (the ability to take in and manipulate new information). These women also had problems holding their focus.[58]

Most importantly, this type of memory loss is temporary in most cases. Within a couple of years, as hormonal levels even out, the symptoms tend to disappear. In the meantime, although the evidence remains insufficient, the strategies in this book (especially exercise and sleep) may help to ease some symptoms.

The hormonal fluctuations of perimenopause can be mistaken for early signs of Alzheimer's disease. Other conditions that can lead to an erroneous diagnosis of Alzheimer's disease include:

Stress: Unrelenting stress can muddle thinking and make it difficult to pay attention. It can also disturb sleep, which blocks the brain's ability to organize memories into the correct neurological filing cabinets, making those memories more difficult to retrieve. If the stress is temporary—say, the stress of job loss—then your memory and brain function will return to normal. If the stress remains chronic, however, the hippocampi can be damaged, increasing your risk for developing Alzheimer's disease. So, while stress-induced forgetting isn't the same as Alzheimer's disease, it can eventually lead to it. This is one important reason to follow the stress-reduction advice in Chapter 6.

Pregnancy: Expectant mothers call it "pregnancy brain" for a reason. During the nine months that your body is making a baby, you undergo a severe hormonal fluctuation that can affect your mental clarity. Leaning on friends and family for support (Chapter 3) can help. Incidentally, often the most forgettable moment during pregnancy is childbirth itself. Perhaps we evolved this biological mechanism so the pain of childhood could be quickly forgotten, and, no matter how long or difficult the delivery, mothers would be inclined to have another child.

Cancer treatment: Chemotherapy and radiation can affect the brain in ways we don't completely understand, bringing on symptoms that are similar to Alzheimer's disease. These are often referred to as "chemo brain." It's still unclear why this happens, but we do know the issue exists, as Ellen Clegg's *ChemoBrain* shows.[59] For some patients, these symptoms resolve after the treatment ends. For others, they persist. A Brain Smart lifestyle like the one described in *Outsmarting Alzheimer's* may offer some benefit.

And there are many other non-Alzheimer's-related memory problems, including an underactive thyroid, vitamin and mineral deficiencies, hormonal imbalances, prescription or over-the-counter drug interactions, lack of sleep that stems from insomnia or another sleep disorder, head trauma, and other health problems such as blood vessel disease.

If you are experiencing problems with your memory, mention it to your family physician. A medical checkup can help you discover whether one of the issues I just mentioned may be causing your symptoms. If it turns out that you do have the earliest signs of Alzheimer's disease, your doctor may help guide you toward risk-reduction measures or suggest a clinical research trial. Your doctor may prescribe medications to treat high blood pressure, elevated cholesterol, or depression. Treatments that modify, reverse, or slow the course of Alzheimer's disease do not yet exist; however, some treatments are available that can modestly reduce the symptoms for a short time.

Protecting Your Brain from Alzheimer's

I want to help you keep your brain healthy for life. Though there is no drug, procedure, or protocol that can cure this disease, scientists are learning more about Alzheimer's every day, and we have discovered an array of ways to prevent it, slow its progression, and reduce its symptoms.

You'll find 80 of these brain-boosting strategies in Part Two of this book. Which strategies you focus on first—and which ones you put off for later—depends in large part on where you are right now. Your current lifestyle and state of health affect which strategies you need right away, which ones you may not need at all, and which ones you can incorporate into your life at a later date.

That's why the first step in outsmarting Alzheimer's involves assessing your health and lifestyle. In the next chapter, you'll find dozens of questions that will help you to determine your current risk level. What you learn in that chapter will guide you during the rest of your *Outsmarting Alzheimer's* journey.

Ready to take the first important step toward better brain health? Turn the page to get started.

CHAPTER 2

Assess Your Alzheimer's Risk

Whether or not you get Alzheimer's disease depends, in part, on the decisions you make every day—about what to eat for lunch, whether to hit the gym on the way home, and how you choose to relax. But there is no one-size-fits-all approach, and that's because everyone's risk factors are different. The most effective brain health program for you will be different than that of your neighbor or your coworker or even your cousin, because your risk factors are not the same. If you have high cholesterol, it's most important for you to cut back on saturated and trans fats, get in some vigorous exercise, and talk to your doctor about cholesterol-lowering medication. On the other hand, let's say your cholesterol and blood pressure are normal, but you suffer from insomnia. Then you'd lean heavily on the advice in Chapters 6 and 8, incorporating strategies to boost mood, lower stress, and improve sleep. Or let's say you want to exercise, but you have arthritis in your knees. Then weight-bearing movements like dancing and jogging might be out of the question, but swimming or yoga may offer what you need. The point is: Your family history, current state of health, and current lifestyle are all important ingredients that help determine the best brain health recipe for you.

In addition to helping you to personalize your plan, the answers to the questions in this chapter will help you to stay motivated. A Mayo Clinic survey of over 4,000 people found that more than 90 percent of them would pursue a healthier lifestyle if they knew they carried one of the Alzheimer's genes.[60] But you don't need to meet with a genetic counselor to fire up your motivation. You'll have a good idea of your risk by the end of this chapter.

How to Calculate Your Alzheimer's Risk

When we use the word *risk* we're talking about your chance of getting Alzheimer's disease. Many different things can raise your risk: how old you are, whether you have high blood pressure or high cholesterol, how well you sleep, and many others. These are your risk factors. The more risk factors you have, the more likely it is that you will develop Alzheimer's at some point in your life.

Some risks you cannot easily change—your family history, for instance, or your education level. Others, such as high blood pressure, diabetes, or other health conditions that raise your risk for Alzheimer's, may require your doctor's help and some time to change. A third category, the lifestyle habits that raise your risk for Alzheimer's, is very much under your control and is the focus of this book. But it's important to know even those risks that you cannot change to understand your overall risk.

To help you get a sense of where you stand, I've created a quick quiz to identify how many risk factors you currently have in each of these three categories. Answer all of the questions and add up your risk score for each of the three sections. That number is not a diagnosis; instead, it provides insight and motivation and gives you an idea of your current risk for developing Alzheimer's disease. Ideally, you want to take as many steps as you are able to get your Alzheimer's risk score as low as possible.

Your Baseline Score

Alzheimer's disease is a long and slowly emerging disease that depends on many different factors, some of which you can change easily and others that you can't change easily or at all. The higher the score, the higher your risk. In this section, you'll start by assessing the risk factors you can't easily change to find your baseline. Because we all carry some risk of getting Alzheimer's disease, begin this questionnaire with 11 points and then add or subtract points as indicated. Your baseline score will then be added to your modifiable risk score to motivate your brain health planning.

QUESTION #1: How old are you?

Age is the greatest risk factor for Alzheimer's disease. Your risk of Alzheimer's doubles every five years after age 65.[61] After age 85, you have a nearly 50 percent chance of developing dementia. Age may increase risk because other risk factors become more likely the older you get. These include high blood pressure, stroke, heart disease, nerve cell changes, and lowered or delayed or impaired immune response. That's why Bette Davis said, "Old age ain't no place for sissies."

Score your age using the numbering system below:

- 64 and younger = 0
- 65–69 = +1
- 70–74 = +2
- 75–79 = +3
- 80–84 = +4
- 85+ = +5

QUESTION #2: How many first-degree family members have been diagnosed with Alzheimer's disease?

Our parents pass thousands of genes on to us, and some of these genes carry small changes in their DNA sequences that raise risk for specific diseases while others lower risk. We've yet to fully identify all the genes involved in raising or lowering Alzheimer's risk, so currently we can only infer whether you have these risk genes by the presence of Alzheimer's disease in a first-degree family member, such as a parent or a sibling. First-degree family members do not include grandparents, cousins, aunts, uncles, and other extended family members.

Researchers at Duke University Medical Center recently found that people with first-degree family members with Alzheimer's are more than twice as likely as those without a family history to develop silent buildup of beta-amyloid plaques.[62] That said, by incorporating the lifestyle changes recommended in this book, you can reduce the influence of your genetic heritage.

Use the following to assess how your family history affects your score.

- No family history of Alzheimer's disease = 0
- Your mother was diagnosed with Alzheimer's disease = +1
- Your father was diagnosed with Alzheimer's disease = +1
- Neither of your parents was diagnosed, but one or more siblings were diagnosed with Alzheimer's disease = +1

Note: Your highest possible score for this question is 2. Do not add extra points for every additional sibling diagnosed, for extended family members who were diagnosed, or if parents *and* siblings were diagnosed.

QUESTION #3: Have you experienced any severe stressors?

Severe prolonged stress during your 30s, 40s, and 50s can boost your risk of developing Alzheimer's disease 10, 20, or more years later in life by 21 percent. By "severe prolonged stress," I'm not talking about the average daily hassles that we all face when sitting in traffic, working with annoying people, or standing on the slow line at the grocery store. Severe, unavoidable stress goes on for months and even years, and it's unrelenting. For example, maybe you've heard that the stress of going through a divorce is like getting in a serious car accident every day for an entire year. *That's* the kind of stress I'm talking about here.

And the more severe stressors you've faced, the higher your risk of developing Alzheimer's.[63] It's thought that these types of stressors affect us for years, taxing the neuroendocrine system and stressing the brain. Stress hormones remain elevated, disrupting the central nervous system and immune system, among others. This may raise levels of hormones and inflammatory molecules in the brain that damage the hippocampus. The following is a list of common severe or chronic stressors.

- Divorce
- Death of a spouse
- Serious illness of a child
- Serious health or behavioral problems with a child
- Mental illness of a child
- Learning that one of your children has been abused
- Mental illness in a spouse or first-degree relative (parent or sibling)
- Alcohol abuse in a spouse or first-degree relative
- Physical illness in a spouse
- Loss of a job for you or your spouse
- A serious long-term and unsolvable interpersonal work-related issue that threatens your livelihood

Give yourself a +1 if you have one of these and +2 if you have two or more.

Note: the highest score you can get for this question is a 2 and the lowest is a zero. There may be other causes of long-term stress not included on the list. If you feel you've undergone a chronic stressor that isn't listed, still count it as one stressor.

QUESTION #4: Have you ever suffered a concussion or any other brain injury?

Serious or repeated head injuries cause beta-amyloid plaque deposits and neurofibrillary tangles to form in the brain.[64] This may explain why so many football players and boxers go on to develop dementia symptoms. A study by the National Institute for Occupational Safety and Health found that brain and nervous system disorders were three times higher in football players compared to the general population, and that those players had a four times greater chance of developing Alzheimer's disease than did nonplayers.[65] The same may be true of other contact sports such as hockey and soccer.

Score yourself as follows:
- You've been diagnosed with a concussion at some point in your life = +1

- You played a contact sport and sometimes got hit hard enough to temporarily lose consciousness, get confused, or feel dizzy = +1

- You have never suffered a concussion or played contact sports = 0

QUESTION #5: What's your highest level of education?

A high educational level might protect against Alzheimer's disease in two ways. First, learning new information seems to create connections between brain cells. The more connections you start with, the more you can lose before you experience symptoms. Second, a high educational level packs your brain with knowledge. So as you lose the ability to recall some information—for instance, not being able to remember the word *genetic* —you have a rich source of other information to call on. Instead of saying the word you are looking for, you might instead recall a slightly different one, such as *inherited*.[66] These increased brain connections serve as a reserve pool. In addition to the number of years you spent in school, you may have built *brain reserve* through musical training, becoming fluent in two or more languages, or developing a lifelong habit of reading and learning.

Though you can modify this particular risk factor by going back to school, we've listed it under "risks you can't change," because your educational status is most often formed during early life.

Add or subtract points based on your highest level of education.

- Less than a high school education = +1
- High school education = 0
- Two-year associate's degree, four-year bachelor's or advanced degree = −1

QUESTION #6: Have you learned a second language?

In addition to schooling, other types of knowledge can help keep the brain sharp. A second language can include fluency in Spanish, French, Chinese, and other spoken languages or musical languages (such as the ability to read and play music), or computer languages (such as HTML programming language), among others.

Subtract up to one point if you are fluent in any of the following:

- A second spoken language other than your native language;
- A musical language such as the ability to play the piano or saxophone;
- A computer language.

Note: Do not subtract extra points for additional spoken languages if you know more than two. The maximum number of points you can subtract is 3.

* * *

Every single one of us—regardless of our age, health, or family history—has some risk for developing Alzheimer's disease, so no one begins with zero. Instead, you start with an initial score of 11. Then, from 11, add or subtract based on your answers for each question in this section.

For example, if you are a 45-year-old woman with one big life stressor, one family member with Alzheimer's, and an advanced degree, your math would look like this:

11 (initial score)

   + 1 (one stressor)

   + 0 (age 45)

   + 1 (one family member with Alzheimer's)

   + 0 (no history of concussions)

   − 1 (an advanced degree)

   + 0 (no second language)

   Baseline score: 12

This baseline score is *not* a diagnosis. Nor is it a prediction of whether you definitely will or won't get Alzheimer's disease. Rather it's an estimate of your current risk for developing Alzheimer's disease. It is also the first number you need as you proceed through this assessment. Remember, we are all at risk for this disease and your score will reflect that. For simplicity the test assumes that various risks are similarly weighted; a more refined estimate would weight each risk. The higher your baseline score, the higher your risk. Though your baseline score for this section will not change dramatically over time, it can provide you with motivation to ensure your scores in the next two sections are as low as possible. If your score raises concerns beyond the scope of this book, please consult a physician.

Your Health Score

The healthier your body, the healthier your brain. It's important to know your numbers and do everything you can to get them under control. If you don't know your blood pressure and other readings, you can skip this section for now. But I strongly encourage you to make an appointment for a well visit and know your numbers so you can complete this section. Now fully covered under the Affordable Care Act, regular well visits include blood pressure, cholesterol, and blood sugar monitoring.

QUESTION #7: What's your blood pressure?

What is blood pressure? It's the measure of the force of blood against your artery walls. The top number in the reading is called *systolic pressure,* and that's the force against the artery walls as your heart beats. The bottom number, called *diastolic,* is the force as your heart relaxes between beats.

Research has found that high blood pressure, also called *hypertension,* during your 40s and 50s increases the risk of developing dementia after age 70, possibly by damaging the blood vessels in the brain.[67] This finding has been replicated many times, and the evidence is so overwhelming that it would be foolhardy to ignore it.

Get your blood pressure checked at least once a year. Better yet, purchase a good blood-pressure cuff and learn how to check your blood pressure at home. The first time you measure your blood pressure, you may want to bring the instrument to the doctor's office and see if you get the same blood pressure as the doctor does. Be wary of blood-pressure measurements available in pharmacies; sometimes their accuracy is questionable. When you check your blood pressure at home, be sure that you are seated in a comfortable position and completely relaxed. It is normal for blood pressure to vary, rising when we're exercising or under stress and dropping when we're relaxed or asleep. What is important is whether you can get your blood pressure into the normal range when you are relaxed.

(A notable caveat when treating hypertension in the elderly: Blood pressures drift upward as we age, and lowering the blood pressure of an elderly individual with mild hypertension can be dangerous if medication drops the pressure too precipitously. Less elastic blood vessels in the elderly make it even more important for a physician to monitor carefully any pharmaceutical treatment for hypertension.)

Score yourself based on the following:
- 120/80 or lower (low blood pressure) = –1
- Between 120/80 and 130/85 (normal blood pressure) = 0
- Between 130/85 and 139/89 (high blood pressure) = +1
- 140/90 or higher (very high blood pressure) = +2

QUESTION #8: What is your cholesterol level?

A type of fat, cholesterol circulates in the bloodstream with the help of protein carriers, such as high-density lipoprotein (HDL) and low-density lipoprotein (LDL). When *total* cholesterol (all types of cholesterol added together) or LDL cholesterol (sometimes referred to as the "bad" or "unhealthy" cholesterol) are elevated, the artery walls can thicken, choking off blood supply to certain parts of your body, including the brain. Not only can this lead to stroke and heart attacks, but also to vascular dementia, during which brain cells slowly die off from lack of nutrients.

A review of 18 different studies of more than 14,000 participants found that high total cholesterol levels at midlife (in their 40s) increased risk for Alzheimer's disease and dementia several decades later, in their 70s.[68] High levels of *low-density lipoprotein* (LDL) cholesterol increases risk for both vascular dementia and Alzheimer's disease, while elevated levels of *high-density lipoprotein* (HDL) are protective.[69]

Get your cholesterol checked once a year.

Calculate your score using the information below:

HDL Cholesterol

- 38 mg/dl or lower (low HDL cholesterol) = +1

- 38–46 mg/dl (normal HDL cholesterol) = 0

- 46 mg/dl or higher (high HDL cholesterol) = –1

LDL Cholesterol

- 100 mg/dl or lower (low LDL cholesterol) = –1

- 100–129 mg/dl (normal LDL cholesterol) = 0

- 130–159 mg/dl (high LDL cholesterol) = +1

- 160–189 mg/dl (very high LDL cholesterol)= +2

- 190 mg/dl or higher (extremely high LDL cholesterol) = +3

QUESTION #9: What is your fasting blood glucose?

It's important to bring blood sugar under control for many reasons, including the health of your brain. Often measured along with a standard cholesterol panel, your *fasting glucose* is a measure of the glucose (or sugar) present in your blood after you've gone without food or liquid (except water) for eight hours. Elevated fasting glucose levels are a sign of diabetes. Having either type 1 or type 2 diabetes doubles your risk of dementia, possibly by damaging the blood vessels in the brain as well as by encouraging the formation of beta-amyloid plaque.[70]

Use this information to add up your score:

- 100 mg/dl or lower (normal fasting blood glucose) = 0

- 100–125 mg/dl (prediabetes) = +1

- 126 mg/dl or higher (diabetes) = +2

QUESTION #10: Are you overweight?

Excess body weight raises your risk for high blood pressure, diabetes, and other health problems that raise your risk for Alzheimer's disease. Excess body fat can also raise levels of inflammation throughout the body, which can damage brain cells. A study of more than 8,000 people that spanned several decades found that people who were overweight or obese in their 40s were more likely to develop dementia in their 60s and 70s.[71]

There are many methods to calculate ideal body weight. For these purposes, we'll use your *body mass index* (BMI), a result that is calculated based on your weight and height. To calculate your BMI, you can use the Centers for Disease Control and Prevention's Adult BMI Calculator (*cdc.gov healthyweight assessing bmi adult_bmi english_bmi_calculator bmi_calculator.html*) or several others available on the Internet. Or look up your BMI on this chart:

Body Mass Index (BMI) Chart

WEIGHT lbs	100	105	110	115	120	125	130	135	140	145	150	155	160	165	170	175	180	185	190	195	200	205	210	215
WEIGHT kgs	45.5	47.7	50.0	52.3	54.5	56.8	59.1	61.4	63.6	65.9	68.2	70.5	72.7	75.0	77.3	79.5	81.8	84.1	86.4	88.6	90.9	93.2	95.5	97.7
HEIGHT in/cm		Underweight			Healthy					Overweight					Obese						Extremely Obese			
5'-0" 152.4	19	20	21	22	23	24	25	26	27	28	29	30	31	32	33	34	35	36	37	38	39	40	41	42
5'-1" 154.9	18	19	20	21	22	23	24	25	26	27	28	29	30	31	32	33	34	35	36	37	38	39	40	41
5'-2" 157.4	18	19	20	21	22	22	23	24	25	26	27	28	29	30	31	32	33	34	35	36	37	38	39	40
5'-3" 160	17	18	19	20	21	22	23	24	24	25	26	27	28	29	30	31	32	32	33	34	35	36	37	38
5'-4" 162.5	17	18	18	19	20	21	22	23	24	24	25	26	27	28	29	30	31	31	32	33	34	35	36	37
5'-5" 165.1	16	17	18	19	20	20	21	22	23	24	25	25	26	27	28	29	30	30	31	32	33	34	35	35
5'-6" 167.6	16	17	17	18	19	20	21	21	22	23	24	25	25	26	27	28	29	29	30	31	32	33	34	34
5'-7" 170.1	15	16	17	18	18	19	20	21	22	22	23	24	25	25	26	27	28	29	29	30	31	32	33	33
5'-8" 172.7	15	16	16	17	18	19	19	20	21	22	22	23	24	25	25	26	27	28	28	29	30	31	32	32
5'-9" 175.2	14	15	16	17	17	18	19	20	20	21	22	22	23	24	25	25	26	27	28	28	29	30	31	31
5'-10" 177.8	14	15	15	16	17	18	18	19	20	20	21	22	23	23	24	25	25	26	27	28	28	29	30	30
5'-11" 180.3	14	14	15	16	16	17	18	18	19	20	21	21	22	23	23	24	25	25	26	27	28	28	29	30
6'-0" 182.8	13	14	14	15	16	17	17	18	19	19	20	21	21	22	23	23	24	25	25	26	27	27	28	29
6'-1" 185.4	13	13	14	15	15	16	17	17	18	19	19	20	21	21	22	23	23	24	25	25	26	27	27	28
6'-2" 187.9	12	13	14	14	15	16	16	17	18	18	19	19	20	21	21	22	23	23	24	25	25	26	27	27
6'-3" 190.5	12	13	13	14	15	15	16	16	17	18	18	19	20	20	21	21	22	23	23	24	25	25	26	26
6'-4" 193.0	12	12	13	14	14	15	15	16	17	17	18	18	19	20	20	21	22	22	23	23	24	25	25	26

Then add to your score as follows:
- 24.9 or below (normal) = 0

- 25–29 (overweight) = +1

- 30 or above (obese) = +2

* * *

As you add up your score for this section, don't forget to combine it with your previous score from the baseline section. So, for example, let's say that the hypothetical woman we mentioned earlier has normal blood pressure, high HDLs, and normal LDLs, glucose, and weight. The math would look like this:

12 (baseline score)

  + 0 (normal blood pressure)

  −1 (high HDLs)

  + 0 (normal LDLs)

  + 0 (normal glucose)

  + 0 (normal BMI)

  Health score = 11

Due to her good health, so far, she's already gotten her score to 11, even without taking steps to change her lifestyle.

How to Decide If a Medicine Is Worth the Risk

You may remember from the introduction that most of the medicines that have been developed specifically to treat Alzheimer's disease offer little benefit beyond short-term, symptomatic relief in some patients. On the other hand, a number of medicines on the market very effectively treat the medical conditions—high blood sugar, high blood pressure, high blood cholesterol—that raise your risk for Alzheimer's disease. But all medicines possess side effects. Some of these side effects are mild; others more severe. Some are common, and others are quite rare.

When deciding whether to take a medicine, it's important to weigh the benefits of helpful effects against the possibility of harmful side effects. For instance, if a medicine offers the possibility of avoiding Alzheimer's, you may be willing to tolerate some risk, such as mild flushing, itching, or headaches. Talk about the benefits and risks with your doctor. Find out how common undesirable side effects really are and whether you can reduce their likelihood. In the end, only you can decide what risks you are willing to take to achieve a desired benefit.

Your Lifestyle Score

If all of us improved what we ate, exercised regularly, made strides to reduce stress, developed a rich web of friendships, and stimulated our brains regularly, we could prevent a third or even half of Alzheimer's disease cases.[72] Our lifestyles can help us lessen the likelihood of facing preventable health problems like obesity and diabetes, too.

QUESTION #11: Do you accumulate at least 150 minutes of exercise every week?

Arguably, regular physical activity is the most important gift you will ever give your body and brain. The evidence for exercise is overwhelming; even the most hardcore skeptic cannot refute it. Researchers from the Cleveland Clinic asked 100 older men and women to undergo brain scans. About half of the older adults were genetically at high risk for developing Alzheimer's due to the presence of the *ApoE4* gene mentioned earlier. The other half were not. When the researchers repeated the scans 18 months later, they found that sedentary participants who carried the *ApoE4* gene had lost volume in the hippocampal regions of their brains, whereas study participants in the other groups had not. Most striking, the brains of active people with *ApoE4* appeared similar to the brains of older adults without the gene, showing almost no shrinkage at all.[73]

Regular physical activity may protect brain volume by ensuring your brain gets good blood flow. Activity encourages the formation of new brain cells and reduces the risk for many of the diseases that are known risk factors for Alzheimer's disease (including high blood pressure, obesity, and diabetes). It's important to do both aerobic exercise (which benefits the brain by increasing oxygen consumption) and strength training.

Accumulate at least 20 minutes of aerobic and/or strength-training activity most days of the week, or at least 150 minutes a week.

Score yourself as follows:

- If you get no exercise = +1
- If you get some exercise, but less than 20 minutes on most days = 0
- If you accumulate 20 or more minutes of exercise most days of the week = –1

QUESTION #12: How many servings of fruits and vegetables do you consume a day?

The phytochemicals in fruits and vegetables may protect against inflammation and *oxidation*, the rusting of our cells and tissues that erodes our brain health over time. Plant foods that contain antioxidant vitamins seem to protect the brain.

For a few days to a week, keep a tally of your intake of fruits and veggies. One serving equals 1 small piece of whole fruit, ½ cup chopped fruits or vegetables, 1 cup raw leafy greens, or ½ cup berries or grapes.

If you:
- Consume fewer than one daily serving of fruits and vegetables = +1
- Consume one to five servings of fruits and vegetables a day = 0
- Consume more than five servings of produce a day = –1

QUESTION #13: How often do you challenge your brain?

You've probably heard the expression, "Use it or lose it." This seems to be true with the brain. Various studies show that mentally stimulating activities boost brain reserve, in part by developing more cell-to-cell connections. Some research even shows that seniors who took on 15 hours of mentally stimulating volunteer work a week were able to increase the activity in the parts of their brains involved with attention.[74]

Mentally stimulating activities can delay the onset of Alzheimer's disease by up to 10 years. They include anything from taking courses and learning and playing instruments to reading challenging material, playing cards and Scrabble, doing crossword puzzles, and knitting.[75]

If you:
- Do mentally challenging activities less often than once weekly = +1
- Do mentally challenging activities about once a week = 0
- Do at least one mentally challenging activity most days of the week = –1

QUESTION #14: How restful is your sleep?

As you learned earlier in this chapter, sleep is important for the health of your brain. Our brains flush out toxic compounds, including beta-amyloid protein, as we sleep. Lack of sleep might prevent this detoxification process, causing mental fog in the short term and Alzheimer's disease in the long term. Researchers at Duke have also found that the less we sleep, the faster our brains shrink as they age.[76]

Our needs for sleep vary considerably, however. Some people can function well on as few as four or five nightly hours of shut-eye, whereas others need more than double that. So rather than going by how many hours of shut-eye you get, instead consider how you feel during your waking hours: fatigued or energized.

If you:

- Feel rested when you wake each morning and rarely tired during the rest of the day = −1
- Feel somewhat rested = 0
- Feel chronically tired = +1

QUESTION #15: Have you been diagnosed with sleep apnea?

Sleep apnea—a serious disorder that develops when breathing repeatedly stops during sleep—can be especially harmful.[77] Symptoms include excessive daytime sleepiness, loud snoring, abrupt awakenings accompanied by shortness of breath, awakening with a dry mouth or sore throat, and morning headaches. If you think you might have sleep apnea, see a sleep specialist who may either observe you as you sleep overnight in a lab or ask you to wear a device that monitors your heart rate, blood oxygen levels, and breathing as you sleep at home. If it turns out that you do have sleep apnea, your physician will prescribe an oral appliance or a pressurized device called a *Continuous Positive Airway Pressure (CPAP)* machine to help your airways stay open as you sleep.

If you:

- Have been diagnosed with sleep apnea, but are not using a recommended therapy to treat it = +1
- Have been diagnosed with sleep apnea and are successfully using a CPAP or other treatment = 0
- Have not been diagnosed with sleep apnea = 0

QUESTION #16: What do you do to manage stress?

When you are under stress, levels of the hormone cortisol rise. Produced in the adrenal gland, short-term elevations of cortisol help to improve short-term memory and help us fight or flee dangerous situations.

Chronic, unrelenting stress—such as the ongoing stress of a job loss or a serious health problem—can erode memory, possibly shrinking the memory areas of the brain. This is especially problematic if you don't practice stress reduction to help you mitigate and recover from the stress. Stress is considered chronic if it lasts for more than a week. It's unrelenting if you spend more than an hour a day feeling tense, anxious, or concerned about it. Though you can't always take steps to reduce the number of stressors you face, you can take steps to change your reaction to those stressors. That's where resilience-building techniques come in. Activities such as yoga and meditation can help you to feel calm in the midst of an ongoing crisis, lowering the risk stress poses to your brain health.

If you:

- Practice stress relief (yoga, mindfulness, laughter, and the like) regularly and feel calm and collected most of the time = −1

- Do not practice stress relief, and occasionally feel mildly to moderately stressed = 0

- Feel severe stress regularly and don't practice any form of stress relief = +1

QUESTION #17: How rich is your social network?

A study of 2,173 adults aged 65 and older found that feelings of loneliness increased risk of dementia three years later[78] and adults with larger social networks scored better on memory and other cognitive tests, even if their brains already showed evidence of plaques and tangles.[79] It's thought that rich social networks help to exercise the brain, keeping it sharp even as plaques and tangles might be forming. They also may help you reduce stress.

If you:

- Feel close to many friends or relatives and/or rarely feel lonely = −1

- Feel close to one or more friends but still feel lonely sometimes = 0

- Have no close relationships and/or often feel lonely = +1

QUESTION #18: Do you smoke?

Smoking more than doubles your risk for developing Alzheimer's disease and other forms of dementia, possibly because it increases inflammation and oxidative stress in the brain.[80]

If you:
- Don't smoke = 0
- Smoke less than a pack a day = +1
- Smoke more than a pack a day = +2

* * *

Any +1 or +2 answer from this section is an opportunity for improvement. Consider tackling the risks with the +2 answers first, then work on the +1 answers. Eventually, you may benefit from addressing the zeros, too.

In addition to looking at your answers for the individual questions in this section, tally up your answers from all three sections to arrive at an overall Alzheimer's risk score.

Again, using the same woman as a hypothetical example, let's say she doesn't smoke or have sleep apnea, she does exercise and has a rich social network, but she feels chronically stressed, does little to challenge her brain, and feels tired much of the time. She also eats some vegetables, but there's room for improvement. Her math would look like this:

11 (health score)

−1 (regular exercise)

+ 0 (one to five servings of veggies)

+1 (does not challenge her brain)

+ 1 (feels fatigued)

+ 0 (no sleep apnea)

+ 1 (feels stressed)

−1 (lots of friends)

+ 0 (doesn't smoke)

Overall Alzheimer's Risk Score = 12

How might she go about lowering her score? Stress relief and sleep are big areas for her, and good places to start. Taking steps to reduce her stress could theoretically help her to sleep better at night, giving her more energy to improve her diet. All told, these steps could, over time, lower her score by three points. She may not ever score a perfect zero, but every step in that direction is a step away from an Alzheimer's diagnosis.

On the following pages, we've provided a score worksheet to make it easier for you to record your Alzheimer's risk score. Photocopy it so that you can fill it out at different points in time.

Jot down the number you get today. Then, after you spend 21 days with the personalized plan in Chapter 9, take the quiz again. You may be pleasantly surprised to find that your score has dropped several points. As you continue to incorporate Brain Smart activities into your life, take the quiz periodically to see how much you've improved.

Remember that although this score provides an opportunity to help you reduce your risk, it's not a medical diagnosis. It does not tell you whether or not you will get Alzheimer's disease. The goal is simply to get your total risk score from all of the sections as low as possible.

In Part Two of this book, you'll find chapters devoted to helping you reduce your overall *Outsmarting Alzheimer's* score. There you'll find chapters devoted to most of the lifestyle risks you can change, with just one exception. Though you won't find a chapter devoted to smoking, it's important to quit. Talk to your doctor about a prescription medication that can help, and use the support of 1-800-QUIT-NOW, a free telephone support quit line. You'll also find an abundance of free resources at *smokefree.gov*.

Your Outsmarting Alzheimer's Score Worksheet

Photocopy this worksheet so you can record your Outsmarting Alzheimer's score at different points in time.

Question #1: How old are you?

- 64 and Younger = 0
- 65–69 = +1
- 70–74 = +2
- 75–79 = +3
- 80–84 = +4
- 85+ = +5

Score: _____

Question #2: How many first-degree family members have been diagnosed with Alzheimer's disease?

- No family history of Alzheimer's disease = 0
- Your mother was diagnosed with Alzheimer's disease = +1
- Your father was diagnosed with Alzheimer's disease = +1
- Neither of your parents was diagnosed, but one or more siblings were diagnosed with Alzheimer's disease = +1

Score: _____

Note: Your highest possible score for this question is 2. Do not add extra points for every additional sibling diagnosed, for extended family members who were diagnosed, or if parents and siblings were diagnosed.

Question #3: Have you experienced any severe stressors?

Give yourself a +1 if you have one of these and +2 if you have two or more.

- Divorce
- Widowhood
- Serious illness of a child
- Serious health or behavioral problems with a child
- Mental illness of a child
- Learning that one of your children has been abused
- Mental illness in a spouse or first-degree relative (parent or sibling)
- Alcohol abuse in a spouse or first-degree relative
- Physical illness in a spouse
- Loss of a job for you or your spouse
- A serious long-term and unsolvable interpersonal work-related issue that threatens your livelihood

Score: _____

Note: In other words, the highest score you can get for this question is a 2 and the lowest is a zero. There may be other causes of long-term stress not included on the list. If you feel you've undergone a chronic stressor that isn't listed, still count it as one stressor.

Question #4: Have you ever suffered a concussion or any other brain injury?

- You've been diagnosed with a concussion at some point in your life = +1
- You played a contact sport and sometimes got hit hard enough to temporarily lose consciousness, get confused, or feel dizzy = +1
- You have never suffered a concussion or played contact sports = 0

Score: _____

Question #5: What's your highest level of education?

- Less than a high school education = +1
- High school education = 0
- Two-year associate's degree, four-year bachelor's or advanced degree = –1

Score: _____

Question #6: Have you learned a second language?

Subtract up to one point if you are fluent in any of the following:

- A second spoken language other than your native language;
- A musical language such as the ability to play the piano or saxophone;
- A computer language.

Score: _____

Note: Do not subtract extra points for additional spoken languages if you know more than two. The maximum number of points you can subtract is 3.

Your Baseline Score: _____

Question #7: What's your blood pressure?

- 120/80 or lower (low blood pressure) = –1
- Between 120/80 and 130/85 (normal blood pressure) = 0
- Between 130/85 and 139/89 (high blood pressure) = +1
- 140/90 or higher (very high blood pressure) = +2

Score: _____

Question #8: What is your cholesterol level?

HDL Cholesterol (measured in milligrams per deciliter)

- 38 mg/dl or lower (low HDL cholesterol) = +1
- 38–46 mg/dl (normal HDL cholesterol) = 0
- 46 mg/dl or higher (high HDL cholesterol) = –1

Score: _____

LDL Cholesterol

- 100 mg/dl or lower (low LDL cholesterol) = –1
- 100–129 mg/dl (normal LDL cholesterol) = 0
- 130–159 mg/dl (high LDL cholesterol) = +1
- 160–189 mg/dl (very high LDL cholesterol)= +2
- 190 mg/dl or higher (extremely high LDL cholesterol) = +3

Score: _____

Question #9: What is your fasting blood glucose?

- 100 mg/dl or lower (normal fasting blood glucose) = 0
- 100–125 mg/dl (pre-diabetes) = +1
- 126 mg/dl or higher (diabetes) = +2

Score: _____

Question #10: Are you overweight?

- 24.9 or below (normal) = 0
- 25–29 (overweight) = +1
- 30 or above (obese) = +2

Score: _____

Your Health Score: _____

Question #11: Do you accumulate at least 150 minutes of exercise every week?

If you:
- Get no exercise = +1
- Get some exercise, but less than 20 minutes on most days = 0
- Accumulate 20 or more minutes of exercise most days of the week = –1

Score: _____

Question #12: How many servings of fruits and vegetables do you consume a day?

If you:
- Consume fewer than one daily serving of fruits and vegetables = +1
- Consume one to five servings of fruits and vegetables a day = 0
- Consume more than five servings of produce a day = –1

Score: _____

Question #13: How often do you challenge your brain?

If you:
- Do mentally challenging activities less often than once weekly = +1
- Do mentally challenging activities about once a week = 0
- Do at least one mentally challenging activity most days of the week = –1

Score: _____

Question #14: How restful is your sleep?

If you:
- Feel rested when you wake each morning and rarely tired during the rest of theday = –1

- Feel somewhat rested = 0
- Feel chronically tired = +1

Score: _____

Question #15: Have you been diagnosed with sleep apnea?

If you:
- Have been diagnosed with sleep apnea, but are not using a recommended therapy to treat it = +1

- Have been diagnosed with sleep apnea and are successfully using a CPAP or other treatment = 0

- Have not been diagnosed with sleep apnea = 0

Score: _____

Question #16: What do you do to manage stress?

If you:
- Practice stress relief (yoga, mindfulness, laughter and the like) regularly and feel calm and collected most of the time = -1

- Do not practice stress relief, and occasionally feel mildly to moderately stressed = 0

- Feel severe stress regularly and don't practice any form of stress relief = +1

Score: _____

Question #17: How rich is your social network?

If you:
- Feel close to many friends or relatives and or rarely feel lonely = -1

- Feel close to one or more friends but still feel lonely sometimes = 0

- Have no close relationships and or often feel lonely = +1

Score: _____

Question #18: Do you smoke?

If you:
- Don't smoke = 0
- Smoke less than a pack a day = +1
- Smoke more than a pack a day = +2

Score: _____

Your Lifestyle Score: _____

Overall Alzheimer's Risk Score: _____

PART TWO

Prescriptions to Outsmart Alzheimer's

Now that you have some sense of your risk for Alzheimer's disease, let's introduce the tools you will need to reduce your risk. In the next six chapters, you'll find 80 prescriptions to help you outsmart Alzheimer's. Based on an extensive culling of available research, these prescriptions provide you with a wide variety of suggestions. Find those that apply to you; not all of them will. There is no "one size fits all" approach. Just because a prescription is listed first doesn't necessarily mean it's the best prescription for you. Read through all of them to get a sense of the many different possible solutions. Then choose the ones that work for you, using the information you gathered from the self-assessment in Chapter 2, coupled with the advice in Chapter 9.

Similarly, just because I haven't mentioned a particular strategy doesn't necessarily mean it's not useful. Though this book is comprehensive, it's not exhaustive, and you may come up with ways to bolster your Social, Aerobic, and other Smarts beyond what I've listed.

CHAPTER 3

S = Social Smarts

If you remove an ant from its colony and keep it isolated, it will die within days. This will happen even if you give the ant unlimited access to food.[81]

The same is true of termites and bees.[82]

The insects are not dying of starvation. Nor are they dying from thirst.

They're dying from isolation.

And, when it comes to isolation, humans are not much better at enduring loneliness than your common ant. Despite the popularity of survivalist-themed reality shows such as *Naked and Afraid* and *Out in the Wild,* we humans are social creatures whose mental and physical health tumbles into sharp decline when we're separated from others. Even the most stoic loners among us would not last long if stranded on a desolate island. Even if we managed to protect ourselves from the elements and found a vast supply of food and water, our mental health would unravel and our physical health would not be far behind.

Many of us doubt this. We think we are better survivalists than that, but science just doesn't support the loner survivalist hypothesis. Socially isolated people, one study found, were between two and three times more likely to die over a nine-year period than people with rich social networks.[83] A review of 148 studies found that people with the weakest social relationships were at a 50 percent greater risk of death compared to people with the strongest ones. That's comparable to the life-shortening effects of smoking.[84]

Reports of the damaging effects of social isolation date at least as far back as the 1800s, when prison physicians wrote of the hallucinations, delusions, and dementia that cropped up when prisoners were placed in solitary confinement.[85] Even in less austere conditions, we tend to hallucinate imaginary companions when we lack real ones. Back in the 1950s, Donald O. Hebb, a psychologist at

Montreal's McGill University, paid a number of undergraduates $20 a day to lie on a bed in a small cubicle for 24 hours a day. The students could get up for short periods of time to eat or to use the toilet, but they otherwise had little contact with other living beings.

Sounds like a piece of cake, right? Some of us with hectic work schedules might even consider *paying* someone so we could be a part of that study. Indeed, just before the study, these students admitted that they were looking forward to the downtime.

In reality, the students found that, once isolated from others, they couldn't think clearly. Their performance on cognitive tests of basic math, anagrams, and word associations declined the longer they remained isolated.

They also began to hallucinate. The hallucinations started with dots of light, lines, and geometric patterns. Then the visions progressed. One of the students saw a rock and a tree. Another saw babies. Yet another, rows of little men with black hats. Still another, squirrels marching along and carrying sacks. When our eyes, ears, and skin don't provide sensory input to our brains, our brains compensate for the absence of inputs and create missing information in the form of made-up visions, sounds, and sensations.

Most of the students remained in isolation only a few days before begging to be released from the experiment.[86]

The Social Brain

The human brain has expanded rapidly relative to other primates. Although whales and elephants have larger brains than we do, the density of neurons in our brains is higher than in any other species. This dense matrix of neurons carries a high cost in energy use. While the human brain is only 2 to 3 percent of our body mass, it hogs up 20 percent of our energy use. For many years, this has puzzled evolutionary scientists who wondered: Why did humans evolve to have such large brains?

The advantages provided by social intelligence offer us one possible answer. Robin Dunbar, a professor of evolutionary psychology and behavioral ecology at the University of Liverpool in England, has found that our brains allow us to know about 150 people at any given time.[87] In the age of Facebook and thousands of virtual friends, 150 might, at first, seem like a small number. But compared to other animals, it's really quite large. Most other animals live in small groups of just a dozen or so, so their brains have very few identities to put with faces.

The human social brain allows us to peer into the minds of others and imagine how they might feel, what they want, and what they are likely to do. This trait is called "theory of mind" because we build a theory, or a story, about every mind we meet. Our brains quickly take in sensory data about another person's eye movements, tone of voice, and posture, allowing us to calculate whether he or she is attracted to us, repulsed by us, bored by us, or interested in what we have to say. Just by the shake of a hand or by a quick embrace, we can also intuit someone's mood or intentions, although some of us are better at this than others. This very human ability is diminished in autism as well as in some forms of dementia.

We also can remember details not just about *our* friends but also about their friends and their parents and their parents' friends and even their parents' friends' cousin's baby.[88] This ability comes in handy when we're choosing a restaurant as a meeting place. We might settle on one establishment because we know that the menu offers a vegetarian dish for one vegan friend and steak for another who happens to be a meat lover and salad for our friend's cousin's friend who, we've been told, is always on a diet. It also comes into play when staying in good with the boss at work. You might know, for example, never to complain about the boss to Jane because Jane always tells her friend Stacy everything, and Stacy is the office gossip who is most likely to run straight to John, the office backstabber, who is famous for putting in a bad word with the boss regarding just about everyone in the office.

Our social brains are also what allow us to collaborate and cooperate with scores of other humans on complex tasks, like sending an astronaut to Mars, throwing a benefit event, and finding a cure for Alzheimer's disease.

Your Brain on Isolation

Though humans have the ability to know and remember as many as 150 people, many of us travel in much smaller social circles. An analysis by researchers from University of Arizona and Duke University found that our "core discussion group"—the people we turn to when we want to discuss deeper emotional topics—has shrunk over the past several decades, with the number of adults who say they have not even one confidant tripling between 1985 and 2004.[89]

While some people function just fine in smaller social circles, not everyone does. When a lack of social contact results in feelings of isolation and loneliness, Alzheimer's risk goes up. Chronic loneliness has been shown to reduce our performance on IQ[90] tests and increase our risk for Alzheimer's disease. Bryan James, PhD, an epidemiologist at Rush Alzheimer's Disease Center in Chicago, has found that seniors who frequently spend time with others—by dining out, attending sporting events, playing bingo, volunteering, visiting relatives and friends, participating in senior center activities, and/or attending religious services—had a 70 percent lower rate of cognitive decline over 12 years than did seniors with a lower rate of social interactions.[91] And a study of 2,173 older adults found that feelings of loneliness increased risk of dementia later in life, so much so that the researchers described loneliness as a major "risk factor."[92] Loneliness has also been linked to impaired immunity, accelerated aging, and an increased risk for heart disease, high blood pressure, and high cholesterol—all of which are risk factors for Alzheimer's disease.[93]

Why would loneliness lead to poor mental and intellectual health? Researchers from a number of institutions have been able to show that areas of the brain that contribute to optimal social functioning overlap with areas that are involved in general and emotional intelligence.[94] What you don't use, you lose, and social isolation may allow parts of the brain to wither away just as lack of exercise leads our muscles to shrink and become flabby. So, when the social brain wastes away, the intellectual and emotional brains may deteriorate along with it.

In addition to loneliness, isolation may also harm us by tripping the stress response. When our spouse or roommates are away, we may find we feel anxious at night, and for a good evolutionary reason. We're alone, and our social brains may equate being alone with danger. So we may find ourselves feeling hypervigilant and worried: *What was that strange noise? Didn't I just hear something? Is someone in the house? Or am I imagining this?*[95] This hypervigilance may disturb sleep[96] (Chapter 8) and induce stress (Chapter 6).[97]

The hypervigilant brain may also cause lonely people to perceive the world as a threatening place, expect negative interactions with others, and remember negative information about them. This creates a self-fulfilling prophesy. When we're lonely, we're more negative. When we're more negative, others don't enjoy being around us. When others don't enjoy being around us, we get confirmation of our bias, causing us to believe even more strongly in a negative world.

Your Brain on Friends

When we're involved with a rich, rewarding, and supportive social network, we keep our social brain in shape, continually building a social network of healthy brain cells and connections among them. This intricate and vast web of connections gives us a reserve, one that our brains are able to cash in on as we age.

Our friends also buffer us from stress. They're the people we lean on after a hard day at the office, and the ones who help us laugh our way through an illness. When we're grieving, friends bring us casseroles. Sometimes, they even shovel the snow from our driveways or babysit our kids.

Our friends can also support our efforts to improve our cognitive health. We tend to eat what our friends eat. So if we want to adopt a brain-healthy diet, we might hang out with friends who enjoy eating brain-healthy foods. And if we want to get our bodies in shape, we might make exercise dates with physically fit friends.

Finally, our friends keep us company, helping to lift depression and fend off boredom and loneliness.

Which is better for your brain—to have just one or two close friends or many more friends with whom you're not very close?

To some degree, the size of your social network may depend, at least in part, on what type of person you are. If you are an extrovert who loves conversing with large groups of people, you may thrive within a large social network. If you are an introvert who enjoys spending time alone and in small groups, a smaller social circle may be more comfortable.

The quality of your connections may also matter. A backwoodsman who lives with his beloved wife and converses with few other people can be just as socially healthy as a bubbly party goer whose address book contains the names and numbers of hundreds of people. In fact, if the party goer feels misunderstood and maligned by those hundreds of friends, his or her social health may actually be worse than the woodsman, who adores and feels supported by his spouse.

The variety of your connections may also come into play. After surveying 2,000 people about their closest confidants, Mario Luis Small, a professor of sociology at Harvard, found that, for most people, nearly half of their core discussion network—the people they turn to when revealing important matters—was composed of people with which they didn't feel emotionally close: doctors, coworkers, spiritual leaders, barbers, gym trainers, therapists, tax accountants, and so on.[98] This makes sense when you stop to think about it. Aren't we more comfortable talking about embarrassing health issues with our physicians than we are with our closest friends? Similarly, if we're having issues with a spouse, a spiritual leader or therapist offers a more objective sounding board than does another family member who might feel caught in the middle.

So rather than counting and quantifying your friends, consider how you feel. Loneliness is the distress you feel when you perceive that your social needs are not being met by the quantity or quality of your relationships.[99] Do you often feel lonely and isolated? Or do you feel connected, supported, and part of a larger whole? Are there people you can lean on during times of need? Or do you worry that, if something happens to you, you'll have no one to turn to for help?

If you feel lonely and socially isolated, you're not alone, and you're also not stuck. The prescriptions in this chapter will help.

Social Prescriptions

The beauty of Social Smarts: It's easy to work them into activities that you already enjoy. For example, if you enjoy reading, you can easily make it social by joining a book discussion group or by interacting with others on sites like *GoodReads.com*. You can also bolster Social Smarts while doing other Brain Smart activities such as exercise and healthy eating. Exercise with a partner or sign up for a group class occasionally, rather than always exercising alone. Consider ways to make your current volunteer work more social, too. For example, if you drive a Meals on Wheels route, you might set aside time to visit with each person on your delivery route rather than just dropping off the food and getting right back in the car. The more you integrate your social life into the rest of your life, the stronger your social network and the more your social life will protect the health of your body and brain.[100]

Social Smarts Prescription #1: Throw dinner parties

A dinner party provides many opportunities for you to exercise Social Smarts. Deciding whom to invite, what to serve, and who is sitting next to whom forces your brain to contemplate complex social decisions. *Is Sally likely to get along with George? Would Annette enjoy sitting between Carol and Tom, because all three of them are into travel and gardening? Is it really a good idea to invite Caroline? After all, she tends to get on Annette's nerves, doesn't she? But what would happen if you don't invite her?*

Then there's what to serve and why. Do any of your guests have food allergies? Are any of them on special diets for health, for weight loss, or for other reasons?

If you choose brain-healthy dishes such as those featured on pages 186 to 221, you'll wield your Meal Smarts, too.

Cooking the dishes and ensuring they're all ready around the same time the guests arrive requires a great deal of strategic planning, which is a high-level intellectual skill. With each recipe, you follow step-by-step instructions. If you are doubling portions, then there's also some math involved, and there's plenty of measuring and estimating, too.

And you can even work your Resilience Smarts if you use the dinner party as a way to raise money for a charity. Ask the guests to donate what they would have paid for the same meal in a restaurant to a cause such as Alzheimer's research. Or, instead of bringing a host or hostess gift, ask them to make a donation instead.

A few pointers:

- **To reduce stress, start planning the dinner party at least three weeks ahead of time.** This far out, it's a great idea to contemplate your guest list, send out invites, plan your menu, and check to make sure you have enough serving dishes. A week out, you may wish to shop for non-perishable ingredients. Several days ahead of time, clean your home, and check to make sure you have all your ingredients on hand.
- **Consider what you can prepare or cook ahead of time.** This will give you more time to socialize during the actual party.
- **Ask for help.** Suggesting that a friend be in charge of filling water glasses and another be the official wine uncorker does more than help you reduce stress, it also exercises your Social Smarts.

Social Smarts Prescription #2: Play interactive games

Many games—ranging from bridge to Chinese checkers to Pictionary to charades—cause us to exercise Social Smarts along with intellectual ones. (See Chapter 7 for more on brain-boosting games). In addition to using our brains to strategize and, at times, to do math, such games force us to contemplate what other players are likely to do and likely to think. They can bring us closer to others, and often can stir up a good conversation on an otherwise dull evening. Even video games may strengthen your social brain if you play them interactively with at least one other person.[101]

A few pointers:

- **Pick games that you enjoy and find fun.** The more you enjoy a game, the more stress you'll shed as you play. Once you get used to a game, switch to a new one. This will help you to improve your Train-Your-Brain Smarts while you also exercise your social ones.
- **Consider playing for a cause.** Foldit is a multiplayer game designed by computer scientists at the University of Washington, and it enables non-scientists to work with others to solve challenging prediction problems concerning protein folding. One day this game may help us understand how tau proteins misfold in the brain.[102] Another game, Nanocrafter, allows you to build everything from computer circuits to nanoscale machines using pieces of DNA.[103]

Social Smarts Prescription #3: Connect online

As we age, it can become increasingly difficult to see our friends in person, especially if we develop health conditions that stop us from driving. This is where computers can help us stay socially connected. One study found that seniors who used computers regularly were less lonely and less socially isolated than seniors without access to computers.[104]

A few pointers:

- **If you can't connect in real life, set a goal of virtually connecting with at least one person a day.** You might write an email, do a video chat, or respond to Facebook updates.
- **Be generous.** While on social networking sites like Facebook or Twitter, there is a tendency toward self-aggrandizing. As David Brooks recently said in *The New York Times*: "We live in a culture of the 'Big Me.' The meritocracy wants you to promote yourself. Social media wants you to broadcast a highlight reel of your life." Resist the urge to compare yourself to others. If you find yourself envying your more active friends who recently went somewhere exotic and expensive on vacation, see if you can shift your focus and rejoice for them instead.
- **Notice how you feel as you are interacting with social media.** If you start to feel tense, negative, frustrated, or isolated, it might be time to take a break from the computer. If you feel overwhelmed by a steady barrage of incoming messages, then reassess what might be going on. What about social media brings you joy? And what do you find isolating, depressing, or stressful? Do more of the former and less of the latter.

Social Smarts Prescription #4: Talk to strangers

When we're seated next to a stranger on a bus, plane, or train, most of us clam up and keep to ourselves. Yet, research from the University of Chicago Booth School of Business has found that many of us overestimate the difficulty of connecting with strangers and underestimate the rewards of doing so. Before engaging in the study, participants predicted that engaging with strangers would reduce their well-being. But when they went ahead and struck up a conversation with the person seated next to them, the opposite happened. They felt better than when they sat in solitude.[105]

A few pointers:

- **Be considerate of your seatmate, and use your social brain to read body language.** If the person next to you keeps tapping on his laptop or trying to insert ear buds, he may not want to talk.

- **Appear cheerful.** A smile and relaxed posture can go a long way to making others feel comfortable.

- **Practice.** It's easier to strike up conversations the more often you do it. Start with just a smile and a hello when you see a neighbor on the street. You might advance to offering short, helpful, encouraging commentary, such as telling a neighbor "I love your garden" or a waitress "I see you're really busy tonight. Thanks for getting our food out so quickly."

- **Become a regular.** That way you'll get to know the teller at the bank, the checkout person at the grocery store, and the clerk at the post office. Whenever possible, actually walk into such establishments and conduct business in person rather than using the drive-through. In addition to providing you with a moment of face-to-face interaction, this gives you a short burst of movement, which is also good for your brain.

Social Smarts Prescription #5: Exercise with others

Set a challenging fitness goal and rally friends to join you. Depending on your level of fitness, consider forming a team and competing in a tough event—ranging from a Spartan race to a walk-a-thon—as a group. It allows you to exercise your physical smarts along with your social ones.

A few pointers:

- **Sign up for events that raise money for charity.** This will help you firm up your Resilience Smarts along with your social ones. Or, to reduce stress as you build friendships, do something challenging and also fun, such as a "color run," during which volunteers throw colored powder onto racers, and you finish looking more like a rainbow than a human being.

- **Flex your intellectual smarts, too.** Some events, such as many adventure races, include problem-solving obstacles and orienteering.

- **Sign up for group training.** Even if you exercise together at the gym—perhaps by sharing a trainer with a friend or taking a group class—you can bond over the experience. Or, join a walking club, perhaps one organized by the Alzheimer's Association.

Social Smarts Prescription #6:
Create or join a discussion group

Gather like-minded friends to talk about hot topics, current events, movies, or another topic.

A few pointers:
- **Look for existing clubs within your community.** Search the Internet, inquire at your local library, or check out the community events pages for local news outlets to see what's available near you. You might, for example, find a lecture series that brings in experts for presentations for the audience to discuss later.
- **If you can't find a club in real life, form one.** See if your local library, place of worship, or community center is willing to host it and help you spread the word.
- **If you can't join a real-life group due to mobility issues, consider joining one online.** You can find online discussion boards and forums devoted to a range of issues.

Social Smarts Prescription #7:
Take advantage of social network principles

We tend to say and do the things our friends say and do, and the way we cluster ourselves in social groupings according to shared interests or habits is a fundamental feature of social networks. These groups exert a great deal of influence over our behavior. Adherence to group norms has been called *peer pressure,* and it can be used to foster healthy behaviors as easily as it can be used to encourage bad habits.

So if you need motivation and support in adopting Brain Smart eating or fitness, pay attention to whom you hang out with and put energy into finding and befriending people practicing behaviors and lifestyles you wish to emulate.

A few pointers:
- **Sign up for health-focused group activities.** Whether it's a cooking class, yoga, or hiking club, you'll have the ability to befriend others with Brain Smart interests that are similar to your own.
- **Attend community events with a healthy focus.** Whether it's a health fair, charity walk, or something else, you're bound to meet others who are also trying to stay fit and healthy as they age.
- **Look for the mavens within your community.** Every community has at least one. These are the opinion leaders—the people everyone else consults for trusted information. They greatly influence the behavior of

the group, and they're easy to spot and befriend because they tend to be friendly and outgoing. If you are unsure, ask others, "Who is the best person to ask about . . ." and "Who might point me in the right direction or help me get started?"

- **Stay in touch with existing friends.** Just because your current friends do not practice a Brain Smart lifestyle, it doesn't mean you have to ditch them. You can become the maven of your current social circle, using your good example to encourage others to exercise, eat more healthfully, and reduce stress.

Social Smarts Prescription #8: Talk to your pet

If you don't own a pet, you may want to skip over this piece of advice. If you do own one, then you may be pleased to know that your pet may serve as social glue that helps you to get to bond with your neighbors and also helps you to feel less lonely.[106]

Our pets really are part of our social network. They sleep in our beds, are pictured in our family portraits, and often earn a great deal of space in our holiday letters. They also, in many cases, listen attentively to our problems. Some surveys show that our pets are better listeners than our spouses.[107]

A few pointers:
- **If you own a dog, get out of your backyard.** You'll meet and chat with more neighbors by walking your dog than you will by only letting your dog out in the backyard.
- **Form a dog-walking group.** As you get to know the other dog owners in the neighborhood, consider walking your pets together. Or stop by one another's homes for pet playdates.
- **Walk for charity.** Various shelters organize walks to raise money for homeless pets. By raising money and walking, you'll meet other pet owners as well as feel good about doing good (see Prescription #11 in Chapter 6).
- **Take a pet-themed class.** Anything from basic obedience training to agility will allow you to interact with other pet owners.
- **Post photos of your pet.** Arguably, nothing is more popular on the Internet and other social sites than dog and cat photos. By proudly posting your own photos, you'll quickly find the other like-minded pet lovers in your social network.

Social Smarts Prescription #9: Travel with a group

If you love to travel, then group trips can do more than help you make friends. They can enable you to continue to do what you most love. As we age, travel can become more and more difficult. As our bodies grow weaker, carrying luggage becomes a burden, driving in foreign cities may feel more stressful than fun, and you may generally feel safer in a group.

Many different organizations plan trips for older adults: Road Scholar, Eldertreks, and several others.

A few pointers:

- **Consider carefully with whom you decide to travel.** You'll be together a lot during travel: touring, eating meals, perhaps sleeping in the same quarters, or sharing a bathroom. Some people make more compatible travel companions than others. This is especially important if you will be sharing rooms.

- **Talk about your expectations ahead of time.** Before deciding on whom to travel with, ask a lot of questions. Make sure you are all on the same page regarding your sleep/wake schedules, how much time you'll spend together, and other important concerns. Also make sure you're in alignment on a daily budget, the type of cuisine you will and will not consume, the tourist attractions you plan to visit, and how much time you'll spend together versus apart. Now is also a good time to find out if someone has food allergies, a serious snoring problem, or other health limitations that you may want to plan around.

Social Smarts Prescription #10: Create a public hangout

Maybe you frequent the same coffee shop each morning. Or perhaps, once a week you have breakfast out at the same diner or lunch at the same deli. By frequenting the same establishment over and over, you'll do more than get to know the staff. You'll also get to know the other patrons. Over time, rather than only getting coffee or only getting breakfast, you'll feel as if what you are really getting is social time with friends.

A few pointers:

- **Make eye contact and smile.** This will make you appear more approachable, making it easier for others to strike up a conversation.

- **Reveal a little about yourself.** Rather than just answering "good" or "fine" when others ask you how you are doing, consider sharing a short highlight about your day.

Social Smarts Prescription #11: Never use a drive-through

By getting out of your car and going into a bank, pharmacy, or restaurant, you get in a little exercise as well as some social time. If you frequent the same businesses over and over again, you'll find that the staff eventually remembers your name, and you remember theirs. In this way, your acquaintances eventually become your friends.

A few pointers:
- **Look at name tags and refer to staff by their first names, if possible.**
- **Ask staff about their day, about the weather, or about upcoming holidays, and share a little about yourself as well.**

Advice for Caregivers

As Alzheimer's disease progresses, it can become harder for people to remain socially connected. For example, at some point, a physician might recommend that the person you are caring for stop driving. Even before a physician intervenes, you may worry that your family member will become lost if he or she goes out alone.

This is one reason it's so important to help your family member develop and lean on strong social networks before the disease progresses too far. He or she will need the help of many friends in order to remain independent for as long as possible, and you'll need their help for your own peace of mind.

Stay in touch with neighbors, and try to overcome the embarrassment of asking others for help. If your family member meets friends once a week over lunch, ask if one of them might consider driving. Or maybe a neighbor wouldn't mind taking your spouse for a drive to see holiday lights or fall foliage. As you'll learn in Chapter 6, by allowing your neighbors to help, you're giving them a gift. Altruism is good for their health.

Hired help and adult day care are also options. Get leads on potential in-home caregiving help through friends, family, coworkers, physicians, your faith community, and your local senior center. Thoroughly interview potential candidates. Rather than feel guilty about it, know that you are helping your family member by ensuring that he or she socializes with others beyond just you. It's important for your family member to get out and about, and adult day care provides a safe option, allowing you to run your errands worry-free.

However, adult day care does not work for everyone. Ask if the center near you offers a free visit or two. Attend the first visit with your family member, and see how he or she reacts. Then, if you have the option of a second visit, attend for part of it, and see how he or she reacts when you leave as well as when you return.

Even if your family member embraces the idea in the beginning, remain vigilant. Pay attention if he or she refuses to go, and ask staff about any adjustment issues.

In addition to day care programs, you might sign your family member up for community programs based on his or her personal interests. Perhaps your family member might enjoy the gardening club, a knitting circle, or a car club.

Time Banking may also ease your burden. In a Time Bank, community members agree to earn and spend Time Bank hours as a group. So, for example, you might earn time credit by watching someone's children or driving someone to a doctor's appointment. Then you might cash in your credit hours by asking for help at a later date, and the person you helped or someone else in the Time Bank will help you. The website *timebanks.org* offers a directory of Time Banks around the United States.

Or you might consider a support group. Support groups are a great way to meet others and talk about the one thing you share in common: Alzheimer's disease. The Alzheimer's Disease Education and Referral Center can direct you toward a support group near you. Visit *www.nia.nih.gov/alzheimers* for more information.

Finally, know that a dog or cat can be a wonderful companion for someone with Alzheimer's disease, and a pet might ease your mind when you are away from home. The Pets for the Elderly Foundation (PFE) helps to match appropriate shelter animals with seniors, often paying adoption fees and initial veterinary costs.[108] One study done in Germany found that weekly therapy sessions that included dog visits improved attentiveness and talkativeness in nursing home residents with dementia.[109] In some countries such as Israel and Scotland, some dogs have even been specifically trained to assist people with Alzheimer's disease. These service dogs are trained to lead their handler home, preventing someone with Alzheimer's from getting lost. If something should happen to the person with Alzheimer's, the dog is trained to remain with him or her and call attention by barking.[110]

CHAPTER 4

M = Meal Smarts

One dietary pattern could win the award as the top diet for poor brain health and, unfortunately, if you live in the United States, it may very well be the dietary pattern you are following.

It's the typical American diet.

Indeed, American eating offers countless examples of what not to eat for optimum brain health: fast food, fried foods, soft drinks, fatty red meats, processed meat such as bacon and hotdogs, blood-sugar-spiking refined "white foods" such as white bread, snack chips, desserts, and foods that are so fake and contain so many artificial colors and flavors that it's hard to actually refer to them as "food."[111] Together, this assortment of fatty, sugary, salty, fake foods induce inflammation and oxidation, both of which raise the risk for a host of diseases, including Alzheimer's disease.

If not the typical American diet, what should you eat instead? It depends on your lifestyle and food preferences. There is no one best dietary pattern when it comes to eating for optimum brain health. Nor is there one magical food or supplement. Instead, a wide range of eating patterns—Asian eating, the MIND diet, the Mediterranean diet, vegan eating—has been shown to protect your brain. Although those eating patterns vary—for example, some include meat, others don't; some place a heavy emphasis on fish, others suggest no fish—they all tend to have one thing in common: a preponderance of antioxidant-rich plant foods.

Plants manufacture antioxidant chemicals to protect themselves from ultraviolet light and disease. When we eat these plants—in the form of fruits, vegetables, beans, nuts, seeds, and grains—we consume this built-in protection, and their antioxidants can then protect our cells from disease, too.[112] This includes disease protection for cells in the brain, and we know this, in part, thanks to beagles.

Spinach Helps Old Dogs Learn New Tricks

Few humans eat the same foods day in and out, which makes studying how nutrition affects our health a bit difficult. We know, for example, that people from certain cultures and geographic locations are, generally speaking, healthier than people from others. But figuring out what, in particular, makes them so healthy is much harder to tease out. Is it because of their rich network of social support? That they remain active throughout life? Their genes? Or what they eat? And if it's at least partly because of what they eat, what foods in particular help them to live so long?

Thankfully, unlike humans, most dogs don't consume thousands of foods over a lifetime. In fact, many of them are happy to consume just one: kibble.

Carl Cotman, a professor of neurology at the University of California, Irvine, and other researchers have studied how kibble enriched with tomatoes, carrots, citrus, spinach, and antioxidant supplements (vitamins E and C, lipoic acid, and carnitine) affects the brains of beagles. He and his team divided the dogs into four groups. One control group ate a regular diet. A second group ate the enriched kibble that included the equivalent of six servings of fruits and vegetables. A third group ate regular kibble but were offered the canine equivalent of daily school education: an abundance of exercise, playtime with other dogs, and access to novel toys. The final group ate the enriched kibble and went to dog school.

As the study progressed, the researchers repeatedly tested the dogs with increasingly difficult learning problems. In one, the dogs had to learn whether a treat was hidden under a black or a white block. Overall, the dogs in the combined group—the ones who played, exercised, and ate fruit-and-veggie-packed kibble—did the best on the learning tasks. No surprises there, as playtime and intellectual enrichment are just as powerful Brain Smarts as good nutrition. But even the dogs who only ate the enriched kibble and who were not offered extra playtime performed better than the dogs who only ate regular kibble. Sixty percent of them were able to continually find the hidden treat, whereas only 25 percent of the dogs who ate regular kibble could do the same.[113]

Now, you might argue that humans and dogs are not the same. And, sure, in some fortunate ways, you're right.

But, neurologically and biologically speaking, dogs are more similar to humans than many of us might assume. Dogs are susceptible to many of the same age-related diseases as humans, including age-related brain degeneration. This is why we have the saying, "You can't teach an old dog new tricks."

As Cotman's research shows us, though: Old dogs *can* learn new tricks as long as they eat antioxidant-rich fruits and vegetables throughout their lives. And the same may be true of humans.

The Elements of Smart Meals

Antioxidant-rich foods are just one important component of a Brain Smart eating pattern. In addition to antioxidants, many foods also contain substances that lower inflammation throughout the body and brain, as well as nutrients needed for cells to do their jobs.

All of these nutrients seem to work together to create good health. It's for this reason that there is no one food or beverage to consume for good health. Brain Smart eating isn't about gorging on just blueberries or chia seeds or some other healthy food du jour. It's not even about just *one* specific eating pattern. It turns out that many different foods and different dietary patterns have been shown to protect us from Alzheimer's disease, and this is great news for all of us. It allows us the freedom to tailor our Brain Smart food choices to our personal tastes and lifestyle.

Consider embarking on one of the following Brain Smart eating patterns—or perhaps even a combination of them.

The Asian diet: The residents of many Asian countries, such as Korea and Japan, enjoy a diet that is high in antioxidant-rich vegetables and fresh herbs and low in inflammation-boosting saturated fats (from animal products) and trans fats (from partially hydrogenated oils). Among the cuisines of these Asian countries, Japanese food has been the most studied.[114] Rich in fish and plants—including soybeans, seaweeds, vegetables, and fruit—Japanese dishes are often steamed rather than fried, and staples include yams, green tea, cruciferous vegetables, and shiitake mushrooms. Interestingly, as people in Japan have switched to a more Americanized diet that includes more fatty meats and processed foods, Alzheimer's prevalence has gone up.[115] Korean diets offer an as yet relatively unexplored wealth of unusual vegetables that likely have health benefits. For Asian dishes loaded with brain-boosting foods, see Thai Noodles with Cashews and Stir-Fried Vegetables (page 213) and Bok Choy, Tofu, and Mushroom Stir-Fry (page 210).

The Mediterranean diet: Several studies show that the Mediterranean diet preserves cognitive function and overall health.[116, 117, 118] People in countries near the Mediterranean Sea (Spain, Portugal, southern France, Greece, and Italy) tend to consume diets rich in fruits, vegetables, whole grains, potatoes, poultry, beans, nuts, olive oil, and fish. Fat tends to come from olive oil rather than butter, and fish makes a more regular appearance on the dinner table than red meat. On this diet, nearly every meal and snack includes plant foods (fruits, veggies, nuts, legumes, seeds, herbs, whole grains), and fish is consumed at least twice a week. Try Lentil and Rice Paella with Clams (page 207) or our Mediterranean Salad with Edamame (page 197).

The DASH diet: Originally developed by the US National Institutes of Health to lower blood pressure, the Dietary Approaches to Stop Hypertension (DASH) diet contains a high intake of plant foods, fruits, vegetables, fish, poultry, whole grains, low-fat dairy products, and nuts, while minimizing the intake of red meat, sodium, sweets, and sugar-sweetened beverages. In a four-month-long randomized clinical trial of 124 participants with elevated blood pressure, people who followed the DASH made greater improvements on tests of memory, reasoning, learning, planning, and problem solving than did people not on the diet.[119]

The MIND diet: A blend of the Mediterranean and DASH diets, the MIND diet was designed by a nutritional epidemiologist at Rush University Medical Center in Chicago. It showcases 10 brain-healthy foods (leafy greens, vegetables, nuts, berries, beans, whole grains, fish, poultry, olive oil, and wine) while severely restricting red meat, butter and margarine, cheese, sweets and desserts, fried food, and fast food. Among the brain-healthy foods, the diet recommends you consume three whole grain servings, a salad, and at least one vegetable every day, beans every other day, poultry and berries twice a week, and fish once a week. One study found that it lowered risk of Alzheimer's disease by as much as 53 percent.[120]

Plant-based diets: Vegetarian diets have been shown to drop blood pressure,[121] inflammation,[122] and body weight,[123] as well as improve longevity.[124] Also, results from the Adventist Health Study found that heavy meat-eaters were more than twice as likely to develop dementia than were vegetarians.[125] Eco Atkins, a type of vegan diet that restricts refined starch and sugar, has been shown to drop blood cholesterol by roughly 10 percent and speed weight loss, two outcomes that could potentially reduce Alzheimer's risk.[126] And if you are not quite ready to give up all of the meat in your life, simply moving toward a plant-based diet may offer some benefit. One study found that people who consumed a diet rich in nuts, fish, tomatoes, poultry, cruciferous vegetables (such as cauliflower, cabbage, and broccoli), fruits, and dark and green leafy vegetables and who minimized high-fat dairy, red meat, organ meat, and butter were at the lowest risk for Alzheimer's disease compared to people who consumed less produce and more fatty animal products, organ meats, and red meats.[127]

Though they have yet to attract the attention of researchers, many other healthy-eating patterns—ranging from raw diets to the Ornish diet to low-glycemic diets—may also be protective.[128] So rather than rigidly fixate on just one eating pattern, put your focus on eating more real plant-based foods and fewer artificial foods that are full of fat, starch, sodium, and/or sugar. Our brains thrive when we feed them food that is rich in fiber and antioxidants. The prescriptions in this chapter, along with the recipes in Chapter 10, will help you do just that.

Which is better for your brain—aluminum foil or cling wrap?

The answer is: Neither.

Many people avoid aluminum foil based on speculation dating back to the 1960s and 1970s about it possibly playing a role in Alzheimer's disease. Since then, more than three decades of research and scores of studies have failed to find a connection between the everyday exposure to aluminum—whether from foil or cooking pots or antiperspirants—and Alzheimer's disease. The link between dietary aluminum and Alzheimer's has been thoroughly repudiated, and there is no reason to fear using aluminum cooking pots. Despite this, people still continue to worry about aluminum, making it one of the most persistent health myths to penetrate the public consciousness.

On the other hand, bisphenol A (BPA)—a chemical used to make cling wrap, as well as plastic water bottles and the linings of some food cans—is thought to mimic estrogen in the body, disrupting the endocrine system and raising risk for cancer, diabetes, obesity, and heart disease, any of which can raise your risk of Alzheimer's, too.[129] Luckily, many cling wraps and other plastic products (including Ziploc bags, Saran wrap, and Glad wrap) are now BPA-free.[130, 131] Unfortunately, the most common BPA replacement is a chemical called *bisphenol-S* (BPS), and new evidence suggests that this chemical may also be harmful. One test-tube study found that every plastic compound had the potential to leech into the body and disrupt the endocrine system.[132] Follow-up studies done on various types of animals have corroborated those findings.[133]

What to do? Plastics are most likely to bleed chemicals into food when they are exposed to heat. So, even if the packaging claims to be "BPA-free," don't use "boil-in-a-bag" or "steam-in-a-bag" products. Remove microwave meals from their packaging and cook them on a plate. Remove cling wrap from leftovers before cooking in the microwave, and avoid drinking out of plastic water bottles that have been left in a hot car or in sunlight.[134]

Whether you need to take additional precautions by storing your food in stainless steel or glass containers is still a matter of debate and requires more data. Such concerns underscore the importance of ongoing scientific research to fully understand the health risks in our environment.

Smart Nutrition Prescriptions

The prescriptions in this chapter will help you move toward a whole food, plant-based diet and away from fake, highly processed foods that are rich in fat, starch, sodium, and/or sugar. As with other chapters, you'll find a range of prescriptions and some may apply to you more than others. Choose what works best for you.

Though nutritional change may initially feel daunting, it's often easier than many people assume. Brain Smart meals can be just as delicious as unhealthy ones, especially when you flavor your meals with an array of herbs and spices (see prescription #5). They also can be quick to prepare and easy on your monthly budget. And they offer a powerful side benefit: In addition to boosting your brain health, these prescriptions will result in more energy, less bloating, improved heart health, and a slimmer body.

As you incorporate these prescriptions into your life, consider how you can combine them with your Train-Your-Brain, Social, and Resilience Smarts. Perhaps you offer to cook for community fundraisers, which can help you flex your Resilience Smarts by providing a strong sense of purpose. Maybe you exercise as you cook. While you wait for water to boil, for example, do one or more of the moves from the seven-minute circuit routine (page 222) in the Aerobic Smarts chapter. Simply following the steps of an unfamiliar recipe helps you use Train-Your-Brain Smarts, and doubling or tripling that recipe so you can cook for a crowd flexes those smarts even more.

Meal Smarts Prescription #1: Fill up on fewer calories

As we mentioned in Chapter 2, obesity in your 40s and 50s is associated with Alzheimer's disease in your 70s and beyond.[135] Filling up on fewer calories allows you to shed pounds, which can help reverse other risks for Alzheimer's disease, including sleep apnea, high blood pressure, and diabetes.[136] Cutting your daily intake of calories by 30 to 50 percent also reduces your metabolic rate and therefore slows oxidation throughout the body, including the brain. It lowers blood glucose and insulin levels, too.[137] This is true even if you are not overweight. To reduce your daily intake, however, you don't have to go hungry. You need only swap calorie-dense foods for lower-calorie ones. This allows you to consume the same size portions—and possibly even larger ones!—while slashing your calorie intake.

A few pointers:
- **Start your meals with a serving of vegetables.** They're rich in fiber and water, both of which can fill you up quickly, but they're low in calories. An entire head of lettuce, for example, contains only 53 calories. An

appetizer of salad or steamed vegetables can take the edge off, causing you to automatically consume less of the higher-calorie main course.

- **Fill up on beans and lentils.** In a Spanish study of 30 obese men and women, study participants who ate four weekly 1-cup servings of lentils, chickpeas, peas, or beans had lower levels of inflammatory markers than those who cut calories without eating legumes. The bean-eaters also lost more weight, probably because the beans filled them up on fewer calories.[138]

- **If you are a stress eater, try doing a few minutes of deep breathing before meals and snacks.** Also create a list of soothing and enjoyable distractions. Instead of eating, try snuggling with someone special, taking a brisk walk on a beautiful day, or listening to music.

- **Combine any efforts to cut calories with efforts to improve your sleep quality.** Lack of sleep generally causes us to feel hungrier, and it also increases cravings for high-calorie, fatty, and sugary foods. See Chapter 8 for advice on getting a good night's sleep.

- **Join a weight-loss community.** Programs like Weight Watchers and the Dean Ornish program are so successful, in part, because they include group support. The power of the group can help you stay true to your goals and motivate you when you're feeling overwhelmed or discouraged.

- **Use smaller plates and glasses.** Brian Wansink and his colleagues at the Cornell Food and Brand Lab have done dozens of studies looking at how our environment influences our eating. He's found that we automatically eat less when we serve ourselves smaller portion sizes of food on smaller plates. (Place just two handfuls of chips on an appetizer plate, for example, instead of eating them straight from the jumbo-sized bag).[139]

Meal Smarts Prescription #2: Cook your own food

One of the swiftest ways to cut back on calories: Eat in rather than out. Restaurant portions are notoriously supersized, providing much more food than most of us need. And, as Brian Wansink's research shows, the more food on our plate, the more food we eat.[140] As a result, a review of nearly 30 studies found that people who ate out the most tended to weigh more than people who ate out the least.[141]

Restaurant fare is also rich in saturated and trans fats, both of which can raise your risk for heart and Alzheimer's disease. And these dishes are generally loaded with salt, which increases blood pressure in salt-sensitive people. Restaurants have another unhealthy trick—they leave you waiting at your table with a basket full of tempting bread. White bread, skinless potatoes, and other starchy foods tend to digest quickly, stimulating your appetite. This is why many of us eat slice after slice of bread before a meal. Three dinner rolls can add up to 300 calories, and you're still hungry for more.

Of the various types of restaurant fare, fast food is especially problematic. According to researchers from Ohio State University as well as the University of Texas at Austin, the more fast food elementary and middle schoolers consumed, the lower their test scores in reading, math, and science.[142] And mice fed a "fast-food" diet for nine months developed more tau tangles.[143]

Eating in, on the other hand, allows you to prepare your meals with more spices (see Prescription #5) and vegetables (see Prescription #3), and less blood pressure–raising salt. By trying new recipes, you'll also challenge your brain, which is a nice way to flex your Train-Your-Brain Smarts (Chapter 7). Make it social by inviting people over or cooking with a friend, and you flex your Social Smarts (Chapter 3), as well. For great Brain Smart recipes, see Chapter 10.

A few pointers:

- **Start with what you can handle.** If you currently eat out most of the time, it's not realistic to expect yourself to eat in from now on. Setting such a lofty goal may even cause undue stress, and as you'll learn in Chapter 6, stress can harm the brain, too. A more realistic goal: Cook one more meal each week than you are currently cooking. Once that feels easy, add another, and then another.

- **Take cooking classes.** Cooking classes allow you to strengthen your Social Smarts while you learn to cook healthier or more intellectually challenging recipes.

- **Choose fresh ingredients over processed ones.** Three-fourths of the salt we eat comes packaged into the food we buy, and this is especially true of the processed foods found in the middle aisles of the grocery store.

- **Shop for ingredients at farmers' markets when available.** Many of us can't get ourselves out of a grocery store quickly enough. But most farmers' markets offer a different experience entirely. Many are situated outdoors in pleasant locations, and some even include live entertainment, such as folk bands and other music. As a result, shoppers tend to linger and socialize with each other and the farmers. You can also find out more easily how and where the food was grown, helping you to avoid buying foods treated with pesticides. Conventionally grown crops that have been treated with pesticides may contain chemical residues that have been shown to increase risk for Alzheimer's disease. Though all of your foods do not necessarily need to be organic, you'll definitely want to shop organic when it comes to the following foods, whose conventionally grown counterparts are most likely to contain pesticide residues, according to the Environmental Working Group: apples, celery, cherry tomatoes, cucumbers, grapes, nectarines, peaches, potatoes, snap peas, spinach, strawberries, bell peppers, hot peppers, kale, and collard greens.[144]

Meal Smarts Prescription #3:
Eat at least five servings of fruits and vegetables daily

Remember those older beagles who learned new tricks? They were eating the equivalent of five or six servings of fruits and vegetables a day.

Vegetables especially can help you to fill up on fewer calories and more easily reap the benefits of Prescription #1.[145]

Higher vegetable consumption was associated with slower rate of cognitive decline in 3,718 people aged 65 years and older who participated in the Chicago Health and Aging Project. Study participants filled out food logs and agreed to undergo tests of their cognitive abilities periodically for six years. All of the study participants scored lower on cognitive tests at the end of the study than they did at the beginning, but those who consumed more than four daily servings of vegetables experienced a 40 percent slower decline in their abilities than people who consumed less than one daily serving.[146]

Antioxidant-rich vegetables include dark, leafy greens, artichokes, okra, Brussels sprouts, beets, bell peppers, broccoli, red cabbage, tomatoes, eggplant, corn, onions, sweet potatoes, winter squash, and most other vegetables that are brightly colored.[147] For cooking ideas, see Cock-a-Leekie Soup with Kale (page 204), Braised Mixed Greens with Dried Currants (page 216), Spinach and Goat Cheese Omelet (page 192), Summer Greens Scramble (page 192), Spinach Salad with Chickpeas (page 195), and Spinach, Sweet Potato, and Shiitake Salad (page 196).

Among fruits, dates, figs,[148] dried plums,[149] berries,[150] apples, oranges, grapes, plums, cherries, and pomegranates are standout sources of antioxidants[151]that may protect the brain from oxidation.[152] See Fig, Apple, and Cinnamon Compote (page 219), Nutty Muesli (page 188), and Grilled Salmon Salad (page 199).

A few pointers:

- **Choose the brightest of the bunch.** The pigments that lend bright colors to many fruits and vegetables are especially powerful sources of antioxidants.

- **Eat a variety.** Don't limit yourself to the few fruits and vegetables that have captured the headlines. We need a variety of antioxidants for total body health. They work as a team to minimize damage and locate repair mechanisms.

- **Use vegetables to transform not-so-healthy dishes.** When chopped or pureed, vegetables can be added to just about any dish to reduce the fat and calories and boost the overall nutrition. For ideas, see Spinach-Stuffed Meat Loaf (page 206) and Macaroni and Cheese with Spinach (page 212).
- **Eat fruit for dessert.** Fruit is naturally sweet. Sprinkle a little cinnamon on top of berries for a simple, low-calorie brain booster. Or puree berries, watermelon, and other fruits, and freeze them. Try Pomegranate Ice (page 221).
- **Eat whole fruits and vegetables rather than processed ones.** Many of the antioxidants in fruits and vegetables are concentrated around the skins and the seeds. Tomatoes, for example, contain potent antioxidant chemicals in the yellow fluid around tomato seeds—the part of the tomato that is often thrown away before tomatoes are processed into salsas, sauces, and soups.[153] For ways to use the whole fruit with the skin, see Hot Cereal with Apples and Dates (page 189) and Fruity Brussels Sprouts (page 214).

Meal Smarts Prescription #4:
Eat whole foods, not artificial foods

The best foods for our overall health are easy to trace to their original source. It doesn't take a degree in botany, for example, to know that apples come from apple trees. On the other hand, it's not so easy to guess where Apple Jacks come from.

The more highly processed a food, the more likely it is to contain one of the following:

Processed starch: When wheat is ground into white flour, most of its nutrition and fiber is lost. Foods made from refined wheat fiber—ranging from white bread to snack chips—are rich in calories and blood-sugar-raising carbohydrates and low in fiber and nutrients.

Sugar: Processed foods are rich in added sugar, and this sweetener makes its way into a surprising array of foods. You wouldn't, for example, expect to find sugar in pasta sauce. But the average jar of processed red sauce contains 12 grams of sugar per half cup. That's 3 teaspoons of sugar in every half cup of sauce—a lot of sugar for a food that few of us think of as "sweet."

The consumption of excess sugar leads to weight gain and insulin resistance (a precursor for diabetes), both of which can raise your risk for Alzheimer's disease.[154] High blood-sugar levels may damage blood vessels throughout the body, including those in the brain. High blood sugar also leads to greater oxidative stress, which may render beta-amyloid protein more toxic to the cells lining the blood vessels in the brain.[155]

Sodium: Sodium intake has become controversial, with new data that questions previous advice on the necessity for lowering salt consumption. The most important reason to lower sodium intake is its link to high blood pressure. However, not everyone is susceptible to blood-pressure elevation with a high salt intake. If your blood pressure is high, then it is worth assessing whether trying a low-salt diet can lower your numbers. If you have a family history of high blood pressure, restricting salt intake may help you to avoid hypertension later in life. A good rule of thumb here is moderation: Neither excessive salt nor severe salt restriction is recommended. However, the devil is in the details, and for your specific salt intake recommendations, consult with a nutritionist.

Nitrites: The nitrites added to preserve foods like hot dogs and lunch meat convert to nitrosamines when they are heated to high temperatures (such as by frying or flame broiling). This also happens when nitrites meet amines in the acidic confines of the stomach.[156] Nitrosamines are chemical compounds used to make pesticides; they are thought to be carcinogenic and may also contribute to Alzheimer's disease, though more research is needed to fully understand this connection.

Whole, unprocessed foods—such as fresh fruits and vegetables and uncured animal products—are naturally low in these additives.

A few pointers:

- **To cut back on processed starch, choose whole grain foods over processed ones.** In other words, choose brown or wild rice instead of white, 100 percent whole wheat bread and cereals instead of those made from refined white flour. Also experiment with quinoa, bulgur, barley, and millet—all of which are sold in their most unrefined versions.

- **Avoid processed foods that list sugar within the first few ingredients.** The following ingredients all count as "sugar": cane juice, cane syrup, corn sweeteners, high-fructose corn syrup, fruit juice concentrate and nectars, honey, malt syrup, molasses. Ingredients that end in "ose" (such as dextrose and maltose) are often chemical names for types of sugar.

- **Look for "sodium nitrite" on the ingredient labels of processed foods.** You're most likely to find this listed on cheeses, smoked foods, lunch meat, sausages, and bacon, and you'll want to avoid foods that contain it. Whenever possible, it's better to consume fresh meat rather than cured or deli meat.

Meal Smarts Prescription #5: Use spices liberally

Herbs and spices add flavor to food, allowing you to cut back on butter, oil, and salt. Because they come from plants, many herbs and spices also contain antioxidants and offer many healing benefits, including Alzheimer's prevention.

The following spices have all been shown to promote good health.

Curry and turmeric: These spices contain the antioxidant curcumin, which is what lends them their bright colors. Several different studies show that curcumin helps to reduce the risk of cancer, arthritis, depression, and Alzheimer's disease.[157] For ideas on cooking with curry and turmeric, see Chicken Curry Soup (page 203), Curried Chicken Salad Sandwich (page 200), and Curry-Seared Scallops (page 209).

Cinnamon: Just a quarter teaspoon of the spice twice a day has been shown to reduce fasting blood sugar up to 29 percent in people with type 2 diabetes. This is important, because type 2 diabetes can raise your risk for developing Alzheimer's disease. The spice has also been found to reduce blood cholesterol and inflammation, both of which can further reduce your risk for Alzheimer's.[158] Cinnamon can help you to add some sweetness to foods without using sugar. Sprinkle it on oatmeal, fruit, pancakes, and coffee, and experiment by adding it to other main course dishes like chili.

Rosemary: This herb contains antioxidant and anti-inflammatory compounds that may protect brain health. In one small study, 28 seniors who drank a tomato drink spiked with 750 milligrams of dried rosemary—somewhat more of the spice than you might typically ingest through normal culinary flavoring—performed better on a memory test given six hours later than seniors who did not ingest the spice.[159] Although such small studies are never definitive, they do point the way toward larger studies. Another caveat: More rosemary is not more potent. Seniors who took a supplement that contained more than six times as much dried rosemary performed worse on the same memory test.[160] Even just smelling the herb may offer some benefit. Study participants who sat inside a cubicle that was infused with the scent of rosemary were able to solve a series of math problems more quickly than when they weren't surrounded by the scent. It's thought that rosemary may boost brain function by preventing the breakdown of a key neurotransmitter in the brain.[161] Keep a potted rosemary plant in your kitchen, and use the herb to flavor everything from soups to roasted vegetables. Puree some with olive oil to create a pesto. You can also use the rosemary branch to skewer shrimp for grilling.

Meal Smarts Prescription #6: Soak potatoes before cooking

Generally speaking, potatoes are a healthy food, and they can count as a serving of fruits and vegetables. That said, they contain an amino acid called asparagine that, when exposed to high heat, changes into acrylamide, a neurotoxin.[162] Acrylamide binds to the ends of our axons, making it tougher for brain cells to communicate with one another.[163]

Frying is most likely to trigger the creation of acrylamide, so minimize your intake of French fries and potato chips, which are also rich in trans and saturated fats, two types of fat that are bad for the brain. Water protects asparagine, so soaking potatoes before cooking them can stop it from transforming into acrylamide.

A few pointers:

- **Avoid frying as much as possible.**[164] According to the Food and Drug Administration, frying produces the most acrylamide, followed by roasting and baking. Boiling or microwaving does not produce acrylamide.[165] Whenever possible, boil or steam potato products instead of roasting or frying. Try New Potatoes with Nori (page 217).

- **If you must roast potatoes, soak raw potato slices in water for 15 to 30 minutes before doing so.** Drain the potatoes and blot them dry before cooking.

- **Experiment with cooking potatoes at a lower oven temperature and for shorter periods of time.** By cooking roasted potatoes to golden yellow rather than crispy brown, you'll cut down on acrylamide.

- **Sprinkle turmeric on your fries.** A bioactive ingredient in this spice is capable of latching onto and neutralizing acrylamide. Other foods with similar compounds include apple skins and wine.[166, 167] Rosemary may help, as well.

- **Do not store potatoes in the refrigerator.** Cold temperatures break down the starches. Not only does this render the potatoes unpleasantly gritty, it also can make them more likely to produce acrylamide during cooking, according to the FDA. Instead store them in a cool, dark place, such as a pantry.

Meal Smarts Prescription #7: Marinate meat before cooking

Acrylamide isn't the only toxin capable of forming on cooked foods; another one is *advanced glycation end products (AGEs)*. These compounds form when fat, protein, and sugar react with heat. They are found in particularly high levels in bacon, sausages, processed meats, and fried and grilled foods.

And much like acrylamide, the consumption of high amounts of AGEs has been shown to cause harmful changes in the brain.[168]

But there's an easy way to slash your AGE consumption: Make your food (especially meats) as moist as possible. By boiling, braising, poaching, or marinating meat and fish before grilling or broiling, you allow moisture to permeate their flesh, dramatically reducing the AGEs.

A few pointers:

- **Avoid store-bought marinades.** Most contain high-fructose corn syrup, which can cause AGEs to proliferate. For a great marinade recipe, see Barbecued Flank Steak (page 204).

- **Marinate for at least an hour before cooking.** This will allow the moisture to fully penetrate the meat.

- **When cooking, add more moisture by poaching** (creating a tent with foil that prevents the steamed juices from escaping) or braising (searing the meat just until it browns and then adding liquid such as wine or juice and boiling it covered inside the oven).

Meal Smarts Prescription #8: Eat coldwater fish once a week

Fish that swim in cold waters tend to develop a layer of fat to keep them warm. Called omega-3 fatty acid, this type of fat has been shown to reduce inflammation throughout the body when consumed by humans. In a study of 815 people, people who consumed fish at least once a week reduced their Alzheimer's disease risk by 60 percent compared to people who rarely or never ate fish.[169] High omega-3 standouts include anchovies, Atlantic mackerel, canned light tuna, herring, salmon, and sardines.

A few pointers:

- **Trade in farmed salmon for wild.** Wild salmon consume plankton and small crustaceans, whereas farmed salmon are given concentrated feed made from anchovies and herring that has tested high in PCBs, an industrial pollutant, carcinogen, and neurotoxin. Farmed salmon have tested eight times higher in PCBs than wild salmon.[170, 171, 172]

- **Use these recipes for ideas on cooking coldwater fish.** Try Salmon and Fennel Lettuce Wraps (page 201), Salmon Cake Sandwiches (page 202), Grilled Salmon Salad (page 199), Poached Salmon with Cucumber Dill Sauce (page 208). For sardines, try our Open-Faced Sardine Sandwiches (page 202).

- **Minimize your consumption of larger, predatory fish,** as these are likely to be high in the neurotoxin mercury. Fish and shellfish to avoid are shark, swordfish, king mackerel, tilefish, albacore tuna, sea bass, bluefish, grouper, halibut, lobster, marlin, red snapper, pike, orange roughy, Spanish mackerel, and walleye.[173]

- **If you don't consume fish, try getting your omega-3s from nuts and seeds (and check out the next prescription).** Walnuts, flax, chia, and hemp seeds, and, to a lesser degree, green vegetables such as Brussels sprouts, kale, and spinach, all contain this important fat. Just 1 ounce of chia seeds contains 4,900 milligrams of omega-3s, and 1 ounce of flaxseeds, 6,300 milligrams; both of these are many times more omega-3s than the same amount of wild salmon. But it's a different type of omega-3 than is found in fish. Plant foods contain the omega-3 alpha linolenic acid (ALA), while fish contains docosahexaenoic acid (DHA) and eicosapentaenoic acid (EPA). Some brands of eggs also contain small amounts of ALA due to the flaxseeds and/or fish oil fed to the hens. It's thought that EPA and DHA are the true omega-3 stars while ALA plays a more supporting role, but more research is needed, and nuts and seeds and other ALA foods are healthy for many other reasons (see next prescription).

Meal Smarts Prescription #9: Snack on nuts and seeds

As you've learned, nuts and seeds are a rich source of omega-3 fatty acids. Nuts and seeds also provide a good dose of selenium and vitamin E, two other nutrients that may promote brain health. Walnuts may be a particularly potent source of edible brain protection. In addition to omega-3 fatty acids, walnuts are rich in antioxidants that have been shown to reduce Alzheimer's disease in mice.[174]

A few pointers:

- **Consume 1 to 1.5 ounces (about a handful) of your favorite nuts and seeds a day.**[175] This amount comes loaded with omega-3s and other brain-healthy nutrients but is a small enough serving to keep your weight in check.
- **Sprinkle nuts and seeds over salads, puree them into pesto sauces, or make a trail mix with them.** A trail mix of nuts and dried fruit offers a perfect snack to eat before exercise (see Prescription #14).
- **Don't go overboard.** Nuts and seeds are rich in calories, so consuming too many of them could result in weight gain.

Meal Smarts Prescription #10: Drink several cups of tea a day

Black and green tea are rich sources of antioxidants called catechins that may fend off oxidative damage throughout the body, including the brain.[176] Green tea is also a rich source of epigallocatechin-3-gallate (EGCG), which has been shown to reduce beta-amyloid plaque and tau tangles in mice.[177] Tea has also been shown to drop blood pressure[178] and cholesterol levels.[179]

A few pointers:

- **Drink the tea you enjoy.** The jury is still out on whether green tea outperforms oolong and black when it comes to good health. So drink whichever variety you enjoy the most.

- **Some herbal teas offer some benefit, too.** For example, hibiscus tea has also been shown to drop blood pressure.[180]

- **Brew it yourself.** Commercially available bottled teas have been shown to contain few, if any, of the protective substances of freshly brewed green or black tea.[181]

Meal Smarts Prescription #11: Enjoy coffee in the morning

As you'll learn in Chapter 8, caffeine consumed too late in the day may disturb your sleep. But coffee consumed in the morning and perhaps the early afternoon, depending on your personal caffeine sensitivity, may reduce risk. Coffee contains a chemical called eicosanoyl-5-hydroxytryptamide (EHT) that, in studies done on rats, has been shown to protect against Alzheimer's disease.[182] The caffeine itself may also be protective: Mice developed fewer tau tangles in their brains when their drinking water was infused with caffeine.[183] In humans, Johns Hopkins researchers have shown that 200 milligrams of caffeine—the amount in one strong cup of coffee—can help us consolidate memories and more easily memorize new information.[184]

Coffee consumption may also reduce your risk for Parkinson's disease,[185] as well as improve insulin sensitivity[186] and liver health,[187] and protect your eyesight.[188]

A few pointers:

- **Overcome the jitters with decaf.** Decaf coffee may provide at least some of the benefits of regular. So if caffeine makes you feel nervous or keeps you up at night, decaf may be a good option.[189] Note, however, that even decaf coffee still contains small amounts of caffeine, about 6 to 12 milligrams per cup.

- **Drink your coffee as close to black as possible.** Many drinks from commercial coffee houses contain so much sugar and fat that they are essentially liquid donuts. A 24-ounce Starbucks Frappuccino with whipped cream contains more than 500 calories, 16 grams of fat, and 83 grams of sugar.[190]
- **Skip this tip if you have high blood pressure.** Coffee and other caffeinated beverages may not be the best option for you, as caffeine can spike blood pressure substantially. If your physician has suggested you avoid caffeine, then this prescription isn't for you.

Meal Smarts Prescription #12:
End dinner with dark chocolate—not chocolate cake

Most desserts are rich in blood-sugar-spiking sugar, and recent research has linked high blood sugar levels with oxidative damage as well as an elevated production of beta-amyloid protein plaque.[191] While this doesn't mean you can never enjoy a cookie, slice of pie, or cake, it does mean that you want to make most desserts a rare treat rather than a regular indulgence.

Chocolate, however, may be one exception. Chocolate contains antioxidant chemicals called *flavonoids,* protective substances also present in many brightly colored fruits and vegetables. Baby boomers who consumed chocolate-rich drinks twice a day for three months performed as well on memory tests as did people a few decades younger.[192] In part of the same study, tests revealed that the chocolate drinks also seemed to improve blood flow to the hippocampi regions of the brain. One caveat: Caffeine levels in chocolate can induce insomnia in some people when taken before bed.[193]

A few pointers:
- **Watch your portion size.** Chocolate is still rich in calories and sugar. One 1-ounce square of dark chocolate runs you 170 calories and contains 6 grams of sugar.
- **Experience it with all your senses.** Smell it. Take small bites, savoring each one as it melts in your mouth. This will help you to enjoy the experience, reducing the likelihood of eating several squares rather than just one.
- **Dip fruit in melted chocolate.** This allows you to consume a larger portion while reaping the benefits of two antioxidant powerhouses. Strawberries, for instance, house vitamin C as well as phenols, both potent antioxidants. They're also only a few calories per berry. See Chocolate Fondue (page 219).

- **Mix it with other healing foods.** For example, when creating chocolate desserts, consider adding walnuts for an additional brain boost. See Chock-Full Chocolate Chip Cookies (page 218).

- **Make your own hot cocoa rather than using store-bought options.** Many commercially available hot chocolate mixes contain mostly sugar and very little cocoa. The same is true of commercially available chocolate milk. And it's also true of most commercially available "chocolate" dips and spreads, including Nutella, which only contains 7.4 percent cocoa powder by weight. The main ingredient in Nutella and other spreads like it: sugar. But you can make your own cocoa drink at home by mixing 1 tablespoon 100 percent cocoa powder with 1 tablespoon sugar and 2 teaspoons of water until you form a paste. Then add nonfat milk and either heat it or drink it cold, depending on your preference. It won't have as much cocoa as was used in the study, but it will still provide some benefit.

Meal Smarts Prescription #13:
Hold yourself to just one daily serving of wine or beer

You may have heard that beer and wine are good for your health. Both contain health-boosting antioxidants that help to lower blood cholesterol and improve heart and brain health. In wine, resveratrol and other polyphenols have been found to diminish plaque formation.[194] In beer, hops used to brew beer contain an antioxidant shown to boost cognitive function in mice.[195]

So why is our advice to limit wine and beer? While beer and wine contain protective antioxidants, the alcohol in these drinks is toxic in high amounts. Heavy drinking (more than two drinks a day) has been shown to speed up the development of Alzheimer's disease by accelerating brain cell death.[196] It also may contribute to breast cancer. So, if you enjoy beer and wine, one or two daily drinks may be good for you, but more than that amount could do you harm. And if you don't currently drink, there's no reason to start. Just use any number of the other Meal Smarts tips in this chapter.

A few pointers:
- **Watch your portions.** Beer comes in handy, one-serving, 12-ounce bottles that can help prevent you from over-imbibing, as can the standard pint glasses that we tend to pour beer into. Leave about an inch of space between the beer and the top of your pint glass, and you'll pour a 12-ounce serving every single time. Wine, however, is a different matter. Wine glasses come in many shapes and sizes, making it difficult to

easily judge your portion size. As a result, many people over-pour wine, serving themselves much more than a standard 5-ounce serving.[197] We're especially likely to over-pour, the research found, when the wine glass is wider (for example, created for red wine) and when it's on a table instead of being held in our hand. To help limit yourself to just one serving, consider marking off the 5-ounce spot on one favorite glass. Some glasses are sold with the pour line already marked. For those that are not, you can simply measure 5 ounces of a fluid using a measuring cup. Then pour it into your favorite glass and mark off a pour line.

- **Pay attention to what you eat while you drink.** Alcohol has a tendency to lower our inhibitions, causing us to consume fatty, crunchy, or sugary foods.

Meal Smarts Prescription #14:
Fuel up for exercise with brain-healthy foods

A wide array of foods—sports drinks, sports bars, sports gels—has been developed for endurance exercise. Most are made from glucose, a fast-digesting sugar, and are designed to boost blood sugar levels during long bouts of exercise that span more than an hour.

For most workouts, you really don't need one of these sports products. Your body has enough stored energy to get you through 30, 45, and even 60 minutes of exercise. But if it's time to exercise and you happen to be ravenous, then a snack may be in order. Otherwise, hunger is likely to derail your exercise efforts. You want a snack that isn't going to weigh down your stomach, causing cramping and discomfort during exercise, but instead will fuel your body with brain-healthy nutrients found in veggies, fruit, and whole grains rather than empty, blood-sugar-spiking glucose. Good options include a banana smeared with peanut butter, a trail mix of nuts and dried fruit, a make-at-home fruit smoothie (fruit, ice, and a little yogurt are all you need), plain nonfat yogurt mixed with fruit, or oatmeal.

A few pointers:
- **Go for easy-to-digest fruit** if you are going to be doing a bouncier type of exercise such as running or trampoline-jumping, rather than foods that contain fat or protein. The latter are likely to cause stomach discomfort during exercise. Even among fruits, you may find that some, such as bananas, digest more easily than others, like apples.
- **Give yourself time to digest.** You may wish to time your snack an hour or two before exercise to prevent stomach discomfort.

Meal Smarts Prescription #15: Air-pop your popcorn

Generally speaking, popcorn is a healthy, low-calorie food. Four entire cups of air-popped corn run you only 124 calories.[198] Popcorn is also considered a whole grain, one rich in fiber (each cup offers a whole gram of it) as well as antioxidants.[199]

But it's easy to adulterate a good thing, and popcorn is no exception to this rule. Microwave popcorn contains many different potential health hazards. For one, most bags of microwave popcorn are lined with perfluorooctanoic acid (PFOA), a chemical thought to raise risk for cancer (though the jury is still out).[200]

Many microwave varieties with a "buttery taste" contain partially hydrogenated soybean oil, or trans fat. Research has linked a high consumption of trans fats to Alzheimer's and heart disease, and the evidence is so strong that the FDA is considering banning the fat.[201] In some brands of popcorn, the buttery flavoring also comes from diacetyl, a chemical that has been linked to lung disease.

Then there's movie-theater popcorn, which is popped in copious amounts of oil. Thanks to the added oil, a small popcorn, without butter, will run you more than 200 calories and 11 grams of fat. A large? Depending on the chain, that generally adds up to more than 1,000 calories. Then, the yellow, greasy "butter" (aka soybean oil) that you add to it totals 130 calories a tablespoon.

A few pointers:

- **Embrace DIY popcorn.** It's easy. Even if you don't own an air-popper, you can make microwave popcorn by placing popcorn kernels inside a plain brown paper lunch bag. Fold the top down a few times. Then heat it up for two to three minutes, until the popping starts to abate. Voilà. Microwave popcorn without the trans fats and chemicals.

- **Skip the butter and salt.** Instead flavor your popcorn with healing spices such as cayenne pepper, turmeric, nutritional yeast, or some other spice of your choosing.

- **When you do choose microwave popcorn, read the label carefully.** Some brands have done away with trans fats as well as diacetyl, and they also offer PFOA-free bags. Many of them state as much on the packaging.[202]

What's better for my brain—healthy foods or an arsenal of supplements?

While the evidence in favor of eating real, whole foods is quite strong, the evidence in favor of specific supplements is not. That's partially because food comes packaged with a vast array of nutrients that no supplement can duplicate and partially because we've studied food more extensively and for much longer than we've studied supplements.

To date, we have few well-designed studies showing any benefit for supplements touted for brain health. This doesn't necessarily mean they offer no benefit at all. It only means that, at this time, we don't know much about them. We currently don't know how much of them you might need to achieve the desired effect. Nor do we know whether they interact with other medications you might be taking or pose other undesirable side effects.

Also, unlike the prescription drug industry, the supplement industry is unregulated. Repeated studies by the consumer watch group ConsumerLab.com[203] have found that many supplements lack the active ingredient claimed on the bottle, and others contain impurities ranging from insect parts to lead.

Bottom line: The jury is still out on most of the supplements purported to bolster brain health—and it may be out for many years to come.

There is an exception. Unlike most supplements touted for brain health, one in particular has been extensively studied: gingko. One of the best-selling herbal supplements, initially gingko seemed promising because it was thought to open up blood vessels, possibly safeguarding against ministrokes. But years and years of repeated studies have found no benefit for this supplement. In high amounts, it may result in bleeding if you are already taking a blood thinner.[204, 205]

Unlike gingko, a few other supplements may be warranted. Though food sources of omega-3s are ideal, a fish oil or omega-3 fatty acid supplement might be beneficial if you have elevated triglycerides or an inflammatory condition such as rheumatoid arthritis.[206] If you are a vegan or vegetarian, then you probably need a B-12 supplement, because this vitamin is not available from plant foods. And depending on how diligent you are about sun protection, you may want to consider supplemental vitamin D.[207] Everyone's health is different, and whether or not you need any of these supplements depends on many different factors. So talk with your physician to see if they are right for you.

Advice for Caregivers

Whether healthy nutrition can slow down advanced Alzheimer's disease is not clear. Nevertheless, it may be beneficial to encourage your family member to eat more fruits and vegetables and fewer fatty animal products and processed foods. These foods are good for your family member's overall health, including brain health.

Just don't get too pushy. As Alzheimer's disease progresses, you may have to pick your battles. If the person you are caring for refuses to consume healthy foods, it may be better to just let him or her consume favorite foods than to wage war every evening over dinner.

Over time you may notice that your family member picks at his or her food. This, in part, may happen because drugs used to treat Alzheimer's can decrease appetite. It also may be because people with Alzheimer's can lose their sense of smell, causing some foods to lose their allure. If the person you are caring for becomes a picky eater, you'll need to weigh the potential value of good nutrition against the challenge of coaxing an Alzheimer patient to conform to a more healthy food regimen.

Though it's unclear why, in some individuals with Alzheimer's, a craving for sweets may emerge. If this is the case, the only way to limit intake of sweets is to remove them from the kitchen and be sure they are not hoarded elsewhere.

As the disease progresses, the person you are caring for may simply forget to eat, lose the ability to use utensils, or experience trouble swallowing. Gently encourage your spouse or family member to eat, even with his or her fingers. As swallowing problems progress, liquid meals can help.

CHAPTER 5

A = Aerobic Smarts

If there was a medicine that could boost blood flow to the brain, protect existing brain cells and encourage the birth of new ones, and prevent Alzheimer's disease, you'd want to know about it, wouldn't you?

What if this medicine could also help you sleep more restfully and blast away stress, too? Oh, and it's free.

You'd probably consider taking it, wouldn't you?

Well, that medicine exists and you don't need a prescription to get your hands on it. In fact, all you have to do to put this medicine to work is move your body. Study after study has found that exercise ranks as the most potent Alzheimer's protection.[208] Arthur Kramer, PhD, and several colleagues at the University of Illinois at Urbana–Champaign have found a significant relationship between physical activity and a decreased occurrence of dementia. People who exercised at least three times a week for at least 15 to 30 minutes a session were less likely to develop Alzheimer's disease, and this was true *even if the disease ran in their family.*[209]

Even better, the results have been found to kick in quickly—within three months—even if you've been sedentary most of your life.[210]

The Many Benefits of Exercise

Generally, aerobic exercise refers to anything that gets your heart rate up, such as running, swimming, and cycling. Because strength training and stretching have also been shown to protect the brain, this chapter includes prescriptions for all forms of exercise, beyond just aerobic exercise. And in addition to preventing Alzheimer's, physical fitness has been shown to improve your ability to:

Cross the street without getting hit by a bus. The simple act of walking from one side of the street to another requires much more than merely looking both ways. To step onto the street and get to the other side, we must absorb a lot of information at once: *Is there a crosswalk? Is the traffic light red, yellow, or green? Is there a walk sign? Are there oncoming cars?* We also must estimate the speed of oncoming vehicles against our walking speed and the width of the street. All the while, we must remain alert to changing variables, such as a vehicle that is running a red light. These calculations can become more difficult with advancing age, especially as our brain's processing speed becomes more sluggish, which is why people aged 65 and older account for 17 percent of pedestrian deaths.[211] But it doesn't have to be this way. Not only will physical fitness help you with the reflex actions needed to step out from the path of an oncoming car, it can also help ensure you don't end up in the car's path to begin with. Researchers at the University of Illinois at Urbana–Champaign have studied people of all ages—ranging from children to seniors—as they've walked on a treadmill while a virtual reality scene has unfolded on floor-to-ceiling screens in front of and next to them. They've found that physically fit people of all ages tend to make better decisions about when to cross and when not to, compared to less physically fit individuals. Their faster mental-processing speeds and swifter reaction times allow them to quickly step back onto a curb when, say, a speeding car guns it as a yellow light turns red.[212]

Find your way. For many years, Carl W. Cotman, PhD, and his colleagues at the University of California–Irvine, have been studying the effects of exercise and mental stimulation on mice. He and his team have provided some mice with exercise wheels, tunnels, balls, and other mentally and physically stimulating items while keeping other mice alone in boring, bare cages and without access to a running wheel. Then, one at a time, he removes the mice from their cages and places them in a water-filled tub. Just beneath the surface of the water in the middle of the tub is a submerged platform that the mice can't see. The mice don't enjoy the water. Nor do they love to swim. But they have no choice. If they do nothing, they'll drown. So they swim until they find the platform either by happenstance or by process of elimination. He's found that the active mice tend to find the platform more easily on the first try. Then, during repeated swims, they remember it and swim straight to it. On the other hand, the sedentary rodents take longer to find the platform, and they are less likely to remember the platform on future swims.[213]

Few of us (hopefully) will ever find ourselves submerged in a pool, swimming for our lives as researchers watch to see if we can find a platform. We will, however, find ourselves in many other somewhat similar situations. Whenever we're lost or trying to find our way in an unfamiliar area, we must use the same brain skills to find our way as those rats did to find the platform. In such situations, we're searching systematically and keeping track of where we've looked and where we haven't.

Similarly, when we meet new people, the memories of their names are stored with other memories of how we met them. This is called *relational binding,* and it explains why we think of certain people when, as just one example, we hear a song that was playing on the day we met them. This handle on memory retrieval is also how we put a name to a face, and research shows that people who are physically fit tend to score better on tests of relational binding than people who are less physically fit.[214, 215]

Ignore the beeping smartphone. As a general rule, humans are notoriously poor multitaskers, which is why it's never a good idea to text and drive. That said, physical fitness seems to help us multitask somewhat more effectively, possibly because it increases activity in the parts of the brain that are dedicated to attention. In the street-crossing experiment I mentioned earlier, the fit pedestrians were more likely to safely cross the street—even when they were distracted by a smartphone—than were the unfit pedestrians. Fitness may allow the brain to ignore distracting information quickly. For example, fit people may stop texting more quickly and start looking at an approaching car.

Remember what you just read. Physical fitness has been shown to improve your ability to acquire new knowledge and understanding. When 86 seniors with mild cognitive impairment exercised twice weekly for six months, their scores on tests of verbal and spatial memory improved. The seniors were able to remember more words from a 15-word list they'd recently studied than they'd been able to do six months earlier. They were also able to better remember the location and color of dots that quickly appeared and then disappeared on a computer screen.[216]

Stay on your feet. Exercise strengthens your muscles and improves balance. Though neither of those benefits affects your brain health directly, both can prevent you from tripping and falling, an important component in staying alive and protecting your brain from concussions. According to the Centers for Disease Control and Prevention, falls are the leading cause of fatal and nonfatal injuries in older adults,[217] and people with dementia are four to five times more likely to fall than people without it, possibly because they forget to avoid hazards or make poor decisions, such as deciding to tackle stairs they forgot they don't have the dexterity to climb. And once people with mild cognitive impairment end up in the emergency room or ICU, their cognitive problems tend to dramatically worsen. We're not completely sure why this happens, but the stress of injury or the isolation and sensory deprivation of hospital care can bring on severe disorientation, confusion, and other cognitive issues. It's so common that we even have a name for it: ICU psychosis. In some people, these cognitive problems reverse once they are released from the hospital. In others, they persist.[218]

The benefits of exercise are powerful, and they are good to keep in mind as you contemplate starting a physical fitness program. They could provide the motivation you need to maintain this new habit. Indeed, Dr. Cotman has admitted that, throughout much of his life, he wasn't the most active person. But as his lab did one study after another that showed just how powerfully physical fitness affected the brain, he became convinced of its importance, and he took up tennis as a result.[219]

Your Brain on Exercise

How does physical activity keep the brain fit?

In part, it does so by keeping the entire body fit. Remember all the medical risk factors for Alzheimer's disease that you read about in Chapter 2, and how they eroded brain health? Diabetes, high blood pressure, elevated blood cholesterol, obesity; physical fitness can help you prevent, stall, or even reverse nearly all of them.[220] Physical activity can also help you sleep more soundly as well as mitigate the effects of stress, both important Brain Smarts that you'll learn more about in Chapters 6 and 8.[221] Physically fit people may also naturally gravitate toward healthier foods and generally take better care of themselves. For example, one study found that teens who exercised regularly were less likely to smoke or use drugs and more likely to consume fruits and vegetables than teens who were sedentary.[222] A different study on adults found that study participants were 32 percent more likely to consume a healthy diet if they were physically active compared to those who were sedentary.[223]

But physical fitness also affects the brain more directly by:

Improving blood flow to the brain. Increased blood volume to certain areas of the brain may improve the functioning of those areas. Arteries all over our bodies grow stiff with age, but exercise can help to keep them soft and pliable. It encourages the formation of new blood vessels and improves the health of the cells that line those vessels. This can allow blood vessels throughout your body and brain to function as they did when you were much younger. One study from the University of Pisa, for example, found that the blood vessels of older runners, cyclists, and triathletes functioned as well as those of people half their age. The healthier your blood vessels, the less likely they are to rupture or clog, reducing your risk of stroke.[224]

Boosting growth factors. *Brain-derived neurotrophic factor*, or BDNF, is an important growth factor that acts like fertilizer to encourage the growth of new neurons. Research done at the University of California–Irvine finds that exercise boosts levels of BDNF and several other related growth factors, particularly in the parts of the brain in control of learning and thinking and that are vulnerable to Alzheimer's disease. These elevated levels of BDNF and other growth factors help to encourage the growth of new neurons and also protect those neurons from damage.[225]

Protecting neurons where it matters the most. When researchers from the Cleveland Clinic in Ohio used an fMRI machine to scan the brains of 100 men and women who had a family history of Alzheimer's disease, they found that the size of the hippocampal brain regions of fit people remained the same over an 18-month period, even if those study participants were carriers of the *ApoE4* gene (mentioned in Chapters 1 and 2). Their brains looked like the brains of people at low risk for developing Alzheimer's disease. On the other hand, sedentary study participants who were carriers of this gene experienced a 3 percent shrinkage in this area of the brain over the same period of months.[226] Other research finds that exercise may even *increase* the volume of the hippocampi by 1 to 2 percent over one year, which seems to protect the brain from Alzheimer's disease.[227, 228]

Improving connections between neurons. *White matter integrity*—a measure of the pathways between neurons—has been shown to improve within days of starting an exercise program.[229] Exercise may encourage dendrites to grow, neurons to proliferate, synapses to remodel themselves, and signals to pass more readily from one neuron to another.

Reducing plaque formation. Compared to sedentary animals, active mice had 50 percent fewer plaques and beta-amyloid fragments in the cerebral cortex and hippocampal regions of their brains, possibly because regular exercise may change the way the amyloid precursor protein is metabolized.[230]

Which is better for your brain—aerobic exercise or strength training?

As it turns out, neither is better. They're both important, but for different reasons. Much of the Alzheimer's research has focused on aerobic exercise over the years, and this form of exercise is key for maintaining the health of your blood vessels and boosting BDNF, the brain-cell-protecting growth factor mentioned on page 78. It can also reduce your chances of developing high blood pressure and other diseases that raise risk for Alzheimer's.

Like aerobic exercise, strength training can also help to normalize blood sugar levels as well as blood pressure. Strength training is also good for healthy bones, and research done on mice shows that resistance exercise may boost levels of a different growth factor also important for protecting brain cells.[231]

In addition to aerobic and strength exercise, take steps to improve your balance and flexibility. Though a more flexible body and a better sense of balance do not necessarily reduce your risk of Alzheimer's disease, they can help you to feel better, reduce the chance of injury, increase your vitality, and enable you to do other forms of exercise.

Sound like a lot to do? It doesn't have to be. If you're up to the challenge, more vigorous forms of yoga provide all four types of exercise in just one workout. The 7-minute circuit workout (page 222) will help you to improve your aerobic fitness, strength, and balance in just seven minutes. Add a few stretches afterward and you can improve your flexibility, too, all in the same short workout. However you end up putting the four types of exercise together, aim for 150 weekly minutes of exercise, or 25 minutes most days of the week.

How to Use Exercise to Outsmart Alzheimer's

If you already exercise regularly, just read through the rest of this chapter to get a sense of how you are doing and whether there's any room for improvement. Especially consider ways to incorporate the five other Brain Smarts into your current routine. Could you improve your Social Smarts by exercising with a friend or with a group? Or Resilience Smarts by building some relaxing routines—such as yoga or tai chi—into your regimen? Or Meal Smarts by fueling up for your workout with a brain-healthy snack such as a homemade fruit smoothie?

If you are currently sedentary or have an on-again, off-again relationship with exercise, you'll want to start with something you can maintain, slowly working your way up to a minimum of 150 minutes of moderate exercise or 75 minutes of vigorous exercise per week, spread out over at least three days. That comes out to 25 to 50 minutes of exercise per bout.[232, 233] That's the minimum amount of fitness that has been shown, in research, to bolster brain health.

Ideally you'll do more—breaking a sweat every day and building movement into your life: shunning elevators and moving walkways, walking or cycling rather than driving, parking farther from your destination, and stretching while watching television.

On the following pages, you'll find descriptions of several types of exercise with built-in social or intellectual enrichment, along with advice for keeping them as mentally stimulating as possible.

Motivation Smarts: Four Ways to Get Yourself Moving

Think about a time when you were fit and happy. When researchers from the University of New Hampshire asked college students to recall positive memories about exercise, the students automatically worked out harder and more consistently over the coming week than did students who either recalled negative memories or were not asked to recall any memories.[234]

Keep track of your steps, calories, or distance. Women who wore pedometers to track their number of daily steps naturally increased their daily walking over three months by at least 512 daily steps compared to women who did not wear pedometers. Modern technology offers us numerous ways to track our energy use and distance, ranging from cheap pedometers that clip to the waistband to mobile phone apps, high-tech smart watches, and Fitbits and other wearables.

Build in accountability. It's easy to skip an exercise session if you're the only person you're letting down. It's a lot harder to do so if an exercise partner, group, or trainer is waiting for you to show. Here's another way to keep yourself accountable: sign a contract. Office workers who set contractually binding exercise goals increased their physical activity by an average of 20 minutes.[235]

Lean on your friends. Let one or more people in on your promise to get fit. You might even consider posting updates on Facebook or another social media site, so your friends can cheer you along.

Aerobic Smarts Prescription #1: Dance the night away

If brain fitness awards were given to types of fitness pursuits, dance would earn the first-place trophy year after year after year. That's because it combines several brain-health prescriptions into one. If you dance with a group or a partner, you are exercising Social Smarts (Chapter 3). If you are learning new steps, you're also boosting your intellectual fitness (Chapter 7). Dance, by nature, is fun, which helps to reduce stress (Chapter 6). Studies show that it boosts serotonin levels, indicating that it may lift depression, too. It's nearly everything rolled into one.

This isn't just my opinion. There's research to back this up. Ballroom dancers, for example, have performed higher on tests of cognition than did nondancers, and competitive ballroom dancers have scored higher on many different measures of cognitive performance, including reaction time.[236] One study, done by the Albert Einstein College of Medicine in New York City and funded by the National Institutes of Health, followed the health outcomes of 75 seniors for 21 years, finding that dance reduced risk for dementia more than any other type of physical activity—and even more than doing crossword puzzles.[237]

Does it matter what style of dance you perform? We don't yet know, but it seems as if ballroom, salsa, swing, and other styles of complex partner dancing are all probably equally effective. Country line dancing, square dancing, contra dancing, and even Zumba are probably also great for the brain, for the same reasons.

A few pointers:

- **Count dancing as part of your 150-minute weekly goal,** but only count the time you actually spend on the dance floor. Time spent watching other dancers doesn't count.
- **Keep learning new moves.** Once you master one routine or type of dance, start learning a new one.
- **Involve others.** At home, maybe you simply turn on fun music and hold a "dance party" with a spouse, children, or grandchildren. Also look into classes such as Zumba, contra, line dancing, and other options that can help you connect with others as you dance.
- **Enjoy the music.** Many styles of dance are linked to particular types of music. Salsa dancing goes with a Latin beat, line dancing with country, and so on. The more you enjoy the music, the more you'll enjoy dancing, so you'll stay on your feet longer as well as blast away more stress.

Aerobic Smarts Prescription #2: Play active team sports

Many different team sports provide a rich social setting coupled with complex intellectual challenges. Not only must you make repeated split-second decisions—when to catch or hit a ball, when to pass it, how long to run with it, and so on—but you also must exercise your social intelligence. Who will you pass it to and why? Which member on the other team is the weak link? Who can you steal the ball from? The complex decision-making goes on and on and on.

So it makes sense that researchers at the University of Illinois at Urbana–Champaign who studied professional volleyball players found that they performed better on tests of *executive control* (the ability to connect past experiences with present actions so you can better plan, organize, and strategize), memory, and *visuospatial attention* (being able to direct your eyesight and attention to the right object at the right time) than did nonathletes. Though the researchers only looked at volleyball players, there's no reason to assume that other team sports aren't equally good for the brain.[238]

A few pointers:

- **Wear the appropriate protective gear for any given sport, especially a helmet.** This will help to protect your brain from concussions, one of the main risk factors for Alzheimer's disease.

- **Avoid high-contact sports, choosing flag football over tackle,** for instance. Again, this helps to protect your brain from concussions.

Aerobic Smarts Prescription #3:
Train in short bursts of vigorous activity

This prescription can come in handy when life is very busy. Rather than exercise in one long 30-minute session, consider breaking up your exercise into shorter 7- to 10-minute bursts, repeated several times a day. And it combines strength and aerobic training into one session that can firm up your entire body (and, consequently, your brain) in a very short amount of time.

If you decide to break up your exercise like this, make sure to get your heart rate up. Maybe you walk uphill on a treadmill, jog in place, do jumping jacks, skip rope, or do a series of heart-pumping calisthenics like the routine shown on pages 222 to 225.

This kind of training may be ideal for people who have diabetes, a risk factor for Alzheimer's, especially if you do these bursts about a half hour before each meal. Study participants with insulin resistance (a precursor to diabetes) were instructed to do six minutes of vigorous exercise (such as walking uphill on a treadmill or vigorous calisthenics) interspersed with six minutes of recovery exercise (such as slow walking) about a half hour before breakfast, lunch, and dinner. Other study participants just walked for 30 minutes before dinner. Those who did the six-minute vigorous intervals experienced better post-meal blood sugar levels than study participants who did the once daily, moderate session.[239]

Other than a chair, the short circuit routine on pages 222 to 225 in Chapter 11 requires no equipment. You can do it anywhere, even a hotel room. It's based on a routine developed by the Human Performance Institute in Orlando, Florida, and featured in the American College of Sports Medicine's *Health and Fitness Journal*.[240] The whole routine lasts just seven minutes.

A few pointers:

- **Get a thorough checkup.** Because the routine includes intense exercises, check with your doctor before trying it, especially if you have heart disease, joint pain, are very out of shape, or are obese.

- **Keep challenging your fitness.** If you find that the 7-minute circuit feels too easy, repeat the circuit up to three times, either right away or later in the day.
- **Modify the routine, as needed.** If joint problems prevent you from doing one of the exercises, skip it, and march or jog in place instead.

Aerobic Smarts Prescription #4:
Have fun while improving your hand-eye coordination

Many different sporting activities, ranging from horseshoes to shuffleboard to bowling, help you to hone your attention, focus, and aim while you remain social with others. Because these sports are so much fun, they can also help you to reduce stress, and, in some cases, by getting you outdoors and into the sunlight, they may also help you reset your circadian clock, improving sleep.

These fun, moderate forms of exercise may be ideal for people with dementia who may not be able to manage more intense types of exercise. In one study, nursing home patients with dementia participated in two-hour-long, daily therapy sessions that included bowling or croquet, as well as gardening, brain games, and crafts. Patients who participated in these sessions were still able to perform the tasks of daily living, such as eating or using the bathroom, unassisted, after 12 months. Residents who did not participate in the sessions lost ground in their ability to perform these tasks without help.[241] Did the beneficial effect stem from the exercise, the crafts, or the brain games? It's likely that all three are important, which offers yet another reason to include a variety of Brain Smarts into your daily repertoire rather than focusing on just one of them.

A few pointers:
- **Stay as active as possible during play.** When you are not actively bowling or tossing a horseshoe, remain standing rather than sitting. In fact, standing is almost always preferable to sitting for improved physical health. Do it as often as possible, especially if your profession involves lots of sitting. (See Prescription #12 for more advice on standing as a form of exercise.)
- **Relax and have fun.** Focusing too much on your technique or the overall score can generate stress, which is bad for the brain. So be willing to laugh at yourself if and when you miss.

Aerobic Smarts Prescription #5:
Break a sweat while raising money for charity

Many sports can be transformed into opportunities to raise money for good causes—including the cause of Alzheimer's research. When you exercise for a cause, you combine the powerful effects of altruism (see Prescription #11 in Chapter 6) with the effects of physical activity. These events are also social, and they can inspire you to stay motivated and to train harder.

A few pointers:
- **Do some research.** Check the Alzheimer's Association's website for a list of Alzheimer's-focused fund-raising events, such as the Walk to End Alzheimer's and the ALZ Stars. Of course, walking or running for other charities can work equally well.
- **Sign up for the event months ahead of time.** This will provide motivation to train.
- **Consider entering as a team rather than an individual.** This will make the event and the training even more social.

Aerobic Smarts Prescription #6: Join a fitness class

Fitness classes such as Zumba and Spinning allow you to get in shape under the watchful and motivating guidance of an instructor. Many of these classes can also be quite fun, and they provide a nice social outlet as well.

A few pointers:
- **Keep mixing it up.** Once you've grown accustomed to one instructor or one type of class, consider shifting to a new one in order to keep your brain and your body challenged.
- **Break out of your shell and chat with other participants in the class.** The more social the experience, the more benefit to your brain, and the more likely you'll feel inclined to keep showing up for class.

Aerobic Smarts Prescription #7: Stretch out with yoga

Depending on the style you practice, yoga is capable of improving all four types of fitness. Standing poses like Tree Pose and Balancing Stick improve your balance. Many different postures improve your strength, especially Downward Facing Dog, Handstands, Plank, and many more. And of course, yoga stretches you out.

Some styles of yoga may also get your heart rate up. (See the pointers below to decide if these more vigorous styles of yoga are right for you.)

And, thanks to the emphasis on breathing, meditation, and relaxation, yoga calms the mind. It can also be social, especially if you hang out and chat after class. And, as long as you are learning new moves, it can be intellectually stimulating, too. As part of a Wayne State University and University of Illinois study, seniors who took yoga classes three times a week scored better on tests of memory and mental set shifting (the ability to shift their focus quickly from one task to another) after eight weeks than did seniors who took a stretching class.[242]

A few pointers:

- **Consider the best style of yoga for you.** Some styles are more taxing than others. Check with your physician before trying hot yoga or more strenuous styles such as Ashtanga to make sure you are in good cardiac health.

- **Ask a lot of questions.** In some forms of hot yoga, the room is heated above 100 degrees. In other forms, the room temperature is a more moderate 80 degrees. If you wish to try this style of yoga, talk with the instructor beforehand to find out how hot the room will be. If you take a hot yoga class, bring plenty of water, and leave the room if you start to feel faint or dizzy.

- **Take a class rather than doing yoga at home,** for the social benefits.

- **Keep trying new styles.** That will force your brain to learn new movements continually.

- **Get out of your comfort zone.** Balancing postures provide a wonderful challenge to your brain because you must make many quick decisions as you shift your weight back and forth.

Aerobic Smarts Prescription #8: Explore tai chi and qigong

Tai chi is an ancient Chinese martial art that involves a series of movements performed in a slow, focused manner. It's closely related to qigong, another Chinese discipline that is rooted in Chinese medicine. Both have been shown to improve balance, strength, endurance, aerobic capacity, and walking speed, as well as reduce the incidence of falling and stress. Of the two disciplines, tai chi is more studied and has also been shown to lower blood pressure, blood cholesterol, insulin, triglycerides, and inflammation, all risk factors for Alzheimer's disease. [243, 244]

Both practices are gentle and well suited for people who are overweight or who have joint pain and other mobility issues.

A few pointers:

- **Take classes.** This will allow you to see the movements in action as well as to connect with other students.
- **Give yourself time to grow comfortable with the movements.** Because tai chi and qigong are unlike so many forms of exercise, they pose a fairly steep learning curve and initially require a great deal of memorization. It may take several weeks of lessons before you remember the sequence of movements. So give it time. You just may find that, as your familiarity grows, tai chi and qigong grow on you.

Aerobic Smarts Prescription #9: Grow vegetables, plant flowers

The act of gardening can not only help you grow some of those organic fruits and vegetables that you learned about in the Meal Smarts chapter, it can also be more physically taxing than many people assume. It involves lots of crouching, repeated weed pulling, digging, pruning, and more. It raises the heart rate and strengthens muscles in your hands, arms, shoulders, back, and legs.

It can also be incredibly relaxing. This is why so many long-term care facilities include elaborate garden spaces for their residents. Just being outdoors and surrounded by beautiful flowers can relax the mind. Finally, gardening requires intellectual smarts to plant the right seeds in the right places at the right time of year, to prune plants when they need it, and to combat pests and other obstacles.

A few pointers:

- **Alternate using the right side of your body with the left.** For instance, pull 15 weeds with your right hand and then 15 more with your left to prevent muscular imbalances.
- **Consider joining a community garden.** This offers a gardening outlet if you don't have a backyard, and it can also help you connect with other gardeners.
- **Join a gardening club.** This is another way to flex your Social Smarts while you garden.

Aerobic Smarts Prescription #10: Hike for hidden treasure

Hiking is a great form of exercise that gets you out in nature and may improve your balance as you navigate rocky terrain. You can increase the intellectual challenge by going letterboxing or geocaching.

Letterboxing is like a scavenger hunt. You are provided with clues about landmarks—such as, "turn left at the 'wheel of fortune'"—that help you to navigate yourself to a "treasure": a hidden box that contains an ink stamp for your letterboxing passport. Geocaching is similar, but instead of landmarks, you use geographical coordinates. It's estimated that there are at least 2 million geocaches hidden around the world. You sign a logbook and trade treasures, taking one from the box and adding another one in its place.

A few pointers:

- **If you are traveling, head to the visitor's bureau and ask about local geocaching or letterboxing routes.** Many bureaus will sell you maps or clue lists for a small fee or may even provide them for free.

- **Consider joining an online community.** Several communities exist for both hobbies, including *Letterboxing.org, AtlasQuest.com,* and *OpenCaching.com,* among others. On these sites community members share hints, recommend their favorite routes, and offer coordinates and clues.

- **Lean on the help of apps.** You can download a free geocaching app from *geocaching.com* that can suggest numerous caches near where you live or where you might be headed on vacation.

Aerobic Smarts Prescription #11:
Sign your dog or cat up for agility training

If you own a dog or cat, agility training offers an intellectually stimulating form of exercise for both of you. It involves leading your pet through a series of obstacles, ranging from catwalks to hurdles to tunnels. It provides exercise to you both and causes you to think quickly as you shout commands and use your body language to communicate with your pet.

A few pointers:

- **Sign up for a group class.** This allows you to reap even more social benefits as well as continually encourage yourself and your pet to learn new tricks.

- **Keep pushing yourself and your pet to try new challenges.** Once you master a beginner course, try a more advanced one. Or once agility training starts to feel easy, consider different types of competitions ranging from nose work to fly ball.

Aerobic Smarts Prescription #12: Stand every half hour

Though standing isn't technically exercise, it is much more active than sitting. You may have heard the aphorism, "Sitting is the new smoking." If you sit all day at work and then tend to lounge on the couch once you get home, you should follow this prescription to ease yourself into a more active lifestyle.

When researchers asked overweight and obese office workers to use a standing workstation for 30 minutes out of every hour, the workers' post-meal blood-sugar response improved, thus reducing their risk for developing Alzheimer's.[245]

A few pointers:

- **Calculate your average sitting time.** You can do this with a rough estimation (work hours spent sitting plus leisure time spent sitting). Or try a more formal sitting calculator like the one offered at *JustStand.org*. Use this information as motivation, as well as to guide you in your efforts to stand more during the day.

- **Look into a standing desk or one that can adjust back and forth between sitting and standing positions.** Many different styles are available for a range of prices.

- **Set a timer to buzz every half hour.** If you are using an adjustable desk, allow the timer to nudge you to transition from sitting to standing at regular intervals. If you don't have access to an adjustable or a standing desk, then get up and stretch, do some light calisthenics, or go for a short walk for a minute or two before sitting back down. Those one- or two-minute breaks will add up by the end of the day, allowing you to accumulate 16 or more minutes of movement.

- **Make use of every opportunity possible to stand.** Stand when talking on the phone, while waiting for the bus or a plane, and while chatting at get-togethers.

- **Never use a drive-through.** Always get out of your car and walk into the bank, pharmacy, liquor store, and other businesses.

Advice for Caregivers

As Alzheimer's disease progresses, the person you are caring for may become less mobile, making many of this chapter's aerobic prescriptions difficult, if not impossible. In Chapter 11, on pages 226 to 228, you'll find a routine designed for people with mobility issues that was initially developed by the Veterans Administration for people with Alzheimer's disease.

Talk with your family member's physician about appropriate exercise options. You might even bring this book with you to the next appointment, asking, "Do you think he (or she) is up to this?" If not, perhaps your physician can suggest some exercises that are more appropriate.

Also, keep in mind that the person you are caring for may resist your attempts to get him or her moving. In that case, back off. It's better to find activities that your loved one enjoys than to force him or her through the paces of a specific exercise routine.

Though the routine in Chapter 11 may not reverse the physical function your family member has already lost, it may very well slow or stall any further decline. When Finnish researchers followed the outcomes of 210 individuals with Alzheimer's disease and their families, they found that those who took part in a home-based exercise program maintained more independence—continuing, for example, to eat, bathe, and dress without assistance—than others who did not exercise.[246]

If you are caring for someone with Alzheimer's, consider doing this routine together so you can both improve your physical fitness. Do it three times a week, pairing it with 30 daily minutes of cardiovascular exercise such as walking, if possible.[247] Start by doing the routine just once. As fitness improves, restart at the beginning and do it one more time. You can also increase the challenge by holding hand weights or by using ankle weights. Start with one-, three-, or five-pound weights and progress from there.

In addition to doing the routine together, use this advice.

Use music. Music is calming, and it can also trigger memories and lift depression, a negative mood state that becomes more common as Alzheimer's disease progresses. You might try moving to familiar songs that your family member may remember from childhood, including the chicken dance or even the hokey pokey. You may be quite surprised by the way long-forgotten music can activate the brain.

Flip off the television. Though television programming might help you take your mind off exercise, it's likely to distract someone with Alzheimer's, causing him or her to ignore your encouraging words and suggestions.

Hold hands. Balance will become challenged as the disease progresses. Serve as a spotter, or encourage the person you are caring for to place one or both hands against a chair, table, or wall.

Remain consistent. Exercise regularly, and, if possible, at the same time each day. This will help you both to remember to do it and how to do it.

Keep it fun. Verbally encourage your loved one, and keep it interesting. Do things your family member enjoys rather than adopting a one-size-fits-all approach.

Turn your house into a gym. Involve the person you are caring for in household chores such as folding laundry, mixing, mashing, and beating various foods, shucking corn, watering plants, grooming pets, and more.

Split it up. If your family member's endurance declines, try shorter bouts of movement that are repeated over the course of the day.

Move in the morning. This is generally the time of day when people with Alzheimer's disease are least restless and most energetic.

CHAPTER 6

R = Resilience Smarts

Jeanne Calment, the Frenchwoman who lived to age 122, spent her final years nearly blind, deaf, and immobile. Once a year on her birthday, journalists crowded into her room to interview her about her long life, but usually she spent her days alone, confined to the inner world of her thoughts and memories. Just reading about her experience causes many of us to stiffen up with discomfort, thinking "how horrible" and "how sad."

Yet Calment reportedly enjoyed the later years of her life, once telling a researcher, "My sight is bad, my hearing is bad, I feel bad, but I don't suffer, I don't complain. I don't lack for anything. I have everything I need. I've had a good life. I live in my dreams, in my memories, beautiful memories."[248]

Calment's ability to make the best of any situation may very well be one of the traits that allowed her to live so long. In Calment's obituary, *The New York Times* quoted researcher Jean-Marie Robine as saying, "I think she was someone who constitutionally and biologically speaking, was immune to stress."[249]

Another word for an immunity to stress: resilience. When we're emotionally resilient, we're able to bounce back from life's trials and tribulations. We recover quickly from difficulties and this plays a powerful role in total-body health. Chronic negativity, anxiety, depression, and loneliness can accelerate aging throughout the body, including the brain. On the other hand, a joyful, calm, "no worries" attitude like Calment's can serve as a protective balm.

Despite popular belief, the body's stress response—often called the "fight-or-flight" response—offers many benefits. Whenever we're in a life-threatening situation—such as when slamming on a car's brakes to avoid an accident—the fight-or-flight response allows our bodies to react quickly.

During fight-or-flight, the hypothalamus (a part of the brain that controls automatic functions such as breathing and sweating) tells the adrenal glands to release the stress hormones adrenaline and cortisol. These hormones affect cells and organs all over the body. They cause the heart to beat faster and blood pressure to surge. Our vision sharpens. Pain perception drops. The liver releases sugar for muscle cells to burn. Memory and mental clarity improve. Blood flow is diverted from the stomach and sex organs and to the working muscles and the brain. The blood itself becomes thick and sticky, ready to clot if there's an injury. With the help of the fight-or-flight response, we now have a tremendous amount of physical energy and strength, as well as the ability to see, think, and make quick decisions. Our vision intensifies, and our focus becomes nearly single-pointed and our thinking lucid.

Stress, in small doses, can also help us in other situations that are not life-threatening. For example, we need at least a little bit of stress to motivate us out of bed in the morning. The fight-or-flight response allows us to think clearly when solving work challenges. It's what gives us that "pumped" feeling when we are performing at our peak, allows us to quickly scoop up a toddler who is about to walk into traffic, and spit out the right answer when playing Trivial Pursuit or another competitive game. Researchers at the University of California at Berkeley have found that these types of moderate, short-lived stressors may actually improve the performance of the brain, encouraging the formation of new brain cells over time. In their studies done on rats, brief stressful events caused stem cells to proliferate into new neurons in the hippocampus, the part of the brain that is most affected by Alzheimer's disease. These new brain cells allowed these rats to perform better on memory tests.[250]

Relaxation is just as lifesaving as stress. Our ancient hunting-and-gathering ancestors did not always have the ability to eat every day. The brain's relaxing chemicals allowed them to rest and digest after a hunt, burning as few calories as possible until their next eating opportunity.

You might think of stress and relaxation as two ends of the same seesaw. Neither is better or worse than the other, and both processes are needed to keep the body in balance. When the seesaw remains balanced, you're resilient. Problems develop, though, if one end of the seesaw is much heavier than the other. When the parasympathetic (calm-inducing) nervous system is too heavy, we suffer from fatigue, listlessness, and depression. When the sympathetic (fight-or-flight) nervous system is too heavy, we feel frazzled, anxious, and fearful.[251]

For the vast majority of people, it's the sympathetic nervous system that is too heavy, and the prescriptions in this chapter will help remove some of that heavy load and bring you into balance. When you get to Chapter 7, you'll discover an assortment of intellectual pursuits that will allow you to keep your sympathetic nervous system engaged just the right amount, so you'll feel alert and lucid, but not anxious and scatterbrained.

The Importance of Resilience

Humans seem to be able to deal with stress that lasts for a few minutes to a few hours, but chronic stress is another story. Long-term stress that lasts for weeks, months, or years elevates levels of *glucocorticoid* stress hormones, which suppress the formation of new neurons in the hippocampus, providing the opposite effect of short-term stress.

There are some long-term stressors—such as illness, grief, and financial difficulties—that we can't avoid. But we can change the way we react to those stressors, as well as more short-term everyday stressors like traffic, long grocery store lines, sluggish Internet connections, and nitpicky spouses. For example, not everyone feels stressed when stuck in traffic. What makes the difference? The people who feel anxious tend to focus on the clock and what's going to happen to them when they show up late to wherever it is they are headed. Others, on the other hand, might quickly accept the fact that they're going to be late, call to let someone know, and then relax and listen to a radio program or audiobook. That's resilience: the ability to adapt, overcome, and even grow from a challenge rather than become defeated by it.

When we lack this kind of resilience, the fight-or-flight response remains flipped on day in and day out. Blood sugar, pressure, and inflammation stay elevated, and now this high-pressure, fast-flowing blood continually rages like a stream after a big storm. This nicks up the walls of the blood vessels, leading to plaque formation throughout the body, including the brain.

When levels of the stress hormone cortisol remain chronically elevated:

- levels of beta-amyloid protein rise, which in turn triggers stress hormones to rise even more;[252]

- tau fragments are more likely to aggregate into strands that may damage brain cells;[253]

- communication between brain cells is impaired;

- dendrites shrivel and neurotransmitters don't function optimally;

- the production of new neurons is slowed, especially in the hippocampus, causing this part of the brain to shrink.

Stress can cause the hippocampi to degenerate and shrink at any stage of life, even childhood. University of Wisconsin psychologists recently found that people who experienced chronic stress as children—physical abuse, neglect, or poverty—had shrunken amygdalae and hippocampi. Their brains did not fully develop in these areas. And the more stress they braved, the smaller these structures were and the more behavior problems the children had.[254]

In addition, chronic stress can indirectly cause problems by disturbing sleep. Lack of sleep then leads us to self-soothe with unhealthy foods and other unhealthy behaviors such as smoking and excessive drinking.

All of this helps to explain the powerful role chronic stress plays in Alzheimer's disease. A Canadian study found that people with mild cognitive impairment and high levels of stress were at a greater risk of developing Alzheimer's disease than calmer people. Over a three-year period, risk of Alzheimer's jumped 33 percent for people who reacted to stress with mild anxiety, 78 percent for people with moderate anxiety, and 135 percent for people with severe anxiety.[255]

How to Develop Resilience

To become more resilient, we want to do more than simply find ways to relax. Ideally, we'll find that elusive balance—the middle way—between stimulating the mind and stilling it. As you'll learn in Chapter 7, a bored mind is a forgetful one. But so is an overstimulated mind. So, in addition to the prescriptions on pages 99 to 112, use this advice:

Keep stress in perspective. Mind-set is important, and if you see stressors as short-term challenges that will make you stronger and smarter, chronic stress may be less likely to harm your health. This is what researchers at the University of Wisconsin-Madison found when they asked 29,000 people to rate their levels of stress along with their beliefs of how stress influenced their health. Highly stressed people who believed their stress impacted their health for the worse were at a 43 percent increased risk of death. On the other hand, people who were just as stressed but who did not perceive stress to be a major problem were the least likely to die prematurely.[256] So try to shift your thinking from *This is terrible* to *What can I learn from this?*

Care for your body. During and just after a stressful period, it's especially important to practice healthy behaviors. Eat a brain-healthy diet, get plenty of exercise, and do everything possible to keep your sleep habits regular. Use the advice in Chapters 4, 5, and 8.

Hit the pause button. Our brains need downtime, just as our bodies do. What you do to hit the pause button will be unique to you. In the following pages, you'll find many different techniques, all of which can help. No one technique offers a panacea for all people. You may find that one prescription works great, whereas others do not. Or, for you, a variety of prescriptions may work best.

Or, maybe, due to your cool disposition and regular exercise habits, you really don't need resilience prescriptions right now. So experiment, and find what works for you.

Resilience Smarts Prescription #1: Get moving

In Chapter 5, you learned about the powerful ways physical activity protects brain health: improving blood flow, reducing the risk of stroke, boosting brain activity, providing an optimal environment for neurons to grow and flourish, driving down the forming of plaque, and encouraging dendrites to grow.

Here's one more reason physical fitness helps to prevent Alzheimer's: it counters the damaging effects of chronic stress. That's what researchers from Washington University in St. Louis, Missouri, found when they looked at the relationships among fitness, stress, and brain health in 91 older adults. Some of those studied already had been diagnosed with Alzheimer's disease, and some had not. The scientists used fMRI scans to study the brains of the seniors, and they also extensively collected through interviews their exercise habits and stressors they'd experienced throughout their lives. They found that people who'd undergone high amounts of lifetime stress (for example, those who'd survived natural disasters, car accidents, sexual abuse, poverty, and so on), and who exercised very little had more atrophy of the hippocampi and performed worse on memory tests than those with the same amount of lifetime stress who exercised more.[257]

Exercise might buffer stress, in part, by burning off stress hormone levels while boosting levels of *endorphins,* brain and nervous system chemicals that serve as natural painkillers and mood boosters. Regular physical activity may also help by promoting sleep and lifting depression.

A few pointers:

- **Pick an activity you enjoy.** Yoga, weightlifting, walking, running, circuit training, swimming, kickboxing, dancing, and many other activities are all capable of blasting away stress. The more you enjoy doing it, the more likely you'll keep doing it and the more potent the stress relief may be.

- **Do it outdoors.** Outdoor exercise helps you make the best use of one natural stress reducer: nature. You may find that nature is quite restorative. So after a stressful day, consider hiking on a nature trail rather than walking indoors on a treadmill.

Resilience Smarts Prescription #2: Explore Kriya yoga

Unlike the more physical styles of yoga, Kriya is less centered on postures (known as *asanas*) and more centered on breathing exercises (called *pranayama*), meditation, and chanting. Born out of the Kundalini yoga tradition, Kriya involves chanting the sounds *Saa, Taa, Naa,* and *Maa,* coupled with visualization and specific hand movements.

Dharma Singh Khalsa, MD, the president and medical director of the Alzheimer's Research and Prevention Foundation, has spent many years studying how this lesser-known style of yoga affects the brain, and his research has been illuminating. In study participants who'd been diagnosed with some form of memory loss, Khalsa found that just 12 daily minutes of this style of yoga boosted mood, reduced anxiety, and lifted tension and fatigue.[258] Kriya yoga also seems to improve cerebral blood flow and cognitive functioning[259] and may even boost levels of telomerase, important in protecting DNA from aging.[260] Other research has linked this breathing-based meditation with a reduction of post-traumatic stress disorder symptoms in US military veterans[261] and improved cholesterol and other blood lipids in stressed engineering students who were taking final exams.[262]

It's also a great strategy for people who are caring for others with Alzheimer's disease. One study done at the University of California, Los Angeles, found that this brief, 12-minute meditation lifted depression and improved mental health in people who were caring for others with dementia.[263]

And it's easy to learn. You simply chant four different one-syllable sounds (*Saa, Taa, Naa, Maa*) as you touch your other fingers to your thumb. The sounds are ancient Sanskrit words that mean "my true identity" or "my highest self."

A few pointers:

- **Match the right sound to the right finger movements.** As you say the Sanskrit word *Saa*, touch your index finger to your thumb. Then, for *Taa*, touch your middle finger to your thumb. For *Naa*, your ring finger, and *Maa*, your little finger. Use the chart on the next page as a quick reference.

- **Use this visualization:** As you chant each sound, imagine that the sound waves travel down the crown of your head and out your "third eye" (between your eyebrows).

- **Follow this sequence:** Chant the words at a normal volume for two minutes, then two minutes at a whisper, and then two minutes silently. Repeat the sequence in the reverse order, for a total of 12 minutes. For more instruction, check out the Alzheimer's Research & Prevention Foundation website, which offers materials that can help you get started with Kriya chanting, as well as CDs and MP3s available to download by donation.

Sound	Finger Mudra	
Saa	Index finger touching thumb	
Taa	Middle finger touching thumb	
Naa	Ring finger touching thumb	
Maa	Little finger touching thumb	

Volume	Minutes
Normal	Two
Whisper	Two
Silent	Two
Silent	Two
Whisper	Two
Normal	Two

Resilience Smarts Prescription #3: Learn to meditate

In addition to Kriya yoga, several other styles of meditation, ranging from mindfulness to Transcendental Meditation (TM), may be just as helpful for reducing stress and boosting attention and memory. There are many different forms of meditation. Some involve concentrating on mantras (such as om-ah-hum and so-hum). Others teach you to follow the breath. Still others involve holding your attention on short prayers, words, or phrases, beliefs and ideas (such as "people are kind"), and mental states (such as love and patience).

As you bring your attention to what you are meditating on, you'll naturally shift your attention away from the thoughts that may be causing your stress. By disregarding the busyness of your mind, everything will naturally settle and a deep feeling of peace will arise. In addition to helping you to relax, various forms of meditation have been shown to have beneficial effects on the brain. A review of the existing research, done by researchers from several different institutions, found that a wide variety of meditation techniques helped older adults improve memory, attention, executive function, processing speed, and cognition in general.[264] Here's a rundown of the beneficial effects:

Boosted brain performance: Researchers from National University of Singapore found that people who performed Vajrayana meditation—a Tibetan style that involves connecting with and visualizing enlightened beings—experienced improved attention and performed better on cognitive tasks just after their meditation sessions, possibly because the meditation boosted blood flow to their brains.[265]

More creativity: Study participants were better able to brainstorm possible solutions to a given problem after a type of meditation called *open monitoring,* during which they practiced being receptive to their thoughts and sensations.[266]

Sharper focus and improved memory: College students who practiced Zen meditation before their lectures scored better on quizzes related to the lecture content than did students who did not meditate.[267]

Certain types of meditation can also change the way you think, leading you to become more compassionate. In other words, you become more aware of and sympathetic to the suffering of others. This is the opposite of cold indifference, and a compassionate mind-set could improve your interpersonal relationships at home and work, reducing stress and tension.[268]

A few pointers:

- **Try a short meditation right now.** Sit comfortably with your eyes closed. Focus on your breath. Notice how it feels as it comes in your nose and goes back out again. Don't try to control it or change it. Just allow it to come in and out naturally. If you notice other sensations, such as an ache in your back or an urgent thought about something on your to-do list, just keep returning to the breath. Allow distractions to pass through your mind like clouds pass through a sky. Every time you notice yourself following your thinking, just redirect your mind where you want it to go. Every time you return to the breath, you are training your concentration and bringing yourself to the present moment. In addition to following the breath, you can try bringing your awareness to a word (such as *one* or *peace*) or a location in your body (such as your heart). You can also concentrate on an idea or belief, such as a feeling of gratitude, compassion, or love.

- **Do it regularly.** Training your concentration is not unlike training a muscle. It will take some time before your mind stops following every passing thought. In the beginning, it may even seem as if you are experiencing more thoughts rather than fewer ones, but this is probably an illusion. You are just becoming aware of your thinking, and this is an important first step to honing your concentration.

- **Start wherever you are.** Just a few minutes can feel like a very long time if you are first trying to meditate. Set an initial goal of sitting for five minutes. Then, as your concentration improves, extend your session from there, eventually making it your goal to practice 10 to 20 minutes a day.

- **Practice in the morning.** Your concentration will be stronger, and your practice will set the tone for the rest of your day.

- **Pause throughout the day.** In addition to a regular practice of five minutes or more, take short time-outs throughout the day. Maybe you pause before meals. Or perhaps, every hour or two, you take a "breather" from whatever you are doing. Just checking in and noticing your thoughts and state of mind is a form of meditation, and you can do this anywhere you find yourself, even as you are standing on line at the bank or grocery store.

- **Tap into apps.** Many free apps and downloads can help you meditate. If you type "free guided meditations" into your Internet browser, one of the first results will be the University of California, Los Angeles, Mindful Awareness Research Center. Go there and you'll find several free downloads that can help you do various types of meditations.

Resilience Smarts Prescription #4: Relax with yoga nidra

Sometimes called "yogic sleep," yoga nidra is a guided visualization that deeply relaxes the body. A class or DVD usually runs 35 to 45 minutes, and the actual visualization often varies from class to class and teacher to teacher.

In one study, college students who practiced yoga nidra for eight weeks experienced less stress, worry, and depression.[269] In another study of 20 women and men who ranged in age from 18 to 47, yoga nidra lowered heart rate, a sign of relaxation.[270] Other research shows that yoga nidra may also help to keep blood sugar in check. This is an important finding because, remember, diabetes is a risk factor for Alzheimer's disease.[271]

A few pointers:

- **Find a class, if possible.** Not only will a class connect you with others, it will allow you to more deeply relax and let go as the instructor guides you through the visualization. As yoga nidra becomes more popular, you may be able to find a weekly session offered at a yoga studio near you.

- **In lieu of or in addition to a class,** you can also listen to a number of free sessions on the Internet. Psychologist Richard Miller, PhD, offers a free guided imagery session available for download at *iRest.us*.

Resilience Smarts Prescription #5: Breathe deeply and slowly

Deep breathing may lower cortisol and reduce pain through its connection to the vagus nerve. The vagus nerve starts at the brain stem and travels downward with branches that wander to many different organs, including the heart and digestive system. It communicates autonomic functions between these organs and the brain and is responsible for controlling our heart rate, breathing rate, and many other processes that take place without our conscious effort.

It's this nerve that connects our breathing rate to our heart rate. When we breathe rapidly and shallowly, the vagus nerve speeds up our heart rate, causing us to feel anxious. When we breathe slowly and deeply, we stimulate this nerve and produce the opposite effect. Our heart rate slows and we feel calm and peaceful.

And it can all take place in a matter of seconds.

The vagus nerve is also connected to the release of oxytocin, the bonding hormone that is believed to be involved in trust. Women's brains release oxytocin when they are in labor, as it causes the uterus to contract and may later cause mothers to bond with their infants. Some research shows that when you give oxytocin to people as a nasal inhalant, they become more trusting.[272] Because of this, deep breathing may also cause us to feel safer and less fearful.

There are many breathing exercises or practices you can try, all of which help you to blend deep breathing with focused concentration. Not only will they reduce your stress and tension, they offer a side benefit of strengthening your attention. Try different breathing techniques and see if one induces more relaxation than others.

A few pointers:

- **Try alternate nostril breathing.** It helps you to take deeper breaths and doubles as a breathing meditation. Use your thumb or index finger to close off the right nostril. Inhale long and slowly through the left. Then switch so your finger closes the left nostril and breathe out through the right. Then inhale through the right and continue to switch back and forth.
- **Practice belly breathing.** Place one hand on your belly and another on your chest. Fully exhale. Then as you slowly inhale, try to cause the hand on your belly to rise before the hand on your chest. Imagine that

you are slowly filling your lungs from the bottom to the top. First your belly will expand. Then your rib cage will expand, too, both rising and widening. Then your sternum and collarbones will rise. Now reverse your breathing, slowly allowing your lungs to deflate like a balloon. Eventually, once you retrain yourself to breathe deeply, you won't need your hands for guidance.

• **Exhale.** Here's another good breathing technique to try: Reverse breathing by counting the length of your inhales and your exhales and seeing if you can make your exhales longer than your inhales. In other words, if you inhale to a count of four, see if you can exhale to a count of six.

Resilience Smarts Prescription #6:
Snuggle with someone you care for

Deep breathing isn't the only way to stimulate the vagus nerve. Warm, close touch is another.

The skin is our largest organ, and the vagus nerve branches into the skin in order to take care of autonomic processes such as sweating, heat regulation, and goosebumps. By stimulating this nerve, a warm touch can calm tension and trigger a release in oxytocin.

Humans, like many other mammals, are social creatures. Though many other mammals spend a good portion of their day in close contact, we humans have gotten out of the habit. This is especially true in the United States. In the 1960s, Canadian psychologist Sidney Jourard studied conversations of friends in different parts of the world. In England, he found that two friends sitting at a café were likely to carry on an entire conversation without touching at all. In the US, they might touch just twice—perhaps with a quick shake of hands at the beginning of the conversation and then again upon parting. In France, friends touched one another—a tap on the forearm, an arm around the shoulder, a jab in the ribs—110 times per hour. In Puerto Rico it was 180 times.[273]

A lack of touching may lead us to feel isolated and perhaps even anxious and fearful, causing unneeded stress. Dacher Keltner, a professor of psychology at the University of California, Berkeley, and co-director of the Greater Good Science Center, has spent several years studying the health benefits of touch. He theorizes that the vagus nerve is important in helping us interpret the meaning of touch. If someone grabs us and shakes us angrily by the shoulders, the nerve rapidly communicates "danger" to the brain and sets off the fight-or-flight system. But if someone lovingly holds our hand or places a palm against our shoulder, it communicates safety.

And, according to research done in his lab, we're quite good at interpreting the difference. He and other researchers did an interesting experiment where they placed strangers on either side of a barrier. The two strangers could not see or hear one another. Then he asked one person to stick an arm through a hole in the barrier. The person on the other side was then instructed to quickly touch that person's forearm, using that quick touch to communicate an emotion such as anger, fear, disgust, sympathy, or gratitude. Those receiving the touch were startlingly effective at reading each touch's meaning.[274] This ability to read touch may be why a warm embrace or a consoling arm around the shoulder helps us to calm down and feel centered.

Touch is incredibly potent, too. University of Wisconsin psychologist Richard Davidson and Jim Coan, of the University of Virginia, told 16 married women that they were about to be shocked with electricity. In some situations, as the women anticipated the shock, they were holding the hand of their partners or of a stranger. In other situations, the women were alone. All the while the researchers studied what was happening in the women's brains, using fMRI scanners. The fMRIs showed that, when the women held their partner's hands, they remained more relaxed than when they held the hand of a stranger. When they anticipated the shock while alone, their stress response was highest.[275]

A few pointers:
- **Look for ways to connect through touch.** Simple activities such as getting your hair washed or having a pedicure may help you shake off the stress of the day.
- **Try partner yoga.** It's active, and it can help you to connect through touch, too.
- **Hold hands while you walk.** If you walk outdoors while holding hands, you'll reap the benefits of three prescriptions at once: touch, nature, and exercise.

Resilience Smarts Prescription #7: Get a massage

One research review out of University of Miami and Duke University concluded that massage helped to lower levels of the stress hormone cortisol while boosting levels of brain chemicals thought to be associated with positive emotions.[276]

A few pointers:
- **Experiment with different styles of massage.** Many different types of massage exist, ranging from intense deep tissue and sports massage to more relaxing, Swedish styles. Experiment with different types until you find one that works for you.

- **Consider couples massage.** By learning massage with your spouse or a friend, you benefit from the intellectual challenge involved in learning several different massage movements. Plus massage is active and may bring you closer to your loved one.

Resilience Smarts Prescription #8: Turn to spiritual practices

If you consider yourself to be a religious or spiritual person, you may find it comforting to know that your religious or spiritual practices may be beneficial to your health, particularly the health of your brain. Prayer and a variety of other religious rituals may allow you to let go of worries that may be preying on your mind, and gathering with a community of like-minded people helps you to feel less alone. In a study by Israeli and American researchers and funded by the National Institutes of Health, Islamic women who prayed daily had a reduced risk of mild cognitive impairment compared to women who did not pray.[277] A different study by researchers at Arizona State University and the University of Utah found that people who considered themselves to be deeply religious or spiritual, prayed regularly, and attended religious services had lower cortisol responses and lower blood pressure than people who were less religious.[278]

A few pointers:
- **Join with others.** If you attend a place of worship, consider getting more involved, perhaps by volunteering during services. This will allow you to meet people as you engage in contemplative practices. And you'll also reap the benefits of "giver's high" (Prescription #11).
- **Do it regularly.** There are many different ways to experience the benefits of prayer, and you don't necessarily need to belong to a religious organization to do so. For one person, it might be a short prayer before meals, during which you reflect on how fortunate you are. For another, it might be a much longer reflection on how little we know about the universe. How you pray may be less important than how often and how consistently you do it.

Resilience Smarts Prescription #9: Single-task

Though many of us may believe we're quite good at multitasking, we're probably only fooling ourselves. Switching back and forth between tasks—such as checking email repeatedly as you complete a work project—actually wastes time and makes you less efficient and productive. Every time you take a break from what you are doing, you have to start the task at hand over mentally. This mental re-start can take anywhere from a few seconds to many minutes.[279]

More than just ruining our efficiency, multitasking can cause us undue stress. Our brains struggle to pay attention to more than one thing at a time. This is why, when we're navigating dense traffic, many of us turn down the car radio. Even though the music on the radio seemingly has nothing to do with being able to see where we are going, sound really does interfere with our ability to concentrate. In a silent car, we can put all of our attention on navigating the car, reducing mental stress.[280]

A few pointers:

- **Think of attention in the same way you think of money—it's a limited resource.** If you spend your attention all at once, you'll feel depleted.

- **Feel free to multitask if one task is ingrained.** It's easy to carry on a conversation while you are tying your shoes because you don't have to think about tying your shoes. You've tied your shoes so many times that the task has become a habit. Similarly, you can probably chew gum while you type an email or listen to a book on tape while you walk on the treadmill. On the other hand, some of the toughest multitasking challenges arise when the same part of the brain must oversee two or more similar tasks. Can you talk and read? Not easily, because both those tasks involve the language center of the brain and neither is automatic.

- **Turn off email and text alerts.** Check your phone or email once an hour or once a morning rather than allowing either to interrupt you while you are working.

- **Create a firm rule: Never talk, text, or email while driving.** This even includes hands-free and voice-to-text options.

- **When you are crossing a street, try to be as mindful of your surroundings as possible.** Slow down and do what you taught your children and grandchildren to do: look both ways.

Resilience Smarts Prescription #10: Laugh

Whenever she was asked for her secrets for longevity, Jeanne Calment, the Frenchwoman who lived to age 122, often answered, "Always keep your sense of humor. That's what I attribute my long life to. I think I'll die laughing." Then she often told a joke, "I've never had more than one wrinkle, and I'm sitting on it."[281]

A good belly laugh produces a chemical reaction that elevates your mood, reduces pain and stress and blood pressure, and boosts immunity. Allan L. Reiss, MD, and his colleagues at Stanford University have traced laughter to a region of the brain called the *nucleus accumbens*. This is the brain's reward center, and it releases dopamine, a natural opiate, when it's activated by anything pleasurable such as food, winning a card game, or sex.

Humor therapy may be as effective as some prescription drugs at reducing agitation in people with Alzheimer's disease and other forms of dementia. Nursing home patients who were entertained by clowns for two hours once a week were significantly less aggressive and agitated. Even two weeks after the nursing home stopped bringing in the clowns, nursing home patients remained less agitated.[282]

A few pointers:
- **Laugh at your foibles.** Making fun of yourself can help you to overcome the embarrassment and the stress of making mistakes.
- **Hang out with funny friends**. Who has a way of making you laugh? Try to connect with that person regularly, and let his or her sense of humor rub off on you.
- **Check out a "laughter club."** It's no joke. Laughter clubs exist all over the country. They're run by "certified laughter leaders"—often psychologists, therapists, and psychiatrists—who are trained in the healing benefits of laughter. These workshops can help you connect with others as you get in a good laugh. Look at WorldLaughterTour, Inc. to find out if there's a club near you.
- **Opt for comedies.** When you spend time being sedentary in front of the TV, opt for comedies rather than dramas. Snuggle with a pet or family member, too, to reap the benefits of healing touch. (See Prescription #6.)
- **Laugh and do yoga**. Another kind of laughter club, Laughter Yoga involves exercises, breath work, stretching, and laughing. In a typical class, you start off with fake laughter, which often turns into the genuine thing.

Resilience Smarts Prescription #11: Help others

When we help others, we also help ourselves.

People who spent time helping others—by driving them to doctor's appointments, running errands for them, providing child care and other tasks—were able to navigate and survive highly stressful life events over five years better than people who didn't.[283] Other research has found that people who volunteer their time have a greater sense of purpose and improved well-being. They also tend to have less trouble sleeping, less anxiety, and less loneliness.[284] It may be that, by helping others, we get a boost in oxytocin or other brain chemicals, which seem to protect us from stress-induced health problems.

A few pointers:
- **Just think about doing it.** Remembering a time when you helped someone in the past or contemplating helping someone in the future is almost as powerful as actually helping someone in the present.
- **Help others in person.** Though any amount of generosity can certainly help you feel more purposeful, you'll get a more robust helper's high if you volunteer in person than you will just by donating money to a cause.[285]
- **Think about how good it felt to help.** Whenever you've helped someone or volunteered, take some time to reflect on the experience. This is like boldfacing and underlining the experience and helps to keep helper's high going a little longer.
- **Find the middle way between helping and overdoing it.** Helping too much can make you feel run-down, exhausted, and taken advantage of. Studies out of East Carolina University and the University of Michigan found that the beneficial effects of volunteering taper off somewhere between 40 and 100 hours a year—or roughly one to two hours a week, and that even just a small amount of volunteering is better than none.[286, 287]

Resilience Smarts Prescription #12:
Cultivate a sense of purpose

In his best-selling book *Man's Search for Meaning*, Viktor Frankl wrote of his time in a Nazi concentration camp, noting that he and his fellow prisoners who survived the traumatic experience tended to maintain a strong sense of purpose. They found meaning in the hardships they endured and in helping each other through their suffering.

Frankl's life story provides inspiration for us all, showing us that purpose really can be found in some of the most trying situations, and research has since added support to Frankl's theory. Researchers at Carleton University in Ottawa surveyed 6,000 people, asking them to rate how much they agreed with statements like, "Some people wander through life, but I am not one of them." Years later, they found that people who'd reported a greater sense of purpose on those surveys tended to live longer than people who were more aimless.

A few pointers:
- **Find meaning in your connections to others**. For example, perhaps you can find a sense of purpose in making others smile or laugh or in making someone's day go a little easier (Prescription #10).

- **Offer your skills to others**. This is an especially potent way to find purpose after you've retired or been laid off from a job. Interestingly, you may also find yourself drawn to volunteer work at this time of life. Research has found that people are less likely to help others when they have a high social status such as an important job title than when they have a lower social status.[288]

Resilience Smarts Prescription #13: Count your blessings

Sometimes our stress stems from what we feel is missing or wrong with our lives. We may feel negative because we can't easily afford a mortgage for a bigger home or because we don't have as much retirement savings as we'd like. Or maybe we're stressed because of our back pain or long work hours. Even missing small things like a party can be stressful for some, so much so that the condition has an acronym: FOMO, or fear of missing out.

But the regular practice of gratitude can help shift our minds away from what's wrong in our lives to what's right.

Robert Emmons, PhD, a professor of psychology at UC Davis, has found that people who keep a weekly gratitude journal are more optimistic. They also exercise more regularly, and a gratitude intervention led to more alertness, enthusiasm, and attentiveness in young adults. We're also more likely to pay it forward and help others (Prescription #11).[289]

A few pointers:
- **Consider how others have been kind to you.** For example, you would not know how to read were it not for your many teachers. And you would not have food to eat if it were not for the farmers who grew it, the workers who picked it, engineers and truck drivers who transported it, and clerks who stocked it on the shelf. There might have even been a person who prepared it for you, too.
- **Keep a journal.** Though it's unclear why, writing down what you feel thankful for may be more powerful than just thinking about it.
- **Set aside time to do it.** A great time to practice: just before meals or before bed. Since you eat every day and also go to sleep every day, pairing the activity with meals and sleep will help you to remember to do it.

Resilience Smarts Prescription #14:
Sign up for a stress-reduction workshop

Stress can become a vicious circle. We go through a hard patch and experience stress. That stress leads to many nights of tossing and turning. The lost sleep causes us to self-medicate with caffeine and sugar. The caffeine and the stress disturb our sleep even more. Eventually the initial stressor is long gone, but we're still walking around feeling anxious and jumpy.

If this sounds familiar, then a class dedicated to stress relief may be in order. Many different programs exist. One of them, Mindfulness Based Stress Reduction (MBSR), was developed by Jon Kabat-Zinn, PhD, in the 1970s, at the University of Massachusetts. It includes a blend of meditation, movement, and group support and has been shown to reduce anxiety, even in veterans with post-traumatic stress disorder.[290] One small study of 34 seniors from Washington University School of Medicine in St. Louis, Missouri, found that the program reduced the severity of worry and also improved memory.[291]

Another program that can help you learn how to reduce stress is the Ornish Spectrum, a program originally designed for heart disease prevention. It includes a blend of nutrition, exercise, group support, and stress reduction and has also been shown to improve cognitive functioning.[292]

In addition to those programs, several other stress-reduction programs and workshops are offered by large and regional hospitals.

A few pointers:
- **Check local hospitals and community centers to see what programs and workshops they offer**. Many large and regional hospitals around the country offer the MBSR, Ornish, and other programs, and some may be completely or partially covered by your health insurance.
- **Stay connected after the program ends**. When you join any workshop—whether it lasts just one day or for many weeks—you develop relationships with others, and that's powerful. This helps you realize that you are not alone. Try to connect with others in your program, and stay in touch with them afterward, perhaps periodically meeting to talk about how your stress-reduction efforts are going.

Advice for Caregivers

Caregiving can be stressful work, so the prescriptions in this chapter may be just as important for you as they are for the person you are caring for. If appropriate and practical, you might even do some of them together. After all, for anyone with any form of cognitive impairment, it may be increasingly difficult to remember to count blessings, practice meditation, or take part in other stress-reduction techniques. But with your help, your family member can simply follow your lead.

Try to find the happy balance between allowing your family member to puzzle through a mild challenge and rushing in to help. Sometimes, depending on the health and cognitive abilities of your loved one, it really might be okay to allow him or her to struggle to remember who someone is or how to operate the ice maker. On the other hand, if this causes your loved one undue stress, then it is preferable to recognize that a function has been lost. Stepping in to do the task yourself can prevent the frustration of struggling with a cognitive handicap.

See if you can read your loved one's mood, using facial expressions, posture, and tone of voice as a guide. For example, if your loved one seems to be getting agitated about not being able to put a face with a name, go ahead and gently say, "You remember, this is Susan, your physical therapist."

How to find that happy medium may, in part, center on the time of day. As Alzheimer's disease progresses, confusion and agitation tend to set in, especially during the late afternoon hours. To reduce late afternoon and evening agitation, use this advice:

Turn off the news. Or watch it when your loved one is not around. The television in general can cause your loved one to stay seated and sedentary for long periods of time, and the news, with its constant parade of crime and destruction, may induce agitation.

Look into massage. When researchers from the Hamamatsu University School of Medicine in Japan provided gentle massage therapy to patients with dementia, levels of Chromogranin A (CgA) dropped, an indication that stress and aggression levels dropped as well.[293] A separate study done at the University of Texas found that slow-stroke massage reduced pacing, wandering, and agitation in nursing home patients with Alzheimer's disease.[294] If you are caring for someone with Alzheimer's, look for a massage therapist who specializes in helping people with dementia. Ask questions like, "How often do you work with people with Alzheimer's? How will you respond if he (or she) becomes agitated or confused? What do you do differently with someone with Alzheimer's?"

Reduce agitation with aromatherapy. Certain scents tend to relax the brain, even in people with a blunted sense of smell. In one study conducted on 28 patients with dementia, 28 days of aromatherapy improved cognitive function.[295] A separate study found that when lavender was added to a hand massage, it reduced aggressive behavior in dementia patients.[296] What scents should you use? In the research, rosemary and lemon essential oils were used in the morning, and lavender and orange in the evening. Consider keeping lavender around the house. Not only will it look nice, the scent may provide some relaxation. You can also spritz lavender essential oil on your spouse's pillow, mix drops into bathwater, or add it to massage lotion.

Play favorite music. Familiar music seems to trigger a positive emotional reaction, especially if our memories of that music are stored with other fond memories. You may find that playing familiar music may help your loved one to recall memories and emotions. When using music to calm:

- Create playlists that feature music familiar to you both from time periods that your family member still remembers. For example, if the person you are caring for can still relive stories from his or her young adulthood, create a playlist of songs popular during that time.

- Consider singing along to classic hits and show tunes together. This improves mental performance and may get you both dancing, too.

- Start playing the music at least 30 minutes before the time of day when the person you are caring for usually gets agitated.

- Pay close attention to your loved one's reaction, especially in the beginning. If your loved one becomes more agitated, stop the music and try a different musical selection.

Which is better for your brain— classical music or hard rock?

It depends on which type of music you enjoy the most. When it comes to relaxation, many of us erroneously assume that certain types of music—especially classical and new age—are better at inducing relaxation than other types of music, such as hard rock. But this isn't necessarily true. Our music memories contribute to music enjoyment. Linda Gerdner, PhD, of the University of Arkansas for Medical Sciences in Little Rock, has conducted research to see what type of music is most likely to allow people with Alzheimer's disease to relax. Her research has found that the most important component for relaxing music is this: whether your loved one enjoys listening to it.[297]

T = Train-Your-Brain Smarts

Have you ever gone through any of the following scenarios?

- *Your computer ran a software update, and now everything on your screen looks foreign. You can't even send an email without getting a headache from thinking so hard.*

- *You are driving in an unfamiliar location. You're not technically lost, but you're also not completely confident you are going in the right direction. You must pay close attention to road signs and landmarks and continually calculate the probability of whether you've missed your turn.*

- *Your children or grandchildren are asking you for help with their homework. Nothing looks familiar. You think, "Did I ever learn this in school?"*

Situations like the ones I just described can sometimes bring out our worst, leading us to feel stressed, anxious, and inadequate. Yet these are precisely the kinds of challenges that provide healthy exercise for our brains. Remember in Chapter 6 how we mentioned that a certain amount of stress is good for us? Our brains need a little bit of stress—in the form of novel, exciting, and challenging experiences—to remain sharp.

When you want to work out your body, you go to the gym. What do you do to give your brain a workout? Get lost in an unfamiliar city, help your grandchildren with their homework, upgrade your computer's operating system, or see if you can put together an entertainment center from IKEA. Such activities force us to slow down and pay close attention to what we are doing. We must read and follow directions as well as absorb and understand new material. The unfamiliar can make us feel uncomfortable, but the more we challenge our brains, the healthier they remain. Without a regular dose of challenging situations, our brains get flabby, in much the same way our bodies get flabby when we don't challenge our muscles with enough exercise. In one study, older adults who frequently took part in stimulating leisure activities such as reading, board games, playing musical instruments, and dancing were less likely to develop dementia over 21 years, compared to older adults who participated less frequently in these activities over the same time period,[298] and several other studies have yielded similar findings.[299, 300, 301] Even study participants who were carriers of the *ApoE4* gene were able to postpone the development of Alzheimer's disease by almost a decade if they spent their adult lives immersed in intellectually enriching activities.[302]

These activities can also help you in daily life. In one study, older adults underwent 10 sessions of brain-training during which they were taught mnemonic strategies to boost their ability to remember lists of words as well as strategies to identify and remember letter and word patterns. They also played computer games designed to improve their reaction time. Compared to people who did not participate in the brain-training sessions, study participants improved their ability to perform a number of tasks including shopping, housework, meal preparation, making change, looking up phone numbers, reacting to road signs, reading and understanding prescription medicine labels, and much more; these effects lasted up to five years after to brain-training sessions ended.[303]

Your Brain on Intellectual Exercise

Exactly why intellectual challenges bolster brain health is a matter of debate. According to one theory, intellectual hobbies create a *cognitive reserve* in the brain. A cognitive reserve is a lot like a large bank of knowledge. If you make continual deposits during middle age and beyond—by learning and acquiring new skills—you'll be able to make more withdrawals during your senior years without overdrafting your cognitive savings account. For example, let's say that, around age 40, you made a New Year's resolution to learn one new vocabulary word a day—and you've kept that resolution ever since. Now, according to this hypothetical example, let's say your brain holds the memories of well over 20,000 words. On the other hand, maybe you have a twin brother named Paul, and Paul really couldn't care any less about his vocabulary. He's spent the second half of his life feeding his brain reality television. As a result, he knows fewer than 15,000 different words—not that he's counted.

According to our story, plaques and tangles begin to form in your brain at the same rate they begin to form in Paul's. In other words, if we put you both in an fMRI scanner and peered inside your brains, your brains would appear to have roughly the same number of plaques and tangles. Yet you have no symptoms, whereas Paul is often at a loss for words. That's because Paul knew fewer words to begin with. So, as the connections between his brain cells withered, he didn't have alternative words to call on. If he couldn't think of the word *grouchy,* then he would just sit there and stare for long moments, feeling befuddled or frustrated that the word just wouldn't come to mind. You, on the other hand, knew more words. So when your brain lost track of the word *grouchy,* it had many other words—*irritable, bad-tempered, cantankerous, petulant, surly, testy, snappy*—to draw from. All these words add nuance to your conversation and musicality to your speech.

So as you can see, the less you know, the less you can afford to lose. The more you know, the more you can afford to lose.

But cognitive reserve may not be the only explanation for the protective power of intellectual challenges. These pursuits may actually encourage the growth of new brain cells and connections between those cells. The hippocampus is one of the only areas of the brain that can grow new neurons. Even during old age, this area of the brain contains residual stem cells capable of birthing new neurons. We suspected this, in part, from researchers who've studied the brains of taxi drivers. To become a taxi driver in London, England, one must pass a series of examinations, proving that one knows all the major routes of the city. This involves memorizing the locations and names of 25,000 streets, 20,000 landmarks, and more than 320 possible routes.[304] That's a lot of information, and it takes most aspiring drivers two years to learn it all.

The process of memorizing, remembering, and using all of this information protects their hippocampi. Two landmark studies—one done in 2000[305] and another in 2006—have found that London taxi drivers have enlarged a part of their hippocampi compared to non-taxi drivers. This part of the hippocampus was bigger than in a comparison group, bus drivers, who only need to memorize a few possible routes rather than more than 320 of them.[306]

One explanation: What brain cells we don't use, we really do seem to lose. Without use, new neurons may die within a month, but intellectual pursuits seem to act like fertilizer, helping new hippocampal cells to mature and stick around.[307]

Intellectual pursuits may also encourage cells to build new connections. When you crawl into bed tonight, you will no longer be the same person—neurologically speaking—as you were when you woke. That's because the brain is continually reorganizing itself. Every new experience and challenge nudges the brain to make new cell-to-cell connections.

Though learning becomes slower and more difficult as we age, our ability to change our brains for the better never ends. Even if our brains are damaged from a stroke or head injury, they can still slowly rewire themselves, forming new paths for information to travel. This is why patients are able to recover after a stroke. At first, they may not be able to talk or move one side of their bodies. But over time, they partially or even completely regain the ability to move, write, and talk, and that's because their brains have built new paths, allowing them to regain access to old information. It's much like traveling a detour when a bridge is out. You can still get to the same destination, but you drive on different roads to get there.

Which is better for your brain—formal brain games or hobbies that you enjoy?

We just don't yet know the answer to that question. It could be that both are equally good for you and that the more activities you use to train your brain, the better. When deciding which intellectual prescriptions to try, consider these questions:

Does the activity transfer benefits to everyday life? Consider what intellectual skills you really need to feel sharp as you navigate daily life. If you are like most people, then those skills might include the ability to remember your computer password, make plans, solve problems, and follow a set of instructions. Some hobbies hone those skills more than others, and other hobbies can be adapted in order to sharpen them.

Does it get you out of your comfort zone? When choosing an intellectual pursuit, embrace activities that differ from your working life. So, for example, if you write for a living, doing more writing during your free time isn't going to do much to help you calculate a tip or put together IKEA furniture. During your leisure time, you might want to gravitate toward hobbies that require math or music or other special skills.[308]

Is it novel? New experiences are particularly stimulating for the brain. When the brain encounters something new, it compares it to past experiences, using the past to make sense of the present. This doesn't mean you need to continually change your hobby, but it does mean that you want to infuse your hobbies with new experiences. Throughout the prescriptions in this chapter, you'll find suggestions for how to do this.

Is it challenging? If something is so easy for you that you can do it in your sleep, then it's probably not challenging your brain. On the other hand, if something is so challenging that you feel stressed and anxious every time you try to do it, you might be taking on too much at once. Try to find the middle way between too easy and too hard. From an intellectual standpoint, the best hobby is one that you can never really master. No matter how good you get at it, there's always room for improvement.

Prescriptions for Training Your Brain

In the following pages, you'll find more than a dozen different ways to challenge your brain. You don't need to try every single one of them in order to keep your brain sharp. Consider which ones seem most enticing, then try them with a sense of experimentation and exploration. Keep in mind that the unfamiliar often feels uncomfortable at first, but that's exactly the point. What gets you out of your comfort zone helps you to really engage your brain. So give new hobbies the benefit of the doubt. With time, your discomfort will likely fade.

As you incorporate these strategies into your life, get creative and look for ways to add intellectual challenges to the tasks you already do every day. Each time you grocery shop, see if you can compare prices and get the best deal on at least one of your purchases. Or compare nutritional labels to see which product contains the least sugar, fat, and/or sodium. Perhaps you start keeping a tally of your gas mileage, and you do personal experiments to see what types of driving and car care can help your car go the most miles for the least gas.

As much as possible, combine prescriptions with advice from other chapters. We've provided suggestions for pairing these intellectual pursuits with Aerobic Smarts, Social Smarts, and more.

Train-Your-Brain Smarts Prescription #1:
Learn to play an instrument

Learning and playing an instrument forces you to sharpen many different cognitive processes, including attention, memory, motor skills, auditory skills, and visual skills. It's no wonder studies have found that playing a musical instrument delays the onset of cognitive decline. When researchers from Emory University tested the cognitive health of 70 older adults, they found that study participants with at least 10 years of musical experience performed better on tests of nonverbal memory, naming, and many other cognitive processes than older adults with less training or no training at all.[309]

In lieu of playing an instrument, you might also benefit from singing in a choir. In one study, older adults who joined a singing group improved their memory and attention.[310]

And it's never too late to learn to do either. Just because you didn't learn an instrument or train your voice when you were a child doesn't mean you can't learn now. In addition to helping keep your brain sharp, music lessons may also allow you to maintain fine motor skills, especially if you learn an instrument that requires complex finger motions. When researchers offered piano lessons to older adults, the study participants were able to improve cognitive abilities—including attention, concentration, and planning—over just six months, compared to study participants who didn't take lessons.[311]

A few pointers:

- **Pick any instrument you think you might enjoy**. It doesn't matter whether it's guitar, piano, or drums. Learning to read music and play the right notes will challenge many different areas of your brain at once, no matter the actual instrument.

- **Keep up what you start.** The benefits of musical training may wear off over time, especially if you stop practicing.[312]

- **If you already know one instrument, consider learning another**. Or challenge yourself by learning how to play an unfamiliar style of music. For example, if you initially learned to play classical music, try jazz or blues.

- **Join a band or amateur orchestra**. In addition to adding a social element, this forces you to work on your timing. Playing music with others provides the extra challenge of coordinating your music with the music of others, and following a conductor for cues. Bonus points if you join a marching band—such as a Shriner's Hobo Band—as this will get you plenty of exercise and also challenge your spatial skills.

Train-Your-Brain Smarts Prescription #2:
Try puzzles and board games

Games of skill—whether they be the Sunday crossword or a weekly chess match—can be a fun way to pass the time and connect with others while you also sharpen your ability to remember and follow rules, plan your next move, remember past plays, and predict what your opponent is likely to do. It's strenuous brain exercise, so it makes sense that these types of activities may keep our brains healthy.

Older adults who regularly played board games and puzzles during their leisure time were more likely to preserve brain tissue and maintain memory and other cognitive functions compared to people who didn't play games, according to a study of 329 people.[313] The results even held true for people who were genetically predisposed to developing Alzheimer's disease.[314]

A few pointers:

- **Choose games that you enjoy and feel challenged to play.** In the study, checkers, crosswords, and card games were all effective. You can even pull out those board games from childhood. Just because you aren't a kid anymore doesn't mean you can't still have some fun while playing them as an adult.

- **Investigate the wide variety of apps that can help you sharpen your brain.** Puzzlejuice and Bonza will challenge you with word puzzles. Bicolor and Quento will do the same with numbers. Trainyard Express and The Heist work your problem-solving skills, whereas Blek will fire up your imagination and Monument Valley will work your spatial and building skills.

- **If your game, by nature, is a solitary one (such as Solitaire), consider ways to involve others.** Maybe you play a game while a friend watches and offers pointers. Or perhaps you keep track of your wins and losses, with the ultimate loser offering to cook a Brain Smart meal for the winner.

- **Keep changing up the games.** It may be better to continually challenge your brain with new games rather than to get better and better at the same game.

Train-Your-Brain Smarts Prescription #3:
Learn a language

When researchers assessed the backgrounds of patients with Alzheimer's disease, they found that patients who were bilingual—fluent in at least two languages—had developed Alzheimer's disease an average of 4.6 years later than patients who spoke only one language. Patients who spoke one language were diagnosed with Alzheimer's disease around age 71, whereas for patients who spoke more than one language, the diagnosis came around age 76.[315]

Just because you didn't learn a second language while you were in grade school doesn't mean you can't learn one now.[316, 317, 318]

A few pointers:

- **If you are homebound,** try learning a new language with the help of online programs designed for seniors. Some, like Speak Shop, will pair you with a tutor in another location who video conferences with you to go over lessons.

- **Combine your language acquisition with travel plans**. So, for instance, if you are learning Spanish, celebrate a big language-learning milestone by visiting Spain or Mexico.
- **Immerse yourself in the food of whatever culture you are studying.** If you are learning French, try healthy French cooking, for example. You'll learn new words as you puzzle out how to make new recipes.
- **Watch movies in the language you are trying to learn, even if they are available in English**. You can do the same with television shows. For example, if you are trying to learn Spanish, try watching Spanish language television channels. You might activate the subtitle button so you can see the foreign words as well as hear them. This enhances your comprehension and learning.
- **Try language learning sites and apps like Duolingo**. This app can help you learn new words and grammar every day and it's free.

Train-Your-Brain Smarts Prescription #4:
Learn how to draw, paint, or sculpt

Artistic pursuits such as painting encourage you to focus your attention. In order to draw a flower, for example, you have to look closely at a real flower or a picture of one—and pay particular attention to the shape of the petals, stem, and leaves. As you draw, you're also making dozens of spatial calculations. For example, how large should the petals be if you want to make sure there's enough space at the bottom of your picture to draw some grass or, in the corner of your picture, to draw a bumblebee? And learning any art—whether it's painting or sculpture—is much like learning a language. In this case, it's the language of shape, light, line, and color.

So it's not surprising that artistic pursuits have been found to protect the brain. Seniors who took up painting, drawing, or sculpting were 73 percent less likely to develop mild cognitive impairment over a period of four years than were people who did not engage in these types of artistic activities, found a recent study of 256 octogenarians by researchers at the Mayo Clinic.[319] Crafting activities—such as woodworking, pottery, ceramics, and quilting—were also beneficial, reducing the likelihood of MCI by 55 percent.

In a smaller study done in Germany, 60- and 70-year-olds who took art classes improved their scores on tests of psychological resilince over 14 weeks, indicating that their ability to cope with stress had grown. Also, fMRI scans revealed that their brains had sprouted new connections in areas that tend to lose connections with increasing age.[320]

A few pointers:

- **Believe in yourself.** You might see yourself as someone who "isn't artistic" or who "can't draw," but that may only be because no one has taught you how. If you take lessons and practice what you learned, you may surprise yourself.
- **Explore classes offered in your area**. Ask for recommendations at your local art museum, artist's colony, or art galleries.
- **Create virtual art**. In addition to classes, you can also use apps to hone your art ability. Tayasui Sketches, ASKetch, Inspire Pro, and Penultimate are just a few of the many apps that are available.

Train-Your-Brain Smarts Prescription #5:
Take acting classes

Acting requires lots of memorization. According to one study, 122 seniors who took twice-weekly acting lessons for four weeks improved their ability to memorize and recall a list of words, remember a series of numbers, read and remember a short story, as well as their performance on many other tests of memory, whereas seniors who didn't take acting lessons did not boost their performance on these tests.[321] In a follow-up study done by the same researchers, the seniors who took acting classes improved their word recall by 19 percent and word fluency by 12 percent.[322]

A few pointers:

- **Look into community theater.** If no classes are available, sign up to help as a stagehand or an extra, slowly learning as you go.
- **Write and star in plays that you put on with other family members,** including children and grandchildren. In addition to stimulating your brain, this can be a fun way to help everyone grow closer.
- **Several local theater groups offer classes specifically for adults and seniors.** Check to see if one is available near you.

Train-Your-Brain Smarts Prescription #6:
Read to learn

Reading may seem like a passive activity, but it has the ability to fill your mind with knowledge. The more knowledge in your mind, the bigger your cognitive reserve. So every time you read, it's like putting memories into an ever-expanding bank. Then, as you age or as mild cognitive impairment begins, you're able to lose more memories before it significantly affects your daily life.

A few pointers:

- **Keep your mind engaged.** Try to strike a balance between reading about things that interest you and challenging yourself with new genres and topics.

- **Consider why you are reading, and remind yourself of your purpose.** This will help motivate you to continually hone your concentration.

- **Take periodic breaks to connect what you've read to what you already know.** This helps to cement the new information in place, giving it a context. Consider the meaning of the text—how does it relate to other stored memories? Or to daily life? What does it mean to you?

- **Highlight as you read.** This helps you to decide which points are important and worth remembering.

- **Consider taking notes as you read.** Make a point of capturing three main points each time you read.

- **Connect with others about what you've learned.** You might join a book club or discussion group. Or you might post your reflections online by writing a review on a site like *GoodReads.com* or sharing your thoughts on a social network like Facebook.

Train-Your-Brain Smarts Prescription #7:
Become a tutor

As you learned in Chapter 6, volunteering can give your life meaning and buffer you from the harmful effects of stress. Volunteering as a tutor adds another component: intellectual stimulation. Women who volunteered 15 hours each week for Experience Corps, a program that pairs senior citizen reading tutors with children who are developing their literacy and problem-solving skills, experienced increased activity in brain regions associated with attention.[323]

A few pointers:

- **Explore the tutoring programs near you.** In addition to Experience Corps, look into Laubach Literacy International, Oasis, and various local programs coordinated through the public school system or your local library.

- **Don't let the "15 hours a week" scare you.** Many tutoring programs ask for only a one-hour weekly commitment. Volunteer the amount of hours that fits your lifestyle.

Train-Your-Brain Smarts Prescription #8:
Explore video games

When we hear the words "video games," we usually think of teenagers and young adults and the advice to cut back on "screen time." Yet, researchers have spent years developing video games specifically for *older adults,* finding that certain electronic games provide a motivating way to exercise one's attention, memory, and other cognitive skills. Until recently, it was thought that the skills learned from video gaming didn't translate into real life. People got better at the games, it was assumed, but they didn't necessarily get better at everyday tasks that involved attention and memory, such as noticing and responding to road signs.

That thinking, however, is starting to change. A growing body of research shows that these games may offer a real benefit, beyond just allowing players to improve their gaming skills. For example, our ability to multitask—cook while talking, watch a movie while browsing the web, drive while listening to an audiobook—drops with age.[324] But one game, designed by researchers at the University of California, San Francisco, may improve the ability of older adults to multitask.[325] Called NeuroRacer, the game is quite simple. You just drive a virtual car, pressing various buttons to navigate and respond to instructional signs that pop up along your route. Seniors played the game 12 hours over a month's time, or about three hours a week. The game was programmed to provide them with increasingly more difficult multitasking challenges. At the end of the four weeks, the seniors had improved so much that they achieved higher scores on the game than did 20-year-olds who were playing it for the first time.[326] More interesting, when the researchers tested the seniors again six months later, the skills remained in place, even though the seniors had not had access to the game during that time period.[327] The study participants also underwent testing to measure their attention and multitasking abilities, and both had improved.

Currently NeuroRacer is merely a research tool and not available to the public, but you may be able to take part in a clinical trial that involves it or a game much like it. Learn more at *AKILIinteractive.com.*

In lieu of NeuroRacer, a wide variety of action games may still offer some limited benefit, as some research shows that action gamers outperform non-gamers on tests of perception and attention.[328, 329]

The same may be true of the widely available brain-training systems such as Brain HQ from Posit Science, Luminosity from Lumos Labs, and a Brain Fitness program from Dakim. These are not as thoroughly researched as NeuroRacer, and we can't say for sure just how much of a benefit you will get from any of them. When I counsel my patients, I tell them that everything that keeps their brains intellectually challenged is probably helpful, and computerized brain-training systems are one option. If you find them interesting and you enjoy playing them, then include them in your Brain Smarts routine. If, on the other hand, you find them boring or even stress-inducing, skip them in favor of any number of other prescriptions suggested in this chapter.

A few pointers:

- **Opt for a challenge.** The more challenging the game, the better. If you get used to a game and it becomes easy, switch to a new one that feels more unfamiliar.

- **Play against other people rather than against other computers.** Many gaming apps allow you to play against others, including strangers. So download Words with Friends, Chess with Friends, Monopoly, The Game of Life, Depict, and any number of other apps, and challenge your friends to a game.

- **Play for a cause.** The University of California at San Francisco is recruiting up to 100,000 people who are willing to share their personal health history and then play video games over time. The games consist of various neuropsychological tests set up as games. Each time you play one, you give the researchers a snapshot of your brain function. You can register online at *brainhealthregistry.org*. It's free. Another free test that involves puzzles and games is offered by Baycrest and available at *cogniciti.com*.

Train-Your-Brain Smarts Prescription #9:
Roam the world

Embrace new scenery as much as possible. Seeing new places and meeting new people continually stimulates all of your senses, and navigating the unfamiliar keeps your brain sharp. And this is a prescription that you can put into place every day—not just once every year or so when you go on vacation. It's just a matter of embracing your inner explorer.

A few pointers:

- **Consider taking a different vacation each year rather than always going to the same spot.** Remember, however, that none of these pointers works for everyone. If you've fallen in love with an annual trip to the shore or somewhere else, consider inviting a group of friends along. In this case the sociality and absence of stress may trump the stimulation of a novel location.

- **Take up a hobby like bird-watching that will encourage you to travel.** As you chase after a rare glimpse of an ibis or a least tern, you'll meet others, expand your memory, and spend lots of time relaxing in pleasant outdoor locations. Similar hobbies include wine tasting and rock collecting.

- **Take a scenic drive once a week.** Maybe you drive through the countryside. Or perhaps you go on a tour of local covered bridges or other sites. As you drive unfamiliar territory, you'll be challenged to find your way, and the new sights will stimulate your senses. Even just taking a different route to work can help take you off autopilot and help you enjoy the scenery around you.

- **Go on walking tours.** They'll help you get in a little physical exercise as you learn about a new place.

- **Hike unfamiliar trails.** Being submerged in nature is naturally calming, helping you to reduce stress. It also encourages you to read a map and follow directional markers on a path.

- **Take the scenic route.** See how many different routes you can find to the same locations.

- **As you explore, take in the new location with all of your senses.** How does the breeze feel on your skin? Stop to smell the flowers or to notice the scent of food from restaurants. Listen to the songbirds, buzzing insects, or laughing children. Watch the sunset or take time to notice how the sky is reflected in a pond or even in a puddle.

Train-Your-Brain Smarts Prescription #10:
Never stop learning

An attitude of continual curiosity can help you continually beef up your cognitive reserve.

A few pointers:

- **Sign up for classes offered at your local colleges**. Sign up for anything that you find interesting. Regardless of the subject, as long as you are learning you're exercising your brain. You might take a random sampling of classes or even go back to school and get that degree you always wanted.

- **Check out the Bernard Osher Foundation**. It supports lifelong learning institutes around the country that offer noncredit classes for people aged 50 plus. There might be one near you. Senior centers and libraries may offer classes as well.

- **Try guided tours**. You'll learn more through a guided tour than you would alone, and you'll get a chance to do so in a group atmosphere.

- **Check out the dozens of online distance-learning programs from accredited universities**. Sign up for one along with a family member or friend.

- **Explore topics that have always fascinated you.** Interested in wine? Go to wine tastings. Want to recognize constellations? Try to see the warriors and animals that the ancients saw in the night sky. Always wished you knew the names of different birds or flowers? Buy an identification guide or download an app, and teach yourself one new bird or flower a day.

- **Take up new pastimes such as stargazing, bird-watching, and flower identification that require you to learn.** See if there is club near you where you can meet with others to talk about your new interest.

Train-Your-Brain Smarts Prescription #11:
Retire to the job you've always wanted

Some adults find retirement quite stressful. They don't know what to do with the free time, and they feel they've lost their sense of purpose. This can bring on loneliness and depression. So rather than seeing retirement as a time to stop working, reframe it as an opportunity to spend the day doing what you really love.

A few pointers:

- **Continue to work in the same career,** but do it part-time or as a freelancer.

- **Check out career centers for older adults.** For example, AARP's "50 Best Employers for Workers Over 50" may offer useful suggestions for a second career.

- **Volunteer to help others.** Maybe you make blankets for the homeless or cook meals for the needy. Or you combine volunteering with physical fitness by offering to lead a walking or hiking group. Or you might offer your professional skills pro bono to nonprofit organizations. For example, you might offer a nonprofit accounting or legal help.

Train-Your-Brain Smarts Prescription #12:
Lean on memorization aids

Tried-and-true memorization aids really do work. To increase the chances of being able to remember important information, try any of these techniques:

- **Repeat it.** To remember someone's name, repeat it to yourself a few times and find ways to say it out loud during conversation. It's the same when you are reading. Stop and repeat main points to yourself and take notes as you go.

- **Elaborate on it.** Elaboration associates new information with other memories, making it more likely you'll be able to store it and retrieve it later on. So rather than only trying to remember someone's name, associate his or her name with something else already stored in your long-term memory. For example, you might remember Jack by thinking, *Jack, like my cousin Jack.*

- **Use mnemonics.** When you use a mnemonic, you transform information into a form your brain can more easily retain. For example, when you were a child, you probably learned how many days were in each month by memorizing, "Thirty days have September, April, June, and November. . . ." This rhyme is much easier to remember than a list of months and numbers. Similarly, if you've ever learned how to read music, then you probably were taught the mnemonic "**E**very **G**ood **B**oy **D**oes **F**ine" to help you remember the order of the notes of the treble clef. So, let's say you need a computer password that contains a series of capital and lowercase letters, at least one symbol, and at least one number. You decide on "At30diS?" How will you remember it? While I encourage you to write it down, another possibility is by considering the question: **A**re there 30 days **i**n **S**eptember?

- **Form word pictures in your mind**. This is particularly helpful in remembering someone's name. If it's Ray, you might imagine a ray of sunshine, for example.

- **Chunk bits of information together**. It's harder to remember a string of random numbers than it is to remember chunks of numbers. Consider the difference between remembering "819379" versus "819-379."

- **Lean on "muscle memory."** This is especially helpful with phone numbers, PINs, and passwords. It may be easier for you to remember the shape your fingers make as they type 4411, for example, on an ATM than it is to remember the actual numbers.

Train-Your-Brain Smarts Prescription #13:
Let your brain serve as your #1 computer

The advent of computers has shifted the way we think and solve problems. Unless we're engineers or statisticians, we rarely do math. We no longer need to remember telephone numbers. We don't read maps because we have a GPS. Though some memory aids can certainly offer peace of mind, some of us may benefit by going old school every once in a while.

A few pointers:

- **Read the paper rather than watch the television news.** Reading is more active and is also more likely to stimulate a conversation.
- **Do basic math in your head.** Calculate a sales price, for instance—rather than always relying on a calculator.
- **Before going on a trip, study a map, and pick out your route.** Then, as you drive, either go without the GPS, or see if you can remember your route before your GPS gives you the right answer.
- **Practice memorizing hard-to-remember information such as computer passwords.** Yes, definitely write them down in case you forget, but also use memory tricks such as mnemonic aids (see page 129).
- **Memorize a poem.** Once you have one poem down, try committing another one to memory. Recite your poem at an opportune moment with friends. They will be surprised and impressed.

Advice for Caregivers

If you live with someone who has Alzheimer's, life can become frustrating as your loved one relies more and more on you to remember important appointments as well as locations of important items, such as his wallet or phone. Meanwhile, you might not have Alzheimer's disease, but you are aging, too—and you may be having a hard enough time keeping track of your own car keys.

This is all the more reason to practice intellectual pursuits with your loved one rather than just tell him to "do puzzles" or "read." By doing them together, you'll both benefit and you'll also laugh and grow closer. For as long as possible, continue intellectual pastimes that you both enjoy, whether it is bridge, checkers, or bingo. As your loved one's memory fails, be encouraging and also gentle. Is it really important to mention that she failed to place a chip down on a bingo letter that was called? Be creative about modifying activities so you both can benefit. Maybe you fill in the crossword but continually read the clues out loud and ask for your loved one's input.

Over time, your loved one may lose the ability to participate in favorite activities. So switch to easier games. You may find that games your loved one played years ago hold a special attraction. This may be especially helpful if your loved one's memory of the past is richer or sharper than her memory of the present. Instead of pinochle, perhaps Go Fish is in order.

Also, try *new* games, perhaps even creating your own. This can really help, especially after your family member can no longer follow the complex rules of typical board games. You might play the first 10 seconds of an old song and ask your loved one to guess the name of the band. Or create a "remember when" game, during which you start a story about a memory and see if he can fill in some of the details.

Also consider board games that have been specially designed for people with Alzheimer's disease. These games often include high-contrasting colors and very simple instructions. Shake Loose a Memory, for example, was developed by gerontologists and it contains questions that help unlock memories. Connect is another board game created for adults with memory problems.

Anything that helps someone remember the past can be helpful. Even just sitting together and organizing or looking at old photos can be stimulating. Flip through an album and ask questions like, "What do you remember from that day?"

Consider compiling a historical record to leave behind for other family members. You can do this by writing down memories or videotaping interviews with your loved one. If you feel you need help with this, a nonprofit service called Life Chronicles interviews older adults and people with serious illnesses about their lives, creating a 60- to 90-minute video that can be shared with loved ones. They can come to your home to do a formal taping, edit footage you send to them, or record you via videoconferencing. The costs are covered by donations. For more information, go to *lifechronicles.org*.

CHAPTER 8

··

S = Sleep Smarts

All creatures sleep, but what actually happens during our slumber isn't well understood. We do know that sustained sleep deprivation can result in death due to the body's reduced ability to fight off infections, but we're still unraveling the answers to many questions: How much sleep do we really need? Why does lack of sleep raise our risk for a variety of diseases, including Alzheimer's? What improves our ability to fall asleep? These unanswered questions can lead to misconceptions and anxieties. In this chapter you will read about some interventions that might improve your sleep habits, but remember: "One size does not fit all." What works for one person may have no effect on another.

The brain's mere three pounds consumes 20 percent of the body's energy. Like any big energy consumer, the brain spews out toxic wastes as it creates thoughts, memories, and chemical instructions. One of these waste products is the amyloid protein thought to contribute to Alzheimer's disease. During the day, amyloid accumulates in the spaces between brain cells.[330] As we sleep, that amyloid and other toxic byproducts are cleared away.

Researchers at the University of Rochester injected a fluorescent chemical into the cerebrospinal fluid of mice. Then they watched as specialized glial cells used their "end-feet" to force the fluorescent fluid into the rodents' brains, flooding and scrubbing the spaces between the cells and pervading every inch of brain tissue, much as the rinse cycle on your washing machine removes soap and debris from your clothing. As the fluid permeated every area of the brain, brain cells temporarily shrank, increasing the spaces between them and allowing the fluid more room to do its job.[331] Then, after this thorough hosing, the waste-filled fluid drained back out of the brain and the brain cells plumped back up to their original size.[332] It's not unreasonable to think that something similar happens in humans, too.

It's also as we sleep that our brain resets, integrating everything that happened during the day. New experiences and insights are consolidated with older memories. Sleeping also helps us to forget unneeded information and unimportant details, such as the fact that it rained last Monday or that you had tuna for lunch last Friday.[333] Sleep is so essential that no drug can make up for skimping on it. When we sleep too few hours or not deeply enough, we not only feel foggy and less alert. We also prematurely age our brains and raise our risk for developing Alzheimer's disease.[334, 335]

Dreaming and Non-Dreaming Sleep

As we sleep, our brains cycle through dreaming (REM) and non-dreaming (non-REM) sleep:

NON-REM SLEEP: During non-dreaming sleep, our brains progress through light, moderate, and deep stages of sleep. During the lightest stages of sleep, we can easily startle and awake. During the deeper stages, breathing and heart rate are at their slowest. It's thought that, in these deepest stages of sleep, the body repairs and regrows tissues.[336, 337]

REM SLEEP: This dreaming sleep is as essential to our well-being as the other sleep stages. REM sleep stimulates the brain regions involved in learning, and when we're deprived of REM, our ability to navigate an unfamiliar location, to prevent ourselves from getting lost, to find a car in a parking lot, and to perform other spatial memory tasks goes down, researchers have found.[338]

When We Don't Sleep Well

Our daily sleep/wake clock (called a *circadian rhythm*) is regulated by sunlight and darkness. Darkness turns on the pea-sized pineal gland in the brain, causing it to produce the hormone melatonin. As your melatonin levels rise, you start to feel sleepy. Your body temperature also cools and your metabolism slows.

Then, after dawn, light switches the gland back off, and melatonin levels fall.

In the morning, levels of the fight-or-flight hormone cortisol and body temperature rise, inducing alertness and wakefulness.[339]

When we sleep in sync with this natural rhythm, we get the most restorative rest. But this rhythm can become disrupted by:

Shift work: Working at night goes against the body's natural circadian rhythms, which is probably why shift workers are more likely to develop heart disease, gastrointestinal problems, and impaired cognition.

Jet lag: When we fly to another time zone, it takes a while before our biological sleep/wake rhythms shift, causing fatigue and other symptoms of jet lag.

Age: As we age, our pupils grow smaller and the lenses thicker, allowing less light to reach the retina and making it harder for our bodies to stay in sync with the natural light and darkness rhythms of the planet. A 60-year-old's eyes absorb only about 30 to 40 percent of the light that a 20-year-old's eyes do, and this doesn't even account for vision problems related to cataracts, glaucoma, and other issues.[340] As a result, our brains produce less melatonin with advancing age.[341] As circadian rhythms get thrown off, our sleep/wake cycle changes. We doze off while watching the evening news only to wake in the middle of the night. Sleep fragmentation is as inevitable with aging as wrinkling of the skin.

Loss of brain cells: A group of neurons in an area of the brain's hypothalamus called the *ventrolateral preoptic nucleus* can degenerate over time, throwing off the brain's sleep switch. If you remember, the hypothalamus regulates autonomic (automatic) functions like heartbeat and body temperature. Research done on rats found that the absence of the nerve cells in the ventrolateral preoptic nucleus reduced sleep by about 50 percent, and the sleep the rodents got was fragmented. Young people have 30,000 of these important sleep cells, whereas 70-year-olds have about half that number and 80-year-olds have fewer than 10,000 of these brain cells. The fewer cells in this area of the brain, the worse you'll sleep.[342]

In addition to circadian disturbances, we're likely to wake for several other reasons as we get older. Aging men with enlarged prostates may wake repeatedly to urinate. During perimenopause, women wake from hot flashes. The pain of osteoarthritis and other conditions can wake us, leading to depression and more pain, which disturbs sleep even more.[343] We also may snore more as we age or find ourselves sleeping next to someone who does, which also disturbs sleep. If the snoring is severe, it may be a sign of sleep apnea (see Prescription #14).

When we don't get enough sleep:

The brain shrinks. A study of 147 adults who ranged in age from 20 to 84 found that insomniacs—people who had trouble falling asleep or staying asleep—experienced a more rapid decline in brain volume throughout their brains over 3½ years than people who slept more deeply.[344]

We make more mistakes. Michigan State University and University of California at Irvine researchers found that people who'd only slept five hours or fewer were more likely to mix up details than participants who'd slept more.[345]

Our risk for developing Alzheimer's disease climbs. According to research done at Uppsala University in Sweden, men who reported not sleeping well were 1½ times more likely to develop Alzheimer's disease over the 40-year study than men who reported normal sleep.[346]

Which is better for your brain: sleeping fewer hours but feeling rested during the day, or sleeping more than eight hours and still feeling sluggish?

Feeling rested is best.

You may have heard that seven to nine hours of sleep is ideal, and that recommendation is based on a Brigham and Women's Hospital study of more than 15,000 women that found that, compared to women who slept seven or eight hours a night, women who slept five or fewer hours at midlife had a worse memory later in life. Interestingly, in the same study, the memory of women who slept nine or more hours was also worse than the control groups.[347] A separate study of more than 7,000 men and women found similar results, with people who slept fewer than six hours or more than eight hours scoring lower on brain function tests.[348]

It's easy to misinterpret those results and assume that all of us need seven to nine hours at night. We don't.

There is no one best amount of sleep that works for all people. A small percentage of people may function well on four to six hours of sleep. Take Marissa Mayer, the chief executive of Yahoo, who averages about that much sleep a night and seems to function extremely well.[349] It's the same with PepsiCo chair and CEO Indra Nooyi, who gets a mere four hours of shut-eye a night, and US President Barack Obama has indicated that he goes to bed at 1:00 a.m. and wakes at 7:00.[350]

On the other hand, there are plenty of other people who sleep just a few hours at night and *don't* feel energized afterward. So they keep themselves awake with copious amounts of caffeine and sugar. For these people, more sleep is definitely in order.

On the other end of the spectrum, there are people who are in bed for nine or more hours at night, but their sleep is fragmented. Maybe they wake repeatedly and toss and turn as they worry about problems at work or at home. Or perhaps they're awoken several times a night by a snoring spouse, restless pets, small children, or their own sleep apnea or back pain. Either way, even though they are getting nine or more total hours of sleep, their brains and bodies are not getting enough rest.

How do you know if you are one of those fortunate few who needs only five or six hours or whether you need seven or eight? Go by how you feel. If you feel alert throughout the day, you may not need more sleep. On the other hand, if you find you are dragging your feet throughout the day or live on caffeine, it's probably a good idea to take steps to sleep longer and better.

Prescriptions for a Better Night's Sleep

The harder you try to fall asleep, the more likely it is that sleep will evade you. You may already know this from firsthand experience, but research supports this advice, too. When Russian researchers told men and women that those who fell asleep the fastest would earn a financial reward, study participants were able to fall asleep, but they startled awake a short time later.[351]

So as you incorporate these prescriptions into your sleep routine, try not to become obsessed with your sleep patterns. See if you can adopt a relaxed mindset, telling yourself that if you fall asleep, great. If you can't fall asleep, then get up and do something boring such as folding laundry. Or try one of the relaxation prescriptions from Chapter 6. Then, once you feel drowsy, crawl back into bed.

Sleep Smarts Prescription #1: Welcome in the morning light

Sunlight is what triggers our brains to flip off the sleep switch and flip on the awake one. Light travels into the retina and influences production of the hormone melatonin, inhibiting its release and helping to reset our sleep clock. When we get sun exposure in the morning, we feel more awake during the day. Then when we avoid light at night, we naturally become sleepy.

A few pointers:
- **Walk outdoors in the morning**. This is particularly helpful during travel, as a brisk morning walk will help to reset your sleep/wake cycle to your new time zone.

- **Check out the various brands of light boxes that are available commercially**. They provide about 30 times more light than your usual lamp, mimicking the effects of natural sunlight. Known as "light therapy," these light boxes can be quite helpful during the darker winter months, and, in addition to improving sleep, research shows that their use may reduce sundowning restlessness in people who already have Alzheimer's disease.[352, 353] You just turn on the box and sit in front of it for a half hour or more in the morning hours. You don't actually have to stare at the light. You can put the box on your kitchen table and light it up while you are eating breakfast. Or, you can bring it with you to work, and turn it on while you are doing paperwork.[354, 355]

Sleep Smarts Prescription #2: Cut back on evening light

At night, you want to do the opposite of what you do in the morning. Minimize light so your brain gets the message that it's time to slow down and fall asleep. This is especially important for so-called "blue" light, emitted by smartphones, tablets, e-readers, and computers, which has been shown to suppress the production of melatonin.[356]

A few pointers:

- **Wean yourself off evening electronics.** You may feel like you need to get more work done in the evening, but for some, this schedule may backfire. One study found that employees who worked on smartphones in the evening ended up getting less done than usual the following day because they were more tired and less engaged.[357] Morning, on the other hand, is a great time of day to work on devices that emit "blue" light. Research from Brigham and Women's Hospital has found that blue light exposure during the day can lift fatigue and improve alertness.[358]

- **Dim the lighting.** Room lighting can suppress melatonin production, as energy-efficient lightbulbs and LEDs also emit this kind of blue light. You don't have to walk around in the dark, but do switch off lights you are not using and dim others as much as possible.[359]

- **Make your bedroom as dark as possible.** This is especially important if you are a light sleeper. Even the glow from power buttons on your alarm clock or radio could potentially disturb sleep. Then, to wake in the morning, consider a natural light alarm clock that slowly illuminates your room. Once you're up, throw open the blinds, and let natural sunlight stimulate alertness even more.

Sleep Smarts Prescription #3: Shower at night

Our body temperature fluctuates throughout the day and the night, varying from one or two degrees below 98.6°F to one or two degrees above. It generally starts to fall during the evening, reaching its lowest point during sleep, and this fall in temperature is one of the mechanisms that causes us to feel sleepy.

You can enhance the sleepiness induced by the body cooling effect by taking a warm shower or bath in the evening. The shower warms you by a degree or two. But then the warming effect wears off. As your body cools back down, sleepiness sets in. In one small study, women who took a long, warm bath in the mid-afternoon to early evening felt sleepier at bedtime and slept more deeply, too.[360]

A few pointers:

- **Shower or bathe at least 90 minutes before bed to experience the best of the cooling effect**. In addition to helping induce grogginess, this can be a great way to unwind and relax away stress.
- **To aid the body cooling effect, you might also consider turning down your thermostat a degree or two at night or sleeping with your window open a crack to allow some cool air in while you sleep**. Experiment with the best temperature for you. Somewhere around 65 degrees may provide the best temperature for sleep, though the right temperature for you may vary.
- **Go to bed as soon as you start to feel sleepy rather than staying up to catch the rest of a television show**. This may require you to go to bed earlier than normal but allows you to sleep in sync with your body's natural drop in temperature.[361]

Sleep Smarts Prescription #4: Exercise regularly

Physical fitness seems to help the body to consolidate sleep, possibly by muting stress. Exercise at any time of day will do this, as long as you exercise at least 150 minutes per week.[362] Here's another way exercise may aid sleep: by heating your body. Then as you cool back down, sleepiness sets in.

A few pointers:

- **Listen to your body**. Some people find that evening exercise—even doing a few exercises just before bed—helps them blast away the stress of the day and fall asleep more quickly. Other people, however, find that exercise is stimulating because, at least initially, it boosts levels of epinephrine. If the latter is true for you, schedule your exercise sessions at least four hours before bed.[363]

- **Go long**. In the research, bouts lasting longer than an hour induced sleep better than those lasting less than an hour.
- **Stay in shape.** As you get in shape, exercise can cause your muscles to feel sore, which can keep you up at night. But once you are in shape, you'll rarely experience post-exercise soreness, allowing exercise to help you to nod off more reliably.

Sleep Smarts Prescription #5: Nap strategically

Some physicians advise their patients to avoid napping, saying that sleeping during the day works against your ability to sleep at night. I'm not one of them. After all, I have a couch in my office. Occasionally, when I'm feeling fatigued, I take a 10-minute nap, and I find it incredibly refreshing. And the research supports this habit, finding that naps can definitely help us feel more alert during the day and help us recover from sleep debt.

Researchers at the Laboratory of Human Chronobiology at Weill Cornell Medical College in White Plains, New York, studied how 22 men and women reacted to varying napping regimens, finding that naps of all lengths enhanced cognitive performance during the day.[364] In another study, Belgian researchers kept study participants awake for most of the night. Then, the following day, the researchers encouraged some of the participants to recover with a 30-minute nap, whereas other study participants were asked to power through. Right after the poor night's sleep, everyone's inflammatory markers were elevated, but for those who napped, those levels dropped back to normal levels.[365]

A few pointers:

- **Choose your nap length based on how long you need a burst of alertness to last**. The benefit of a brief five- to fifteen-minute nap has been shown to fade after one to three hours. After that, the fatigue will catch back up with you. If you nap longer than that amount of time, you may initially feel groggy, an effect known as "sleep inertia." This grogginess will subside within a half hour and, after that, you'll be alert for longer than three hours.[366]
- **Nap in the early afternoon**. This may be the most beneficial time to nap, as this roughly is in sync with natural circadian rhythms.[367] Based on the natural rise and fall of various hormones, alertness fluctuates throughout the day and dips sharply between 2:00 and 4:00 p.m. Napping during your "afternoon slump" allows you to nod off quickly, while napping later than this may make it harder to fall asleep at night.
- **Make it regular**. Though it's unclear why, regular nappers tend to reap more restorative benefits than those who nap only occasionally.[368]

Sleep Smarts Prescription #6: Cut back on late-day caffeine

Caffeine keeps us alert by blocking adenosine receptors in the brain. Caffeine levels peak in the blood 30 minutes after ingestion, and the half-life of any dose is three to seven hours. That means it takes up to seven hours for the caffeine to become only half as effective as it was at its peak. In other words, if you drink two cups of coffee at 9:00 a.m., you'll feel the most alert from that coffee by about 9:30 a.m. and about half as alert by 4:00 p.m. As we get older, caffeine seems to remain active for a longer period of time. So in your 20s, you might be able to drink a cup of coffee or indulge in chocolate late at night and still go right to sleep. But later in life, you may find that having caffeine in the evening causes you to toss and turn.

How much caffeine affects your sleep will also be influenced by your personal sensitivity, metabolism, and dose. Some people can drink a cup of coffee after dinner and sleep soundly all night long. Others can accidentally ingest a small amount of caffeine from a piece of chocolate or decaf coffee (which, surprisingly, contains somewhere between two and twelve milligrams of caffeine per cup) and be up for most of the night.

A few pointers:

- **Experiment with dose.** Tea, coffee, and chocolate all contain caffeine, but these substances are also good for your health. You may not need to abstain completely. Instead, experiment with timing and amount. Have just one cup of tea rather than two, for instance, or mix some decaf coffee beans in with the caffeinated ones, or indulge in chocolate in the afternoon but not after dinner.

- **Drink caffeine earlier in the day**. Consuming caffeine within six hours of bedtime has been associated with disturbed sleep, but note that the equivalent of two to three cups of coffee was consumed in this research.[369] If you think caffeine might be disturbing your sleep, cut yourself off by 3:00 or 4:00 in the afternoon, and see if it makes a difference.

Sleep Smarts Prescription #7: Cut back on alcohol

Though alcohol may cause us to feel drowsy and even nod off, as it wears off, you'll shift from deep sleep to REM sleep, making you more likely to wake. Alcohol also seems to affect how many cycles of sleep you get, causing you to feel groggy in the morning.[370] It can also induce snoring—causing you to briefly wake with a snort—or cause you to get up to go to the bathroom in the middle of the night.[371]

A few pointers:

- **Find what works for you.** As with caffeine, alcoholic drinks can be good for the body and the brain. You do not need to give them up entirely.

You may find that if you have a drink with dinner, you're okay, but if you have a drink right before bed, you toss and turn. Everyone is different, so experiment over time to find what works for you.[372]

- **Hold yourself to just one to two daily drinks.** This is the amount shown to boost health as well as the amount least likely to interfere with sleep. It's also the amount that is good for your brain. (See Meal Smarts, Chapter 4.)

Sleep Smarts Prescription #8: Imagine waterfalls

Research tells us that counting sheep doesn't help us nod off any more quickly than lying in bed and letting our minds wander, but here's a tactic that does seem to help: visualizing a relaxing scene, such as a waterfall. When Allison Harvey and Suzanna Payne of England's Oxford University asked 50 insomniacs to try different distraction techniques on different nights, it was the waterfall visualizations that came out on top. Study participants who pictured waterfalls nodded off 20 minutes more quickly than others who counted sheep or did nothing in particular.[373]

A few pointers:

- **Imagine a scene that you find tranquil and relaxing.** It doesn't have to be a waterfall. Waves crashing against an idyllic beach, a mountaintop with fresh air and wisps of clouds, a wooded area with chirping birds— whatever you think is peaceful.
- **Mentally fill in the details of your imagined tranquility.** How does it smell? Sound? Feel on your skin?

Sleep Smarts Prescription #9: Soundproof your room

Our brains continue to register sound as we sleep.[374] This is why you might fall asleep in front of the TV, only to wake a short time later. The changing pitch and tone of the sound keeps your brain active, so you remain in a light sleep and wake more easily. It might be a brief enough awakening that you don't remember it in the morning, but you'll feel groggy without knowing why.[375]

A few pointers:

- **Mask the noise**. If you live in a noisy environment, you may not be able to stop traffic or get your neighbors to keep it down. But you can use a white noise machine to drown it out. Research shows that white noise reduces the difference between background noise and peak noise such as a door slamming or car horn, allowing you to sleep more deeply.[376]

You can create white noise by running a fan, air purifier, or any other machine that makes a constant hum.

- **Wear earplugs.** Note that not all earplugs will fit your ears. If you find that the first brand you try falls out or fails to drown out noise, keep trying different types until you find a brand that works for you. Our ears also change shape over time, so the brand that worked wonderfully five years ago may not work as effectively today. If you find earplugs uncomfortable, a noise cancellation system may be helpful.

- **Sleep in a different room.** This may allow you to escape a snoring spouse. You may find that some rooms of your house are noisier than others due to their proximity to traffic.

Sleep Smarts Prescription #10: Try sleeping alone

Bed companions—whether they be a pet or a spouse or a toddler—can easily wake us at night. Mayo Clinic physicians have reported that about 10 percent of people who visited their sleep center had sleep issues related to their pets who woke them by snoring, whimpering, wandering, and needing to go outside.[377]

A few pointers:

- **If a small child continually wakes you, consider taking turns with your spouse.** One of you sleeps with the child, and the other sleeps alone one night. Then the next night, you switch. Or, consider putting a sleeping bag, cushions, and/or an air mattress on the floor by the bed. Tell your children that they are welcome to come and sleep *next* to the bed but not *in* the bed.

- **If your issue is your snoring spouse** and you've already gone through every brand of earplugs ever made, consider sleeping somewhere else. Maybe you'll find more restful sleep in the guest room, on the couch, or with one of the kids.

- **If your issue is a pet,** know that it's easier to make your bed off-limits to a new pet than it is to train a pet to stay off the bed once the pet is already accustomed to sleeping on it. To train a pet to sleep somewhere else, be prepared for a few sleepless nights. Set up an alternative sleeping location, one that is as inviting as possible. At night continually lead your pet over to the new sleeping area and, if appropriate, give "sit," "down," and "stay" commands. Then give a "bed!" command, along with a treat. If your pet wanders into your bedroom, just gently lead it back to its sleeping area and repeat the "bed" command with the treat. If your pet is particularly stubborn, you may benefit from the help of a professional trainer.

Sleep Smarts Prescription #11: Eat sleep-friendly snacks

Generally, eating too close to bedtime is more likely to disturb your sleep than aid it. By eating, you're firing up your digestive system, making issues like acid reflux and bloating more likely to keep you awake. And some foods are more likely to disturb sleep than others. Eating acidic foods like tomatoes and citrus too close to bed may trigger reflux, for example. And coffee ice cream contains as much caffeine as a cup of tea. Other foods rich in fat—such as a burger with fries—take a long time to digest, making you feel bloated and uncomfortable.

All of that said, the regular consumption of a few specific foods is thought to improve sleep.

- **Drink cherry juice regularly.** Tart cherries are one of the few foods that contain melatonin and, according to a small, pilot study, fresh tart cherry juice, consumed twice daily, may reduce episodes of insomnia. In the 15 elderly study participants, the cherry juice slashed the time it took them to fall asleep by 17 minutes.[378] The juice used in the study was a proprietary blend not available in stores, and it contained the equivalent of 100 cherries. Look for a tart cherry juice that is all cherries and no sweeteners like sugar. Drink the juice at any time of day—not just in the evening—to benefit from the cherry effect.
- **Snack on kiwifruit.** One study found an improvement in sleep when study participants consumed two kiwis an hour before bed.[379] Though it's unclear why they might help, one theory holds that they are high in serotonin.
- **Try warm milk.** It contains the amino acid tryptophan, the precursor to the brain chemical serotonin. The calcium in the milk also helps the brain to use the tryptophan to make melatonin. A small glass of warm milk might relax you, too, easing you off to sleep.
- **Eat fish and other foods with omega-3 fatty acids regularly.** The omega-3 fatty acids found in fatty fish, algae, flax and chia seeds, and a few other foods may promote sleep by boosting melatonin levels.[380, 381] Other good omega-3 sources include hemp seeds, walnuts, soybeans, and tofu.

Sleep Smarts Prescription #12:
Breathe lavender while you sleep

Research shows that the scent of lavender serves as a mild sedative that can slow heart rate, drop blood pressure, and relax the body. In one study, people who sniffed lavender before bed slept more deeply and felt more refreshed in the morning.[382] A few other small studies have arrived at similar results.[383]

A few pointers:

- **Sprinkle a few drops of pure lavender essential oil on a tissue to tuck under your pillow**. Or just before bed, place two to four drops of the essential oil into a bowl of boiled water. Waft the vapors toward you to inhale.
- **After dinner or early evening, relax with lavender tea**. Steep one or two teaspoons of lavender leaves in one cup of boiled water.

Sleep Smarts Prescription #13: Get hypnotized

Unlike what you might have seen during a stage act, psychological hypnosis is merely a state of inner absorption and focused attention, not unlike meditation. And hypnosis may be one way to control the autonomic brain, the part of your brain that regulates your heart rate, breathing, and other automatic processes.

At the University of Zurich in Switzerland, researchers measured electrical brain activity while study participants slept, looking for the telltale oscillations of slow-wave, restorative sleep. As they dozed off, some study participants listened to a 13-minute hypnosis tape, developed by a sleep specialist to induce deeper sleep. Other participants listened to neutral spoken text.

In the study, women who were considered to be "highly suggestible," based on the Harvard Scale of Hypnotic Suggestibility, experienced 80 percent more slow-wave sleep after listening to the hypnosis tape compared to when they slept after listening to the neutral text. They also spent less time awake. Less-suggestible women didn't experience as much of a benefit.[384] Though the study involved only women, the results probably also apply to men.

A few pointers:

- **Try hypnosis with an open mind, knowing that it may or may not work for you.** It's thought that only about half of the population is "highly suggestible." So if you try hypnosis and experience no benefit, don't blame yourself. Hypnosis may not be for you.
- **Download any number of free apps to try hypnosis at home**. Or you can see a certified hypnotist for a few sessions until you get the hang of it. You can find a certified professional through the American Society of Clinical Hypnosis, *ASCH.net*.

Sleep Smarts Prescription #14:
If you snore, get tested for sleep apnea

Sleep apnea is a serious sleeping disorder. If you have this condition, your airways temporarily collapse as you sleep, causing you to stop breathing repeatedly for short periods of time. Sleep apnea becomes more common if you are overweight or obese, and there's some evidence that the same *ApoE4* gene that raises risk for Alzheimer's disease also raises your risk for developing sleep apnea.[385]

These episodes of halted breathing can last up to 60 seconds, and you may or may not remember them when you wake. Your only symptoms: excessive daytime sleepiness, waking with a dry mouth or sore throat, a morning headache, and trouble concentrating. Others may also complain about your snoring.

Sleep apnea becomes more common if you are overweight or obese, and especially if you carry most of your excess body weight around your abdomen, and it can lead to heart disease, headaches, and depression as well as raise your risk for dementia.[386] A study out of the University of California at San Francisco found that people with diagnosed sleep disorders like sleep apnea were 30 percent more likely to go on to develop dementia than people without these problems.[387]

To find out whether you have the condition, you'll need to see a sleep specialist. Ask your family doctor for a referral or contact the American Board of Sleep Medicine (*absm.org*) for a list of sleep medicine specialists in your area. The specialist will ask you to undergo a sleep study. This can be done either in a lab or at home. During the study, you sleep as you normally would, as medical devices monitor your breathing, brain waves, bodily movements, heart rate, blood oxygen levels, and other vitals.

If it turns out you have sleep apnea, your physician will suggest you wear a CPAP device at night to help ensure your airways stay open as you sleep. This machine comes as a mask or as nose buds and uses continuous ventilation to keep airways open. Physicians at the University of California in San Diego have found that Alzheimer's patients who wore CPAPs at night experienced an improvement in cognitive performance. They were also less sleepy during the day.[388]

A few pointers:

- **Work closely with your sleep specialist to find the best CPAP device for you**. Some people prefer the nose buds, whereas others need the full mask.
- **Be patient.** It can take many weeks to a few months to get used to the machine.
- **Look into other solutions for sleep apnea**. These include weight loss, specially made dental devices, and acupuncture (see next prescription).

Sleep Smarts Prescription #15: Try acupuncture

Acupuncture involves the insertion of thin needles into your skin along your back, ear, and other strategic locations on the body. It may help to improve sleep, possibly by lowering stress hormones and boosting levels of calming brain chemicals.

In one review of the 46 studies that involved acupuncture, Chinese research-ers found that acupuncture helped relieve insomnia even more than some sleep medications.[389] Research by Anaflávia Freire in Brazil also found that the treat-ments helped to strengthen the tongue muscle, which potentially could prevent the tongue from dropping back into the throat and causing breathing problems during sleep.[390]

And a small study out of Hong Kong found that six weeks of acupuncture improved resting and total sleep time in 19 elderly patients with dementia.[391]

A few pointers:

- **Try six to ten treatments and then reassess your stress and sleep.** If your stress levels have gone down and you are sleeping better at night, you may wish to continue, possibly reducing your sessions from weekly to biweekly. If they haven't, you might want to try a different remedy.

- **To save money, consider "community acupuncture."** Rather than being in a private room, you'll undergo the treatment in a room with a few other patients. Payment is usually offered based on a sliding scale of $15 to $50 per session. You can find a community acupuncturist through the People's Organization of Community Acupuncture (POCA).

Advice for Caregivers

As Alzheimer's disease progresses, brain cells are lost in the raphe nuclei, a part of the brain stem. As more of the raphe nuclei is affected, sleep disturbances result.

While over-the-counter or prescription sleep medicines may initially seem like a logical solution, there are several reasons to be cautious. Research done at the Mayo Clinic found that elderly hospital patients were more likely to slip and fall if they'd been prescribed zolpidem, the generic name for Ambien. The most commonly prescribed sleep medicine, Ambien[392] may increase the risk of falling by impairing balance.[393] Falls are a serious matter because they are the leading cause of fatal and nonfatal injuries, according to the US Center for Disease Control. More than 95 percent of hip fractures are the result of a fall,[394] and a hip fracture makes you five times more likely to die within the year after suffering one.[395]

Of the other remedies listed in this chapter, light therapy may hold the most promise. Two and a half hours of morning light therapy—by using one of the light boxes mentioned earlier—may be particularly helpful. In research it allowed people with dementia to sleep 16 minutes longer and fall asleep 29 minutes earlier.[396] Try it for both of you. It will help you to feel more alert during the day and to sleep more deeply at night. Even if it doesn't fully reset your spouse's sleep/wake cycle, research shows that it may reduce sundowning restlessness.[397, 398]

Your sleep is important, too, but it's hard to get a good night's sleep when your spouse or family member is experiencing longer bouts of sundowning. Typical to Alzheimer's disease and some other forms of dementia, *sundowning* is the term we use to describe the confusion, increased arousal, anxiety, aggression, irritability, and pacing and wandering that tends to start in late afternoon and progress into the evening. We don't know what causes it, but fatigue does seem to exacerbate it.

To allow yourself to rest easy, wander-proof your home in the same way you might have baby- or toddler-proofed it years ago. Remove objects that your loved one might trip over from the floor. Lock up medicines. Put grab bars in the bathroom. Install gates across the stairs.

PART THREE

Your Personalized Plan to Outsmart Alzheimer's

Just by reading about the 80 simple and effective prescriptions to reduce your risk of developing Alzheimer's, you have started to improve your chances—because you have already incorporated at least one prescription into your life (Train-Your-Brain Smarts Prescription #6, Read to Learn, page 123). And perhaps you've been inspired to take a quick break to try Social Smarts Prescription #3 (Connect online), Meal Smarts Prescription #9 (Snack on nuts and seeds), Aerobic Smarts Prescription #12 (Stand every half hour), or Resilience Smarts Prescription #5 (Breathe deeply and slowly). That's how easy it is to begin outsmarting Alzheimer's.

In this part of the book, you'll learn how to create a customized program that includes the prescriptions that are most relevant for your interests, lifestyle, and health. You'll also find more than 40 easy and delicious brain-boosting recipes, almost 30 interactive brain-training games, and a simple and effective 7-minute workout.

CHAPTER 9

....

Three Weeks to a Lifetime of Health

Now that you've seen the dozens of prescriptions related to the six key Brain Smarts, you may be wondering, *How do I fit all of this into my life?*

You may be relieved to know that, to outsmart Alzheimer's, you don't have to do everything mentioned in this book. Some prescriptions will apply more to you than others, and some might not make sense for you at all. As I've mentioned, there's no one-size-fits-all approach to outsmarting Alzheimer's. In this chapter, you'll learn how to choose the right prescriptions for you and how to turn them into ingrained habits that require little effort to maintain.

You'll also find a 3-week plan that shows you one way to incorporate all six Brain Smarts into your life every day. It includes the most potent and universal prescriptions from Part Two, and culminates with a dinner party at the end of Week 3. This plan is just a starting point. Depending on your health, lifestyle, and interests, you may decide to follow the plan to the letter, modify it slightly, or merely use it as a general guide in creating your own personalized plan that ultimately looks very different. If you wish to modify the plan, based on your answers to the quiz in Chapter 2, you'll find several pointers to help you do so on pages 173 to 180 within this chapter. You'll also learn how to maintain your progress beyond 21 days.

Before You Start

Read through the plan once, and pay particular attention to the menu suggestions. Make a list and take a trip to the grocery store, if needed, to gather necessary ingredients. Embrace this list making and shopping, as it helps to sharpen your planning abilities. What else might you purchase now—books, apps, magazines, deck of cards, and so on—to make the weeks to come a little less harried?

Also, consider how you will fit the various suggestions into each day. Will you go to bed and get up earlier than usual? Bring a pair of sneakers with you to work so you can take periodic walking breaks? Call a friend or two and tell them about the Brain Smart Plan you are about to try? Perhaps you might even ask a friend or family member to try it with you.

Finally, contemplate how you might modify the suggestions, both to help you succeed as well as to make the plan even more potent. Based on the prescriptions in the previous chapters, what foods might you swap out for the ones suggested here? If you can't do a particular suggestion while you are at work, is there another time of day you can do it? Or is there another prescription you might do instead during that time of day? The plan is set up to start on a Sunday, under the assumption that most people work Monday through Friday. If you work on weekends or don't work at all, you may wish to start the plan on a different day of the week. This creative problem solving is just what your brain needs to reduce your risk for Alzheimer's disease, so make as many modifications as you need to ensure your success.

Once you are done, you're ready to get started.

WEEK 1

Sunday

- **In the morning before breakfast:** Walk outdoors for five minutes or longer. Say hello to anyone you see along the way.

- **For breakfast:** Start the day with a serving of fruit. Mix berries or sliced fruit with 2 to 4 tablespoons of seeds (pumpkin, sesame, chia) and/or nuts. Sprinkle wheat germ on top and mix with nonfat, unsweetened yogurt. Pair your meal with tea or coffee.

- **Throughout the day:** Take frequent breaks from sitting. Stand and stretch, go for a short walk, or march in place. Also, take a look at the meal suggestions for the week to come. What might you shop for now? Which ingredients will you pick up later, perhaps on your way home from work? What can you prep or assemble ahead of time?

- **In the late morning before lunch:** Do one 7-minute circuit (Chapter 11, page 222).

- **For lunch:** Throughout this week, we'll consider ways to add Brain Smart ingredients to the common, everyday salad. For today's salad creation, work in one or more servings of vegetables by having a big salad chock-full of dark greens (such as spinach, kale, watercress, and romaine) and brightly colored veggies (such as red cabbage, bell peppers, tomatoes, and carrots). Top it with canned, wild salmon.

- **Before dinner:** Go for a 20-minute walk. If possible, do this with a friend, neighbor, or family member. If you feel too rushed to do this before dinner, how about after dinner?

- **For dinner:** Make a Brain Smart recipe from Chapter 10. Double or triple the recipe so you can plan to have leftovers for lunch or dinner in the days to come.

- **In the evening:** Visit a friend or snuggle with a loved one (Resilience Smarts Prescription #6, page 105) as you both try your hands at one of the brain games in Chapter 12.

- **Before bed:** Dim the lights and switch off electronics in the last 30 to 60 minutes before bed (Sleep Smarts Prescription #2, page 137). Try to hit the sack early enough to allow for seven to eight hours of sleep. Once in bed, spend a minute or two doing deep breathing (Resilience Smarts Prescription #5, page 104) to relax your body and encourage restful sleep.

- **At any time of the day:** Take a look at your calendar and find a date about three weeks from now that would work for you to host a dinner party. Choose a Brain Smart main course, side dish, and dessert from the recipes in Chapter 10 that you'd like to serve during your dinner party. Plan to do a test run of these recipes later this week, making a grocery list now of needed items. Consider what recipes will challenge your brain without causing too much anxiety.

Monday

- **In the morning:** Walk outdoors for five minutes or longer. If your mornings tend to be rushed and you find you skip your morning walk, do a little problem solving. How might you fit in a morning walk tomorrow? Will you get up earlier than usual, park farther from the office, or walk instead at mid-morning to help energize your mind and boost productivity?

- **For breakfast:** Experiment with a veggie-packed omelet or egg scramble, perhaps trying the Spinach and Goat Cheese Omelet (page 192). Pair your meal with tea or coffee.

- **Throughout the day:** Take frequent breaks from sitting, at least once every 90 minutes. Stand and stretch, go for a short walk, or march in place.

- **In the late morning before lunch:** Get your heart rate up for at least 10 minutes. Maybe you walk around your house or office, head outside, or go up and down the stairs. Bonus points if you do it with a friend, family member, neighbor, or coworker.

- **For lunch:** Continue to experiment with big salads, perhaps trying Spinach Salad with Chickpeas (page 195).

- **Before dinner:** Get your heart rate up for at least 10 minutes by dancing, going for a brisk walk, or doing another form of movement. If possible, do this with a friend, neighbor, or family member.

- **For dinner:** Take one of your favorite recipes and experiment with adding more vegetables to it. Can you puree or finely chop veggies and slip them into a favorite casserole? Or would onions, garlic, or chives add more flavor to a favorite soup? Or might you serve the dish over a bed of spinach or another dark, leafy green?

- **In the evening:** Experiment with Kriya yoga (Resilience Smarts Prescription #2, page 100).

- **Before bed:** Dim the lights and switch off electronics in the last 30 to 60 minutes before bed (Sleep Smarts Prescription #2, page 137). Do a few minutes of deep breathing (Resilience Smarts Prescription #5, page 104) to relax your mind for sleep.

- **At any time of the day:** Look into Zumba, yoga, and other fitness classes near you. Learn as much as you can about how the classes are designed and whether they fit your schedule. Do the same with team sports. Choose one new type of group fitness class or sport that you wish to try. Keep notes on what you learn and decide, but you don't need to actually sign up for anything right now. You'll be investigating several new activities over the next few weeks, and you'll take steps to schedule them into your calendar after you've finished this initial research.

Tuesday

- **In the morning before breakfast:** Walk outdoors for five minutes or longer. If desired, connect with friends on Facebook or another social networking site (Social Smarts Prescription #3, page 49). You might send an "I'm thinking of you" message or respond positively to a few of their updates. Make it your goal to bring some happiness into someone's day just by what you write.

- **For breakfast:** Blend fruit, ice, yogurt or milk, and a dark, leafy green vegetable like spinach or kale for a morning smoothie. Perhaps try Berry Flaxseed Smoothie (page 186). If you don't have time to blend your own, consider a store-bought option. But read labels carefully and ask questions, if possible. Many store-bought smoothies are mostly sugar and light on the fruit and veggies. Have your usual tea or coffee now, or save it for later in the morning.

- **In the late morning before lunch:** Do one 7-minute circuit (Chapter 11, page 222). If you are at work and can't do a circuit now, consider another time of day to pull this off. Maybe you can double the circuit before dinner.

- **For lunch:** Try a different big salad. This time, add beans (black, kidney, chickpea, and the like) for a source of protein and fiber. Use the Mediterranean Salad with Edamame recipe (page 197) for inspiration in creating your own.

- **Throughout the day:** Take frequent breaks from sitting. Stand and stretch, go for a short walk, or march in place.

- **Before dinner:** Do another 7-minute circuit (Chapter 11, page 222).

- **For dinner:** Indulge in leftovers from Sunday, add veggies to a family favorite, or try a new recipe from Chapter 10.

- **In the evening:** Challenge your brain with one or more of the brain game exercises in Chapter 12.

- **Before bed:** Dim the lights and switch off electronics in the last 30 to 60 minutes before bed (Sleep Smarts Prescription #2, page 137). Spend 5 to 10 minutes breathing deeply (Resilience Smarts Prescription #5, page 104).

- **At any time of the day:** Consider ways to give your bedroom a sleep makeover. Over time, how might you reduce sound, darken the room, and enable deeper, uninterrupted sleep, using the advice in Chapter 8 as a guide?

Wednesday

- **In the morning:** Walk outdoors for five minutes or longer and/or play an interactive video game or app such as Words with Friends, Trivia Crack, or Flow Free (Social Smarts Prescription #2, page 48).

- **For breakfast:** Try an unusual whole grain hot cereal with a side of fruit. Oatmeal is great, but there are many other hot whole grain options: cream of rye, multi-grain, oat bran, cream of brown rice, and many others. Or, be adventurous and add an unfamiliar fruit to your hot cereal. Might apples, dates, cranberries, and/or figs liven up slow-cooked oatmeal? Give them a try. Pair your breakfast with tea or coffee.

- **In the late morning before lunch:** Get your heart rate up for at least 10 minutes by dancing, going for a brisk walk, or doing another form of movement. Bonus points if you do it with a friend, family member, neighbor, or coworker.

- **Lunch:** Make a Grilled Salmon Salad, using the recipe on page 199 as a general guide. See if you can add your own signature touch, something that changes the recipe for the better.

- **Throughout the day:** Take frequent breaks from sitting. Stand and stretch, go for a short walk, or march in place.

- **Before dinner:** Get your heart rate up for at least 10 minutes by dancing, going for a brisk walk, or doing another form of movement.

- **For dinner:** Experiment with an easy option that can become your go-to Brain Smart meal on those days when you're in a rush or just too tired to cook an elaborate meal. Maybe you bake boneless, skinless chicken breasts (drizzle the chicken with olive oil, sprinkle with your favorite spices, cover with parchment paper, and bake at 400°F for 30 to 40 minutes) and roasted broccoli and/or other vegetables (toss veggies with olive oil, sprinkle with your favorite spices, and bake uncovered for about 30 minutes, until al dente).

- **In the evening:** Challenge your brain with one or more of the brain game exercises in Chapter 12. If you usually shower in the morning, consider switching to the evening, allowing the warmth of your shower or bath to help induce better sleep (Sleep Smarts Prescription #3, page 138).

- **Before bed:** Dim the lights and switch off electronics in the last 30 to 60 minutes before bed (Sleep Smarts Prescription #2, page 132). Once in bed for the evening, try a relaxing visualization (Sleep Smarts Prescription #8, page 141).

- **At any time of the day:** Head to the store either today or tomorrow to purchase what you need for Friday's dinner party test meal. Also, consider a subject you'd like to know more about. Investigate how you might learn more, such as continuing education, community college classes, lectures, or tours.

Thursday

- **In the morning before breakfast:** Walk outdoors for five minutes or longer.

- **For breakfast:** Repeat a favorite breakfast option from earlier in the week, pairing it with tea or coffee.

- **In the late morning before lunch:** Do one 7-minute circuit (Chapter 11, page 222).

- **For lunch:** Repeat your favorite big salad from earlier in the week. The more you repeat a meal, the easier it is to make over time. This helps to ingrain healthy meal prep and cooking, turning it into a habit.

- **Throughout the day:** Take frequent breaks from sitting. Stand and stretch, go for a short walk, or march in place.

- **Before dinner:** Do two sessions of the 7-minute circuit (Chapter 11, page 222).

- **Dinner:** Have leftovers or go out. If you go out, order Brain Smart foods using the advice you learned in Chapter 4. In particular, try to maximize the vegetables, legumes, and whole grains and minimize the bread, chips, and sweets. Ask for a doggy bag and put half of your dinner in it to enjoy later.

- **In the evening:** Spend time reading about a topic that you wouldn't normally brush up on (Train-Your-Brain Smarts Prescription #6, page 123). For example, if you tend to read novels, then try nonfiction. If you tend to delve into science or math, try English literature. When you're done, connect with someone about what you've just read and learned. Maybe you chat with a family member, call a friend, or email someone.

- **Before bed:** Dim the lights and switch off electronics in the last 30 to 60 minutes before bed. Also experiment with relaxation techniques from Chapter 6, such as meditation (Resilience Smarts Prescription #3, page 101), yoga nidra (Resilience Smarts Prescription #4, page 103), or deep breathing (Resilience Smarts Prescription #5, page 104), to help your mind unwind.

- **At any time of the day:** Consider a place you've always wanted to travel. How might you save up enough money to make such a trip possible? Or, if it's completely out of the question to travel there—due to financial or physical constraints—consider other ways you might experience this location. Could you explore cooking classes that feature its cuisine? Or learn the language spoken there? Or perhaps take art or music classes that relate to that country's culture?

Friday

- **In the morning before breakfast:** Walk outdoors for five minutes or longer.

- **For breakfast:** What Brain Smart foods can you add to your usual cold breakfast cereal? How about infusing it with seeds, nuts, and/or fruit?

- **In the late morning before lunch:** Get your heart rate up for at least 10 minutes by dancing, going for a brisk walk, or doing another form of movement. Bonus points if you do it with a friend, family member, neighbor, or coworker.

- **For lunch:** If you went out to eat last night and took leftovers home, challenge yourself to consider how you might turn those leftovers into a salad. Might you crumble half of a burger over a bed of leafy greens? Or do the same with fish or chicken? If you did not go out, challenge yourself to find a way to make a signature salad from scratch, using your favorite healthy foods. Is there a different topping that you could add? How about dried fruit, artichokes, or olives?

- **Throughout the day:** Take frequent breaks from sitting. Stand and stretch, go for a short walk, or march in place.

- **Before dinner:** Get your heart rate up for at least 10 minutes by dancing, going for a brisk walk, or doing another form of movement. Bonus points if you do it with a friend or family member.

- **Dinner:** Do a test run of your dinner party recipes to make sure you've chosen recipes that you find tasty. Take note of what worked really well and what you might try to do differently. Perhaps you could use a little more spice in your soup. Or you realize you can prep ingredients for your side dish while your main dish is cooking, so you'll be able to get both dishes on the table at the same time.

- **In the evening:** Try more brain games, play a board game, challenge a family member to a card game, or spend time with a Rubik's cube (Train-Your-Brain Smarts Prescription #2, page 120).

- **Before bed:** Dim the lights and switch off electronics in the last 30 to 60 minutes before bed. Also experiment with relaxation techniques from Chapters 6 and 8.

- **At any time of the day:** Plan your guest list for the dinner party. How many people do you feel comfortable inviting? Will that many people fit at your table? If not, how will you accommodate them? Do you have enough plates and flatware? Have you ever cooked for that many before? If this is the first time you've ever held a dinner party, keep the guest list relatively short, to just eight people or fewer. Also think about who you will invite and why. Consider how each guest might interact with the others. Are you choosing guests who tend to light up the room with peace and happiness? Or friends who bring a sour mood and critical tongue to any occasion? Which friends are least likely to back-seat cook, complain about the food, or generally make you feel anxious? Based on your answers to those questions, write out your guest list and gather contact information for those guests.

Saturday

- **In the morning before breakfast:** If this is your day off from work, take a longer morning walk than usual, and consider ways to make your morning walk more social, relaxing, or mentally invigorating. Is there a nature trail nearby? How about walking around a local Main Street or outdoor mall? Or might you walk through a neighborhood as you try to spot a variety of local birds or simply enjoy your neighbors' gardens?

- **For breakfast:** Pretend you are a contestant on a cooking show, and you've been challenged to create an omelet that contains . . . beans. How will you incorporate this ingredient into your omelet? Puzzle it out, and then try it with a sense of curiosity and experimentation. Pair your creation with tea or coffee.

- **In the late morning before lunch:** Do one or two 7-minute circuits (Chapter 11, page 222).

- **For lunch:** Choose your favorite Brain Smart option from Chapter 10, making sure to include a fruit and/or a vegetable.

- **Throughout the day:** Take frequent breaks from sitting. Stand and stretch, go for a short walk, or march in place.

- **For dinner:** Experiment with another easy option that can become your go-to Brain Smart fish meal. Place salmon skin side down in a baking dish. Brush the fish with olive oil and sprinkle with the spices of your choosing. Cover with parchment paper, and bake at 400°F for about 25 minutes, until the fish is completely opaque. Pair with a baked vegetable of your choosing. See Wednesday's dinner suggestion for advice on baking veggies.

- **In the evening:** Go dancing (Aerobic Smarts Prescription #1, page 84)!

- **Before bed:** Count your blessings as you get into bed (Resilience Smarts Prescription #13, page 111). Drift off to sleep as you follow your breath in and out.

- **At any time of the day:** Send out e-invites for your dinner party.

WEEK 2

Sunday

- **In the morning before breakfast:** If you live in a house with a yard, take a walk around your yard and consider small gardening projects that you might do. What needs weeding? Pruning? Raking? Are there plants or bushes in your yard that you might clip and use to create a centerpiece for your dinner party? Even if you don't have a yard, consider ways you might rearrange or de-clutter a room to make it more inviting for your dinner party guests. Or, do an Internet search for ideas on make-at-home centerpieces. Also, think about when you'll have time to do this.

- **For breakfast:** Challenge your mind by making a more involved Brain Smart recipe such as the Mushroom and Bell Pepper Frittata (page 191). Invite a neighbor over for frittata and coffee.

- **In the late morning before lunch:** Walk for 10 minutes or dance to your favorite music.

- **For lunch:** This week, we'll consider ways to add Brain Smart ingredients to the common, everyday sandwich. Try a Brain Smart sandwich, perhaps Open-Faced Sardine Sandwiches (page 202). Serve raw veggies on the side and, if you are still hungry, have an apple, with the skin.

- **In the afternoon:** Take a 5- or 10-minute social break, and check in with a friend. If you are unsure of your centerpiece for the dinner party, ask your friend for ideas.

- **Throughout the day:** Take frequent breaks from sitting. Stand and stretch, go for a short walk, or march in place.

- **Before dinner:** Go for a 25-minute walk, perhaps pushing the pace or even jogging a little if you feel up to it.

- **For dinner:** Make a Brain Smart recipe from Chapter 10. Double or triple the recipe so you can plan to have leftovers for lunch or dinner in the days to come.

- **In the evening:** Consider what you will wear to next week's dinner party. Take a look at what's in your closet. If nothing seems right, flip through magazines for ideas. Or call a friend to talk over some options.

- **Before bed:** Dim the lights and switch off electronics in the last 30 to 60 minutes before bed (Sleep Smarts Prescription #2, page 137). Also continue to experiment with relaxation techniques from Chapters 6 and 8.

- **At any time of the day:** Consider ways you can engage your inner artist. Are there art classes, music lessons, or writing groups you'd like to sign up for or join? Also, if your dinner party test run was a flop, consider different recipes to try later in the week.

Monday

- **In the morning:** Walk outdoors for five minutes or longer. Then play an interactive gaming app with a friend (Social Smarts Prescription #2, page 48).

- **For breakfast:** Choose your favorite Brain Smart option from Chapter 10, making sure to include a fruit and/or a vegetable either on the side or mixed into the dish. Pair it with tea or coffee.

- **In the late morning before lunch:** Do one or two 7-minute circuits (Chapter 11, page 222).

- **For lunch:** Experiment with a new Brain Smart sandwich, perhaps trying the Curried Chicken Salad Sandwich (page 200).

- **Throughout the day:** Don't forget to take frequent breaks from sitting. Stand and stretch, go for a short walk, or march in place.

- **Before dinner:** Do one or two 7-minute circuits (Chapter 11, page 222).

- **For dinner:** Take another one of your favorite recipes and experiment with adding at least two servings of vegetables.

- **In the evening:** Do 12 minutes of Kriya yoga (Resilience Smarts Prescription #2, page 100).

- **Before bed:** Dim the lights and switch off electronics in the last 30 to 60 minutes before bed (Sleep Smarts Prescription #2, page 137). Also continue to experiment with relaxation techniques from Chapters 6 and 8.

- **At any time of the day:** Look into volunteering and charity work. What skills do you have that you might offer to an organization or a person in need? What volunteer programs are already in place near you?

Tuesday

- **In the morning before breakfast:** Walk outdoors for five minutes or longer. If desired, connect with friends on Facebook or another social networking site.

- **For breakfast:** This morning's cooking challenge: the smoothie. Pick one or more fruits (peaches, strawberries, blueberries, kiwis, and such) as your base. Then add a liquid (nonfat milk, yogurt, tea, water). Now for the challenge: add something green. What happens when you add a little avocado? Or how about kale or spinach? Experiment with spices (cinnamon, vanilla extract, cayenne, nutmeg, chocolate shavings, cocoa).

- **In the late morning before lunch:** Dance to your favorite music or go for a walk with a friend or coworker.

- **For lunch:** Experiment with a new Brain Smart sandwich, perhaps wrapping the meat of your sandwich in lettuce instead of bread. See the Beef in Lettuce Wraps (page 205) recipe for inspiration.

- **Throughout the day:** Take frequent breaks from sitting. Stand and stretch, go for a short walk, or march in place.

- **Before dinner:** Go for a 25-minute walk, perhaps pushing the pace or even jogging a little if you feel up to it.

- **For dinner:** Indulge in leftovers, add veggies or beans to a family favorite, or try a new recipe from Chapter 10.

- **In the evening:** Challenge your brain with one or more of the brain game exercises in Chapter 12. Or challenge a family member to a card game. Then spend 5 to 10 minutes breathing deeply (Resilience Smarts Prescription #5, page 104).

- **Before bed:** Dim the lights and switch off electronics in the last 30 to 60 minutes before bed (Sleep Smarts Prescription #2, page 137). Also continue to experiment with relaxation techniques from Chapters 6 and 8.

- **At any time of the day:** Follow up with dinner party guests to see who is coming and who isn't. Ask guests about food allergies and special dietary needs. Think about your centerpiece as well as what else you might need (candles and the like) for a festive-looking table. If you haven't yet decided what you will wear, consider shopping for a new outfit and plan out what you will buy, where you will find it, and when you will shop.

Wednesday

- **In the morning:** Walk outdoors for five minutes or longer and/or play an interactive video game or app with a friend (Social Smarts Prescription #2, page 48).

- **For breakfast:** Try a different whole grain hot cereal (how about hot quinoa?) with a side of a fruit you've never tried before.

- **In the late morning before lunch:** Do one or two 7-minute circuits (Chapter 11, page 222).

- **Lunch:** Try another Brain Smart sandwich, perhaps Tuna and Carrot Sandwich on Rye (page 200). Challenge yourself to add at least one new touch to the recipe to make it even healthier and tastier.

- **Throughout the day:** Take frequent breaks from sitting. Stand and stretch, go for a short walk, or march in place.

- **Before dinner:** Do one or two 7-minute circuits (Chapter 11, page 222).

- **Dinner:** Modify a family favorite to make it more brain friendly, or try a new recipe from Chapter 10. If you are learning to embrace fish, encourage yourself to try a new fish recipe, either from the recipe section in this book or one you find on the Internet.

- **In the evening:** Challenge your brain with one or more of the brain game exercises in Chapter 12, then take a bath or a shower before bed (Sleep Smarts Prescription #3, page 138).

- **Before bed:** Dim the lights and switch off electronics in the last 30 to 60 minutes before bed (Sleep Smarts Prescription #2, page 137). Once in bed for the evening, try a relaxing visualization (Sleep Smarts Prescription #8, page 141) or yoga nidra (Resilience Smarts Prescription #4, page 103).

- **At any time of the day:** Follow up on any travel plans, classes, or workshops that you started to look into. Take a look at your calendar, and decide which ones you'll sign up for in the next few weeks, the next few months, and over the next year. If you feel conflicted about any of these plans, call a friend and talk it over.

Thursday

- **In the morning before breakfast:** Walk outdoors for five minutes or longer.

- **For breakfast:** Try another smoothie challenge. What healthy ingredient can you add to make the smoothie even tastier? What happens when you mix in wheat germ, peanut butter, flaxseed meal, or chia seeds?

- **In the late morning before lunch:** Dance to your favorite music, or go for a walk with a friend, family member, neighbor, or coworker.

- **For lunch:** Continue to perfect your sandwich, focusing, this time, on condiments. Rather than your usual mayo or mustard, what Brain Smart spread could liven up the taste of your usual sandwich? How about mashing avocado or using hummus?

- **Throughout the day:** Take frequent breaks from sitting. Stand and stretch, go for a short walk, or march in place.

- **Before dinner:** Go for a 25-minute walk, perhaps pushing the pace or even jogging a little if you feel up to it.

- **Dinner:** Have leftovers or go out. If you go out, plan to take part of your meal home to eat as leftovers.

- **In the evening:** Spend time reading about an unfamiliar topic. Then connect with a friend over social media, email, or phone about what you just learned.

- **Before bed:** Continue to experiment with relaxation techniques from Chapters 6 and 8.

- **At any time of the day:** Flip through recipe books and dream up ways you could give various options a Brain Smart makeover. Check out Pinterest, a website that allows you to save and organize web content on virtual bulletin boards. Consider making a Pinterest board with your favorite Brain Smart recipes.

Friday

- **In the morning before breakfast:** Walk outdoors for five minutes or longer.

- **For breakfast:** Are you up for another smoothie challenge? If not, switch to an omelet or hot cereal challenge, seeing how many Brain Smart veggies and/or fruits you can add.

- **In the late morning before lunch:** Do one or two 7-minute circuits (Chapter 11, page 222).

- **For lunch:** Can you turn last night's restaurant meal into today's lunch? How might you add more veggies to round out the meal? If you had leftovers yesterday, then take a look through your fridge and pantry and challenge yourself to whip up a meal on the fly, using only what you already have on hand.

- **Throughout the day:** Take frequent breaks from sitting. Stand and stretch, go for a short walk, or march in place.

- **Before dinner:** Do one or two 7-minute circuits (Chapter 11, page 222).

- **Dinner:** If needed, do another test run of your dinner party recipes. Take note of how you can make it better the following week, especially which foods you might be able to prep ahead of time. If your test run went fine, try the same meal again to improve your familiarity. The more you make it, the easier and faster it will be to pull everything together on the night of your get-together.

- **In the evening:** With a friend or family member, flip through photo albums and take a trip down memory lane.

- **Before bed:** Continue to experiment with relaxation techniques from Chapters 6 and 8.

- **At any time of the day:** Connect with a friend by writing a letter, giving someone a call, or stopping by to see how someone is doing.

Saturday

- **In the morning before breakfast:** If enough time permits, download a game and challenge a friend to it (Social Smarts Prescription #2, page 48). Also, don't forget your morning walk.

- **For breakfast:** If this is your day off, make something more involved, such as whole grain pancakes, and invite a friend or neighbor over to enjoy them. See Multigrain Pancakes or Waffles (page 190) for an easy recipe to follow.

- **In the late morning before lunch:** Dance to your favorite music or go for a walk with a friend or coworker.

- **For lunch:** Challenge yourself to create a wrap, using your imagination to fill it with Brain Smart veggies and other ingredients.

- **Before dinner:** Unwind with light stretching, yoga, or an evening walk.

- **For dinner:** Choose your favorite Brain Smart option from Chapter 10.

- **Throughout the day:** Take frequent breaks from sitting. Stand and stretch, go for a short walk, or march in place.

- **In the evening:** Go dancing (Aerobic Smarts Prescription #1, page 84) and thoroughly enjoy yourself.

- **Before bed:** Drift off to sleep with a smile on your face, thinking about how much fun the evening was.

- **At any time of the day:** Call a friend and mention how your Brain Smart efforts are going.

WEEK 3

Sunday

- **In the morning before breakfast:** Walk outdoors for five minutes or longer.

- **For breakfast:** Challenge your mind by trying a new Brain Smart recipe from Chapter 10.

- **In the late morning before lunch:** Walk for 10 minutes, or dance to your favorite music.

- **For lunch:** Try a new Brain Smart sandwich or salad, creating your own or following a new recipe from Chapter 10.

- **In the afternoon:** Connect with one of your dinner party guests, asking him or her to help out in some small way during the party. For example, you might ask your guest if he or she minds arriving early and greeting other guests while you take care of last-minute kitchen tasks.

- **Throughout the day:** Take frequent breaks from sitting. Stand and stretch, go for a short walk, or march in place.

- **Before dinner:** Go for a 30-minute walk, perhaps pushing the pace or even jogging a little if you feel up to it.

- **For dinner:** Make a Brain Smart recipe from Chapter 10. Double or triple the recipe so you can plan to have leftovers for lunch or dinner in the days to come.

- **In the evening:** Watch a comedy with a friend or family member (Resilience Smarts Prescription #10, page 108). Choose among currently popular television shows, or make a nostalgic choice by re-watching one of the classics: *Sister Act, The Pink Panther, Caddyshack, Raising Arizona, When Harry Met Sally,* or another favorite. Enjoy air-popped corn (Meal Smarts Prescription #15, page 75) as you watch.

- **Before bed:** Continue to experiment with relaxation techniques from Chapters 6 and 8.

- **At any time of the day:** Make a shopping list for your dinner party. Check and see what ingredients you have and decide which ones you will purchase today and which others you'll need to buy closer to the end of the week. Also make sure you have enough serving dishes. Also plan out some meals for the coming week. You've experimented with smoothies, sandwiches, cereals, salads, omelets, and more. What were your favorites? When will you eat them in the coming week? What ingredients must you shop for? When will you head to the grocery store to pick up what you need?

Monday

- **In the morning:** Walk outdoors for five minutes or longer. Then play an interactive gaming app with a friend (Social Smarts Prescription #2, page 48).

- **For breakfast:** Make a favorite Brain Smart breakfast based on the planning you did yesterday.

- **In the late morning before lunch:** Do one or two 7-minute circuits (Chapter 11, page 222).

- **For lunch:** Make a favorite Brain Smart lunch, based on the planning you did yesterday.

- **Throughout the day:** Continue to take frequent breaks from sitting. Stand and stretch, go for a short walk, or march in place.

- **Before dinner:** Do one or two 7-minute circuits (Chapter 11, page 222).

- **For dinner:** Take one of your favorite recipes and experiment with modifying it by adding Brain Smart vegetables.

- **In the evening:** Do 12 minutes of Kriya yoga (Resilience Smarts Prescription #2, page 100) or experiment with meditation, perhaps downloading a free audio from the Internet (Resilience Smarts Prescription #3, page 101).

- **At any time of the day:** Consider what you can prepare or cook ahead of time for your upcoming dinner party. Plan when and how you will take care of these tasks so you will have more time to socialize during the actual party. Also consider what time you'll want to start cooking and when certain dishes must go in the oven. Create a schedule to follow so you are mostly done with cooking by the time your first guests arrive.

Tuesday

- **In the morning before breakfast:** Walk outdoors for five minutes or longer. If desired, connect with friends on Facebook or another social networking site (Social Smarts Prescription #3, page 49).

- **For breakfast:** Follow your plan from Sunday. Or, if you are not in the mood, challenge yourself by making up a Brain Smart breakfast on the fly.

- **In the late morning before lunch:** Dance to your favorite music or go for a walk with a friend, family member, neighbor, or coworker.

- **For lunch:** Choose a favorite Brain Smart option based on what you planned earlier in the week.

- **Throughout the day:** Take frequent breaks from sitting. Stand and stretch, go for a short walk, or march in place.

- **Before dinner:** Go for a 30-minute walk, perhaps pushing the pace or even jogging a little if you feel up to it.

- **For dinner:** Indulge in leftovers, modify a family favorite, or try a new recipe from Chapter 10.

- **In the evening:** Challenge your brain with one or more of the brain game exercises in Chapter 12. Then spend 5 to 10 minutes breathing deeply (Resilience Smarts Prescription #5, page 104).

- **At any time of the day:** Consider ways to make your dinner party more social. What topics will you bring up over dinner? Are there fun games to suggest after dinner? How about icebreaker activities?

Wednesday

- **In the morning:** Walk outdoors for five minutes or longer and/or play an interactive video game or app with a friend (Social Smarts Prescription #2, page 48).

- **For breakfast:** Choose a favorite Brain Smart option, following the plan you created on Sunday.

- **In the late morning before lunch:** Do one or two 7-minute circuits (Chapter 11, page 222).

- **Lunch:** Choose a favorite Brain Smart option, following the plan you created on Sunday.

- **Throughout the day:** Take frequent breaks from sitting. Stand and stretch, go for a short walk, or march in place.

- **Before dinner:** Do one or two 7-minute circuits (Chapter 11, page 222).

- **Dinner:** Choose a favorite Brain Smart option, following the plan you created on Sunday.

- **In the evening:** Challenge your brain with one or more of the brain game exercises in Chapter 12, then take a bath or a shower before bed (Sleep Smarts Prescription #3, page 138). Once in bed for the evening, try a relaxing visualization (Sleep Smarts Prescription #8, page 141) or yoga nidra (Resilience Smarts Prescription #4, page 103).

- **At any time of the day:** Pick the music you will play in the background during your dinner party. Do another check for needed groceries. Are there any fresh ingredients that you might purchase today so the end of the week will go more smoothly?

Thursday

- **In the morning before breakfast:** Walk outdoors for five minutes or longer.

- **For breakfast:** Choose a favorite Brain Smart option from Chapter 10, or make your own.

- **In the late morning before lunch:** Dance to your favorite music or go for a walk with a friend, family member, neighbor, or coworker.

- **For lunch:** Choose a favorite Brain Smart option from Chapter 10, or make your own.

- **Throughout the day:** Take frequent breaks from sitting. Stand and stretch, go for a short walk, or march in place.

- **Before dinner:** Go for a 30-minute walk, perhaps pushing the pace or even jogging a little if you feel up to it.

- **Dinner:** Have leftovers or go out.

- **In the evening:** Spend time reading about an unfamiliar topic, then connect with a friend over what you learned (Train-Your-Brain Smarts Prescription #6, page 123).

- **Before bed:** Continue to experiment with relaxation techniques from Chapters 6 and 8.

- **At any time of the day:** Continue to finalize your dinner party plans. Do you have your centerpiece? Will you purchase flowers or any other decorations? If so, when will you take care of this errand?

Friday

- **In the morning before breakfast:** Take a look at your front yard (if you have one) and/or your walkway. How might you make either or both more presentable to your dinner party guests? What might you do to make your home easier for them to find?

- **For breakfast:** Choose a favorite Brain Smart option from Chapter 10, or make your own.

- **In the late morning before lunch:** Do one or two 7-minute circuits (Chapter 11, page 222).

- **For lunch:** Choose a favorite Brain Smart option from Chapter 10, or make your own.

- **Throughout the day:** Take frequent breaks from sitting. Stand and stretch, go for a short walk, or march in place.

- **Before dinner:** Do one or two 7-minute circuits (Chapter 11, page 222).

- **Dinner:** Choose a favorite Brain Smart option from Chapter 10, or make your own.

- **In the evening:** Do any possible prep work for tomorrow's dinner party. Chop veggies and compile as much of your meal as possible. Wash any needed serving dishes and set the table, too. If appropriate, ask family members for some help or do this prep work with a friend.

- **Before bed:** Continue to experiment with relaxation techniques from Chapters 6 and 8.

- **At any time of the day:** Clean your house and do any last-minute shopping for your dinner party.

Saturday

- **In the morning before breakfast:** Walk outdoors for five minutes or longer. As you walk, think about any last-minute plans for the upcoming party. Do a test run in your mind. Is there anything that you may have overlooked?

- **For breakfast:** Choose your favorite Brain Smart option, preferably something quick and easy. Tonight will challenge your brain, so allow breakfast and lunch to be meals you can make almost by rote.

- **In the late morning before lunch:** Dance to your favorite music or go for a walk with a friend, family member, or neighbor. If you walk with someone else, talk about your upcoming party, mentioning any stress you might be feeling.

- **For lunch:** Choose your favorite Brain Smart option, one that is quick and easy to prepare.

- **Before dinner:** Have all the ingredients out and ready before you start cooking. Put them in the order that you will need to use them and chop any remaining ingredients. Do the bulk of the cooking before you get dressed for the dinner party. If possible, wash pots and pans as you cook.

- **For dinner:** Enjoy your dinner party (Social Smarts Prescription #1, page 47)! If there's a mess still in the kitchen from all the cooking you did for your guests, leave it. If one or more details are not quite what you'd originally wanted, let them go. Do your best to enjoy every taste, sound, and feeling. Several times during the meal, put down your fork and take a moment to soak up the good vibes all around you. Not only have you challenged your brain, but now you are offering Brain Smart sustenance to others. Feel good about all you've done.

- **Before bed:** Spend time feeling thankful for good food, good friends, and good times (Resilience Smarts Prescription #13, page 111). Drift off with a smile on your face.

How to Personalize Your Outsmarting Alzheimer's Plan

It's impossible to design one Brain Smart plan that works for all people. Though the plan in the previous pages was designed to be as universal as possible, you'll probably find that you wish to modify and personalize the suggestions. The more you personalize your plan, the more effective your Outsmarting Alzheimer's program will be—and the more likely you'll stick with your new lifestyle long term.

On the next page, we've provided a worksheet where you can write your own personal plan. Photocopy it for as many days as you need.

To personalize your plan, you'll want to create the perfect balance between effectiveness, need, personal interest, and time. Let's take a closer look at each.

Daily Outsmarting Alzheimer's Plan

Photocopy this page so that you can personalize your
Outsmarting Alzheimer's plan to suit your needs and lifestyle.

Week: _____

Day: _____

In the morning: _____

For breakfast: _____

In the late morning: _____

For lunch: _____

Throughout the day: _____

Before dinner: _____

For dinner: _____

In the evening: _____

Before bed: _____

At any time of the day: _____

❏ **Social Smarts**   ❏ **Resilience Smarts**

❏ **Meal Smarts**   ❏ **Train-Your-Brain Smarts**

❏ **Aerobic Smarts**   ❏ **Sleep Smarts**

Effectiveness. The prescriptions from Part Two of *Outsmarting Alzheimer's* were front-loaded for optimum potency. Within each chapter, the solutions appeared from most effective to least, allowing you to see easily which ones offered the highest dose of Alzheimer's prevention medicine. So, for example, when it comes to Meal Smarts, Prescription #1 (Fill up on fewer calories), #2 (Cook your own food), and #3 (Eat at least five servings of fruits and vegetables daily) apply to almost everyone and are also among the most effective nutritional steps you can take to outsmart Alzheimer's. Conversely, the prescriptions listed toward the end of each of the Smarts chapters are less potent, have less research to support their effectiveness, and/or may only apply to some people and not others.

Need. The most effective strategies may or may not be the ones that you most need. Uncontrolled medical risk factors—such as high blood pressure or high blood cholesterol—are especially harmful for the brain. It's important for you to get these risks under control. The Brain Smarts described in Chapters 3 to 8 will definitely help, but you'll also want to work closely with your physician to pair these lifestyle strategies with medications and treatments to bring these risk factors into the normal range. Will you have to stay on medication forever? Not necessarily. Some people find that, once they take steps to improve their diet and physical fitness using the strategies outlined in Part Two of this book, their need for medications to lower their cholesterol, blood pressure, and blood sugar drops. Regular physical activity makes your cells more sensitive to the hormone insulin and causes the muscles to burn up excess fats in the bloodstream, possibly lowering your need for diabetes medications. It's for these reasons and more that, under the direction of a physician, some people are able to get off these medications altogether once they embrace a healthy lifestyle. On the other hand, these medications are safe and effective for most people. If needed, they should be taken regularly to reduce your risk for Alzheimer's and other diseases.

To determine the strategies you most need, take a look at your answers from Chapter 2. What are your medical risks? What lifestyle factors need improvement? Which ones don't? Maybe you eat healthfully, but are currently sedentary. Or perhaps you eat well and exercise, but don't sleep well and are stressed. Congratulate yourself on your strengths, and keep those up. Then zero in on the areas that could use some improvement. For example, if you exercise regularly, you might skip the exercise suggestions from the 3-week plan in this chapter and just keep doing what you are already doing so well. Instead focus on the eating, stress relief, social, and brain-sharpening suggestions.

Personal interests. Making a small change and maintaining it for life is much more effective than making a huge change, but only doing it for a week. And you're much more likely to maintain the strategies that you enjoy. As you embark on the 21-day plan, you might decide to try the suggestions that sound the most interesting and fun. Do, however, keep in mind that it takes some time for any new strategy to feel familiar. In other words, you might hate yoga or dance or a new style of eating for a few weeks, but then grow to love it once you get used to it. So experiment and adopt new strategies with an open mind.

Time. In this busy world, it's hard to fathom that anyone would be able to devote time to exercise, stress relief, healthy eating, brain enrichment, and a social life every single day. If you find you are too rushed to do everything suggested in the Brain Smart Plan, challenge yourself to come up with ways to make a plan that is as well-rounded as possible. Perhaps, instead of walking outdoors by yourself, you go to an exercise class—one that you've never tried before. This helps you to improve your fitness as well as your social and intellectual smarts. It might even serve as stress relief and help you sleep at night. That's five Brain Smarts in just one activity. Also, use the "if you are very short on time" advice below.

In addition to weighing effectiveness, need, personal interests, and time, use these more specific pointers as you embark on the Brain Smart Plan. They'll help you to modify the plan to best suit you.

If You Are Very Short on Time

- Emphasize Meal Smarts (Chapter 4) and Aerobic Smarts (Chapter 5), as the prescriptions in these chapters offer the most protection for the least investment of time.

- Incorporate smart nutritional switches that require little to no prep work. For example, when eating out, ask for a side of veggies instead of a side of pasta (Meal Smarts Prescription #3, page 63). Also, reduce your portion by taking half of your meal home in a takeout container (Meal Smarts Prescription #1, page 61). Similarly, it only takes a second to sprinkle cinnamon, turmeric, or another spice on your meal (Meal Smarts Prescription #5, page 67).

- For exercise, the short circuit workout (Chapter 11, page 222) offers potent results in just seven minutes a day. In addition to this prescription, try to fit activity into your life by using the advice in Aerobic Smarts Prescription #12 to stand every half hour.

- Build Train-Your-Brain Smarts (Chapter 7) into your fitness plan by using a spreadsheet or graph to keep track of your daily fitness accomplishments (number of reps, steps walked, daily minutes spent standing). Build in Social Smarts by posting this information to Facebook or sharing it with another health-minded friend. Many wearable devices and mobile phones now track and graph your activity.

- Practice Social Smarts by connecting with clerks, sales staff, neighbors, and others that you routinely come into contact with every day (Social

Smarts Prescription #4, page 49). This takes very little time, but still offers a satisfying reward.

- Build a variety of Brain Smarts into short snippets of free time. Practice deep breathing (Resilience Smarts Prescription #5, page 104) while waiting in line or sitting on a train or bus. While in the waiting room at the doctor's office, stand rather than sit (Aerobic Smarts Prescription #12, page 92). As you lie in bed at night, visualize relaxing scenes (Sleep Smarts Prescription #8, page 141) or listen to a yoga nidra recording (Resilience Smarts Prescription #4, page 103).

- Create a calming evening routine, as your on-the-go nature may cause you to toss and turn at night. Take heed of the advice in Chapter 8 about "blue" screens at night, and do what you can to optimize your bedroom for sleep.

If You Have Diabetes

- For Meal Smarts, it's especially important to rein in sugar and processed starch by eating whole foods (Meal Smarts Prescription #4, page 65), as overconsumption of these can dramatically raise blood sugar.

- Sprinkle cinnamon on fruit, hot cereal, and other foods, as this spice may help improve your blood sugar control while also reducing risk for Alzheimer's (Meal Smarts Prescription #5, page 67).[399, 400] Because diabetes increases your body's production of advanced glycation end products (AGEs),[401] you'll also want to take special care to minimize the AGEs you ingest in your meat (Meal Smarts Prescription #7, page 68).

- For your Aerobic Smarts, build strength-training exercises into your routine, as lean muscle mass helps to burn off excess blood sugar. The short, 7-minute circuit workout in Aerobic Smarts Prescription #3 (page 86) is a good place to start, as it allows you to exercise in short bursts before meals.

- For Social Smarts, consider shared medical appointments (SMAs), a support group, or another social way to improve your health through the support of others. SMAs in particular have been endorsed by the American Academy of Family Physicians as effective ways to enhance self-care. They're offered by a number of large health care providers, including the Veterans Administration. Ask your health care provider if he or she offers them.

- Also, don't neglect relaxation, as unrelenting stress may raise blood sugar. Deep breathing, healing touch, and the other prescriptions in Chapter 6 can help.[402]

If You Are Very Out of Shape or Frail

- Resilience Smarts (Chapter 6), Social Smarts (Chapter 3), and Train-Your-Brain Smarts (Chapter 7) can allow you to make significant progress, no matter how frail your body.

- Social Smarts may be particularly important, as a rich social network can help you remain independent as your level of frailty increases. In addition to getting to know your neighbors, start looking into services—ranging from meal delivery to lawn care—that allow you to outsource overwhelming tasks. Also, make dates with friends to play cards, bingo, checkers, and other games. Invite friends over for a discussion group or book club, asking them to bring a potluck snack, dessert, or meal. Also connect online with social networks like Facebook.

- For Aerobic Smarts, tai chi (Aerobic Smarts Prescription #8, page 89) and gentle yoga classes designed for seniors (Aerobic Smarts Prescription #7, page 88), along with increased walking, may be the best options for you.

If You Have High Blood Pressure

- Resilience Smarts (Chapter 6) may be most important for you because stress relief may help lower blood pressure, as well as reducing your risk for developing Alzheimer's.[403]

- For Meal Smarts, reduce your sodium intake by cooking your own food (Meal Smarts Prescription #2, page 62) and eating whole foods (Meal Smarts Prescription #4, page 65). Heavy drinking is thought to boost levels of stress hormones that raise blood pressure, so cutting back on alcohol to one serving of wine or beer a day (Meal Smarts Prescription #13, page 73) may lower pressure almost as much as a low-sodium diet.[404, 405] Also consider cutting back on caffeine. In some people, the consumption of caffeine can spike blood pressure, whereas in others it doesn't. To see how caffeine affects your pressure, take your pressure within 30 minutes of drinking a cup of coffee or tea. If your pressure increases five to 10 points, you are probably sensitive to caffeine and may want to cut back.

- For your Aerobic Smarts, you may benefit more from outdoor exercise than from staying indoors. Children who cycled while viewing a film depicting cycling in a forest had lower blood pressure afterward than others who cycled indoors without any visual stimulus.[406] Though more research is needed before we can know whether these results apply to older adults, nature may help drop pressure because it's naturally soothing, helping to relieve stress. Also, sunlight may cause the skin to release more nitric oxide into the bloodstream, dilating blood vessels.[407]

- If your blood pressure remains elevated after taking these measures, work with your physician for guidance on possible prescription medications that may be right for you.

If You Have Joint Pain

- Among your Resilience Smarts, try Kriya yoga (Resilience Smarts Prescription #2, page 100) and meditation (Resilience Smarts Prescription #3, page 101). Just three days of 20-minute mindfulness meditation sessions reduced pain and anxiety in one study out of the University of North Carolina in Charlotte.[408]

- For your Aerobic Smarts, choose low-impact, gentle, or non-weight-bearing exercise. Many people with knee pain find that swimming and cycling don't bother their joints, whereas walking and running (both weight-bearing activities) do. You may also find that tai chi (Aerobic Smarts Prescription #8, page 00), gentle yoga classes designed for people with limited mobility (Aerobic Smarts Prescription #7, page 88), and certain types of dancing, such as low-impact Zumba (Aerobic Smarts Prescription #1, page 84), are also easy on your joints.

- Unhealthy foods can promote inflammation, especially those that are rich in sugar and fat. Vegetables, nuts, and fish may cool inflammation, and therefore, the dietary changes suggested in Chapter 4 may reduce joint pain.

If You Are Caring for Someone with Alzheimer's Disease

- Modify the 3-week plan to include fewer tasks. Gauge your family member's mood and energy level to see how much he or she can handle. Just one or two daily activities may be more than enough.

- Plan to do the bulk of Brain Smart activities in the morning when your loved one is more energetic. This is especially true for exercise, brain games, and social interactions. In the afternoon, sleep and Resilience Smarts may serve as your best options.

- As much as possible, try to do prescriptions together, especially the Aerobic Smarts prescriptions. Walking is a great form of exercise for people with Alzheimer's, and your loved one may really enjoy it. Keep in mind that the person you are caring for may not be able to gauge when it's time to turn around or stop because he may not be aware of how far he has already walked. So you may need to be firm, saying, "It's time to head back," rather than saying, "Tell me when you want to turn around."

- Reduce caregiving stress and instill a sense of purpose by involving your family member in household chores. Perhaps, as you clean the house, you might give your loved one a small task such as dusting a particular piece of furniture, washing a plate, or emptying the trash bins. Don't expect your family member to do these tasks perfectly. Rather, assume that she may leave any job you suggest half finished.

- Participation in social gatherings is particularly difficult for Alzheimer individuals and, depending on the degree of impairment, it may be more comfortable to forego social events except with the closest family members. So, even though the 21-day plan builds up to a dinner party, you may wish to either skip this task or build up to a much smaller event, such as dinner with your adult children.

What to Do Once You Finish the Brain Smart Plan

First, congratulations. In just 21 days, you've taken huge strides toward outsmarting Alzheimer's disease. In the process, you've just gained a delicious taste of what your life can be like when you infuse each moment with Brain Smart activities. At the moment, you may not be able to see the new connections between your brain cells, but new brain imaging techniques are likely to make it possible in the near future to directly visualize new brain connections. Nevertheless, I hope you can notice your improved brain health in other ways. Are you embracing new experiences? Enjoying time with friends? Having more fun? Do you feel less tense and more alive? I hope so.

Now is a great time to go back to Chapter 2 and take the quiz again to see how much your Outsmarting Alzheimer's score has dropped. You may be pleased to find that you've already improved your score by several points.

Don't stop here. Continue to practice what you've learned. Connect with friends, nourish your body with wholesome foods, push your aerobic fitness, and challenge your mind with novel pursuits that put you just outside your comfort zone. All the while take steps to reduce stress and improve sleep. This continued practice is so important. It will help you to take everything you just learned and turn it into a habit.

If you are like many people, you've probably attempted to change lifestyle habits before. Maybe you've gotten in shape for a while, but then skipped one workout routine and then another and another. Eventually you became as out of shape as the day you started. Or perhaps you pledged to give up corn chips or embrace vegetables. You did great for a few weeks or even a few months, but eventually your old way of eating crept back in.

This isn't something to feel badly about. It's incredibly normal. Statistics from the University of Scranton tell us, for example, that 45 percent of people make New Year's resolutions to lose weight, enjoy life more, get fit, and learn something exciting, among many other resolutions. Yet, only 8 percent of people manage to keep them.[409]

Why is it so difficult to ditch bad habits and form good ones?

Ann Graybiel, PhD, a brilliant neuroscientist at MIT, has spent much of her career studying this question. She's found that an area deep in the brain called the basal ganglia plays an important role in our ability to adopt and break habits. Based on her research, we now know that this part of the brain is organized into a series of looped circuits that seem to store habitual patterns. Once a habit becomes ingrained in one of these looped circuits, it's hard to turn that habit off, even if it doesn't benefit us.

Graybiel showed this by training rats to run through a T-shaped maze. As the rats approached the intersection, they heard a tone. When they chose correctly based on the tone, they received one of two rewards—chocolate milk (for turning left) or sugar water (for turning right). She ran the rats through the maze over and over again, so that they linked the various tones to either chocolate milk or sugar water in much the same way Pavlov once trained a dog to salivate at the sound of a bell.

Then she took the rewards away.

The rats continued to let the audible tones guide their path, even though they were no longer rewarded once they arrived at the correct destination.

Then, to get a sense of how difficult it might be to undo a habit, Graybiel mixed lithium chloride into the chocolate milk, but not into the sugar water. This transformed what was once a reward into a punishment. Now when the rats listened to the tones and drank chocolate milk at the end of the journey, they got sick. They didn't get sick when they drank the sugar water.

Now, you might assume that a smart rat would eventually learn to ignore the tone that led it toward the chocolate milk and instead always opt to race through the maze toward the sugar water. This isn't, however, what happened. The rats did grow wise to the milk and stopped drinking it—but they never deviated from the path the tone told them to take. They kept turning left, rather than trying the right path and looking for an alternate reward.[410]

Now, many of us would probably like to think that we are smarter than these rats. But human research tells us that this just isn't true. For example, one study showed that, when inside a dark movie theater, many humans will eat all of the popcorn out of a bucket, even if the popcorn is several weeks old.[411] We get very little reward when we eat stale popcorn. If we eat too much, we feel bloated and ill, not unlike how the rats felt when they drank the lithium chloride–infused milk. And yet what happens? While our brains are occupied with the movie unfolding in front of us, the habitual pattern stored in the basal ganglia tells our hand what to do.

Stored habits are hard to break. About 40 percent of our daily activities are ingrained like this, allowing us to divert most of our attention to other matters. This is why we don't have to choose how to roll out of bed in the morning or consider which hand to use to turn off the alarm. It's also why we don't have to think about how to shampoo our hair or how much toothpaste to put on a toothbrush. And it's why our cars seem to take our bodies to work while our minds are elsewhere.

The question is: How do we make healthy lifestyle habits such as exercise or healthy eating just as automatic as driving to work or shampooing our hair? And how do we make unhealthy lifestyle habits—such as eating cheese doodles whenever you procrastinate—less automatic? Is it possible to break bad habits and form new ones? Indeed it is, especially if you allow neuroscience to guide your way. As you continue to incorporate brain health strategies into your life, keep this habit-forming advice in mind.

Be persistent. In the beginning, when you are learning new habits and breaking old ones, you'll be exerting a lot of self-control, and research done by Roy F. Baumeister, PhD, of Florida State University, shows that self-control is a limited resource that doesn't tend to last all day long.[412] He's found that people do poorly on tests of self-control if they've engaged in a previous act of self-control. So, for example, study participants who were asked not to consume the fresh baked cookies sitting in front of them persevered for just eight minutes when given an impossible puzzle to solve. On the other hand, students who weren't tempted with cookies lasted 20 minutes before giving up on the puzzle.[413]

In real life, self-control depletion explains why we tend to raid the snack cabinet after a stressful day at work, but not after an uneventful one, and why we're more likely to skip an afternoon workout than a morning one.

Here's the good news: You can train your self-control just as you train a muscle. In the beginning of forming a new habit, forgive yourself for your initial backsliding and mistakes, and just keep trying. Over time your self-control will grow as you practice the new habit. In the meantime, you can also try some other strategies. Try adopting new habits in the morning, when self-control is at its peak. Take breaks after doing challenging activities. And avoid unnecessary self-control depletion from hunger and fatigue by eating regularly and even taking power naps if you can.

Form a new habit to replace an old one. Graybiel's rat research offers us good and bad news. The bad news is that once a bad habit is formed, it's always with us. We can't just erase that information from our brains, and certain cues will continually trigger it. The good news, though, is that we can form new habits, and we can cause those newer habits—through repetition—to eventually become stronger than the older ones. To make use of this as you continue to improve your brain health, try to focus on adopting new habits that replace old ones rather than only trying to restrain yourself from bad habits. So, for instance, if you usually hit the couch after work, form a new habit of hitting the gym before you arrive home from work. That way, you might still feel compelled to head to the couch, but you'll go there about an hour later at night than you usually do.

Repeat your new habit over and over. Habits form through repetition, so regularity is important. If you want to form the habit of exercise, for example, try to do some exercise every day. Even if you happen to be having a busy day, doing even just a few minutes of exercise is better than doing none. That way, you are still strengthening the habit. Keep repeating the same experience and, eventually, the habit will form.

Make it memorable. You're more likely to remember to do something if you tend to do it at the same time of day, right after a habit you've already formed. This is why it's so much easier to remember to take medication with meals. It's also why, in the 21-day plan, most of the exercise took place before or after meals. That way, eventually the habit of eating dinner reinforces the growing habit of going for an evening walk.

Make it social. To help you remember your budding habit, try forming habits with a group of friends. Perhaps you form a group at church, at the gym, or in your neighborhood composed of adults, all of whom wish to outsmart Alzheimer's. As a group, adopt habits together. Maybe you all sign up and train for a 5K race. Or maybe everyone in the group downloads Words with Friends or another intellectual gaming app, and you all play against one another. Even if you have differing goals—with some of you focusing more on stress relief and others more on exercise—you can still cheer one another along, helping to cement new habits into place. Further supporting your new resolve is the social pressure that comes from a group, which makes it all the more difficult for one person to bail out.

Build in a reward. If you start new activities you enjoy, the habit of doing that activity becomes its own reward. But let's say you really need to build a few habits that, at least at the moment, you just don't find rewarding. Then build in rewards in some other way. If you dislike exercise, for instance, your reward might be exercising with a friend whose conversation is always engaging. If you are encouraging yourself to cook more often, try treating yourself to a massage after every month of successfully making a predetermined number of new recipes.

Overcome the triggers for your old habits. Our environments often trigger old habits to surface in much the same way those varied tones triggered rats to turn right or left. Sometimes just rearranging or changing your environment can make forming or breaking a habit much easier. Think of how you might have overcome the urge to call an old lover, in part by removing all of the photographic evidence and other reminders of your relationship. With food, you might give yourself a helping hand by putting tempting, unhealthy foods out of sight so they don't cue you to eat them. If you are trying to quit smoking, you might create new routines that, at least for a while, keep you away from the types of places that cue you to light up.

Where Will You Go from Here?

Though you will find several resource chapters after this one—including recipes, workout routines, and brain games to try—you've now come to the end of the program portion of the book. I'd like to leave you with two final pieces of advice:

1. Keep trying.

2. Keep improving.

You might remember them as the two Ks for maintaining healthy habits. How will you put the two Ks to work? What will you do to keep up your momentum? Will you plan another dinner party, this one bigger and more elaborate than the one before? Sign up for more of those classes you investigated during the 3-week plan? Perhaps you go on that vacation you've been putting off for years, start a book club, pledge to try a new recipe every week for a year, or set a goal of playing board games with friends every Friday night. Maybe you take those dance classes your spouse has been begging you to take with her. Or is it finally the time to tackle that long list of activities on your bucket list?

Here's the beauty of the Outsmarting Alzheimer's plan. No matter how you go about doing it, one of the strongest and most persistent side effects is this one: you end up living life to the fullest.

So keep up the momentum, pick a new challenge, and go for it.

....

CHAPTER 10

Brain Smart Recipes

You'll find more than 40 quick-and-easy recipes to help you incorporate a wide range of Meal Smarts into your life. All of the recipes are short on calories (Meal Smarts Prescription #1, page 61) but big on satisfaction. Most lean on just a few ingredients and only a small amount of prep time, making it easier for you to accomplish your goal of cooking more meals at home (Meal Smarts Prescription #2, page 62). Each recipe is also packed full of brain-protecting fruits, vegetables, and other whole foods (Meal Smarts Prescription #3, page 64, and #4, page 65). And you'll find many that include healing spices (Meal Smarts Prescription #5, page 67), fish (Meal Smarts Prescription #8, page 69), and chocolate (Meal Smarts Prescription #12, page 72). One of them even contains tea! (That's Meal Smarts Prescription #10, page 71.)

Enjoy!

BREAKFASTS

Berry Flaxseed Smoothie

Serves 2

Flaxseeds contain healthful omega-3 fatty acids as well as a host of antioxidants and fiber.

- 2 **tablespoons whole flaxseeds**
- ½ **cup orange juice**
- ½ **cup nonfat vanilla yogurt**
- 1 **cup unsweetened frozen mixed berries**
     or blueberries
- 1 **small banana, sliced**

In dry blender, place flaxseeds, cover, and blend until ground into fine powder. Add orange juice, yogurt, mixed berries (or blueberries), and banana. Cover and blend until smooth and creamy.

> **Per serving:** 200 calories, 5 g protein, 36 g carbohydrates, 7 g fiber, 5 g total fat, 0 g saturated fat.

Raspberry-Banana-Oat Smoothie

Serves 4

Adding oats to a smoothie infuses it with fiber and helps you get in a serving of whole grains. Even though this drink is low in calories, it will keep you satisfied.

- 2 **large bananas**
- ¼ **cup rolled oats**
- 1 **cup raspberries**
- 1 **tablespoon honey**
- 2 **cups cold water, divided**
- 8 **raspberries, to garnish**

1. Peel the bananas and cut them into 1½-inch chunks. Put the bananas, oats, and raspberries in a blender. Add the honey and 1 cup cold water. Purée until smooth, then add another 1 cup water and blend for another 4 to 5 seconds.

2. Pour the smoothie into 4 tall glasses. Garnish with 2 raspberries per glass and serve immediately.

> **Per serving:** 150 calories, 3 g protein, 32 g carbohydrates, 3 g fiber, 2 g total fat, 0 g saturated fat

Berry Salad with Passion Fruit

Serves 6

By starting the day with a variety of fruit, you get a jump start on accumulating more than five servings of fruits and vegetables for the day. As a breakfast option, pair this salad with a veggie-packed egg scramble or a bowl of hot cereal. Or mix it with nonfat yogurt.

- 4 cups ripe strawberries, hulled and cut in half
- 1 cup fresh red raspberries
- 1 cup fresh blackberries
- ½ cup fresh blueberries
- ½ cup mixed fresh red currants and black currants, removed from their stalks (optional)
- 2 passion fruits
- 3 tablespoons sugar, or to taste
- 1 tablespoon fresh lime or lemon juice

1. In large serving bowl, combine strawberries, raspberries, blackberries, blueberries, and red and black currants, if using.

2. Cut each passion fruit in half. Holding strainer over bowl of berries, spoon passion fruit and seeds into strainer. Press flesh and seeds with back of spoon to squeeze all of juice through strainer onto berries. Reserve a few seeds left in strainer and discard the rest.

3. Add sugar and lime juice to berries. Gently toss. Sprinkle with reserved passion fruit seeds. Serve salad immediately, or cover and chill briefly.

Per serving: 89 calories, 1 g protein, 22 g carbohydrates, 6 g fiber, 1 g total fat, 0 g saturated fat

Nutty Muesli

Serves 6

Bulgur and oats provide you with a decent dose of fiber to fend off hunger during the rest of your morning, and persimmons, figs, and passion fruit are all rich in brain-protective antioxidants.

½ cup bulgur
1 cup water
1½ cups rolled oats
1 cup apple juice, plus additional if needed
½ cup slivered unblanched almonds
¼ cup pine nuts
2 tablespoons shelled raw sunflower seeds
10 dried apricots, diced
10 dried figs, stalks removed, then diced
¼ cup brown sugar
2 green apples, cored and coarsely grated
1 large or 2 small persimmons, peeled and diced, plus extra for serving
1 passion fruit
   Few drops of pure almond essence (optional)
   Pomegranate seeds or blueberries

1. In large bowl, combine bulgur with water and stir to combine. Cover and soak for 30 minutes to soften bulgur. Drain well in sieve and return to bowl.

2. Add oats, apple juice, almonds, pine nuts, sunflower seeds, apricots, figs, sugar, apples, and persimmon. Fold into bulgur.

3. Cut passion fruit in half. Place sieve over bowl of muesli, and spoon passion fruit pulp and seeds into it. Press until juice has gone through sieve and only seeds are left behind. Discard seeds.

4. Add almond essence, if using, and a little more apple juice if needed to make a moist but not sloppy consistency. Keep, tightly covered, in fridge until ready to eat. It can be kept for up to 2 days. To serve, stir muesli well, then top with pomegranate seeds or blueberries, whichever is in season, plus additional persimmon.

Per serving: 369 calories, 8 g protein, 62 g carbohydrates, 10 g fiber, 11 g total fat, 1 g saturated fat

Hot Cereal with Apples and Dates

Serves 4

Too often, we reserve dates only for snacking. In this recipe, you'll add this antioxidant powerhouse to your morning cereal.

1½ cups low-fat milk
1½ cups water
  1 cup unpeeled chopped apple (¼-inch pieces)
  ½ cup old-fashioned oats
  ½ cup coarse bulgur
  3 dates, pitted and snipped
  ½ teaspoon ground cinnamon

Stir together milk, water, apple, oats, bulgur, dates, and cinnamon in medium saucepan and heat, stirring frequently, until boiling. Cover, reduce the heat to low, and cook, stirring occasionally, for 10 minutes, or until grains are tender.

Per serving: 185 calories, 7 g protein, 37 g carbohydrates, 6 g fiber, 2 g total fat, 1 g saturated fat

Multigrain Pancakes or Waffles

Serves 8

Many commercial pancake mixes are made exclusively from refined flour rather than the whole grain flour that is better for your brain. Why buy expensive commercial pancake mix when you can quickly make up a big batch at home—one that's healthier than anything you could buy at the store? Make up a big batch of the dry ingredients at the beginning of the week to reduce prep time in the mornings.

- 2 cups low-fat buttermilk
- ½ cup old-fashioned rolled oats
- ⅔ cup whole wheat flour
- ⅔ cup all-purpose flour
- ⅔ cup toasted wheat germ
- 1½ teaspoons baking powder
- ½ teaspoon baking soda
- ¼ teaspoon salt
- 1 teaspoon ground cinnamon
- 2 large eggs
- ¼ cup firmly packed brown sugar
- 1 tablespoon canola oil
- 2 teaspoons vanilla extract
- 1 cup maple syrup, warmed
- 1½ cups sliced strawberries or blueberries

1. Mix buttermilk and oats in small bowl. Let stand for 15 minutes.

2. In large bowl, whisk whole wheat flour, all-purpose flour, wheat germ, baking powder, baking soda, salt, and cinnamon.

3. In medium bowl, whisk eggs, sugar, oil, and vanilla. Add buttermilk mixture. Add this mixture to flour mixture and mix with rubber spatula just until flour mixture is moistened.

4. **To make pancakes:** Coat large nonstick skillet with cooking spray and heat over medium heat. Spoon about ¼ cup batter for each pancake into skillet. Cook for 3 minutes, or until bottoms are golden and small bubbles start to form on top. Flip the pancakes and cook for 1 to 2 minutes, or until browned and cooked through. (Adjust heat as necessary for even browning.) Keep the pancakes warm in 200°F oven while you finish cooking remaining batter.

5. **To make waffles:** Coat waffle iron with cooking spray and heat iron. Spoon in enough batter to cover three-quarters of surface. Close iron and cook for 4 to 5 minutes, or until waffles are crisp and golden brown. Keep waffles warm in 200°F oven while you finish cooking remaining batter.

6. Top with maple syrup and strawberries or blueberries. Wrap any leftover pancakes or waffles individually in plastic wrap, and refrigerate for up to 2 days or freeze for up to 1 month. Reheat in a toaster or toaster oven.

Per serving: 292 calories, 8 g protein, 60 g carbohydrates, 3 g fiber, 3 g total fat, 1 g saturated fat

Mushroom and Bell Pepper Frittata

Serves 4

Frittatas offer a simple way to make breakfast for a crowd, and they're quite versatile. For even more brain protection, add even more sliced veggies or finely chopped spinach than the recipe calls for.

  2 tablespoons olive oil
  1 red or orange bell pepper, seeded and cut into 1/4-inch slices
  1 yellow bell pepper, seeded and cut into 1/4-inch slices
  2 cups sliced mushrooms
  8 large eggs
 ¼ teaspoon salt
 ¼ teaspoon ground black pepper
 ⅓ cup grated Parmesan cheese
 10 fresh basil leaves, torn in small pieces

1. In large nonstick skillet over medium-high heat, heat oil. Add bell peppers. Sauté until softened, about 4 minutes. Add mushrooms. Sauté for 5 minutes, or until vegetables are lightly browned. Reduce heat to medium.

2. In medium bowl, stir together eggs, salt, and black pepper. Pour into skillet, spreading evenly. Cook, stirring frequently, for 3 to 4 minutes, or until soft-scrambled. Reduce heat to medium-low. Stir in cheese and basil. Smooth top. Cook for 5 minutes. Cover and cook for 8 minutes, or until eggs are firm and bottom is browned.

3. To serve, loosen frittata around edge with spatula. Invert onto large plate. Cut into 4 equal wedges. Serve warm or at room temperature.

Spinach and Goat Cheese Omelet

Serves 4

Spinach is loaded with brain-protecting antioxidants. Because it shrinks as it cooks, just rinse it, and use it in your morning omelets—no chopping required.

- 2 cups baby spinach, rinsed
- 2 tablespoons crumbled goat cheese or feta cheese
- 1 tablespoon chopped scallion
- 1 large egg
- 2 large egg whites
- ¼ teaspoon hot red-pepper sauce, such as Tabasco
   Pinch of salt
   Pinch of ground black pepper
- 1 teaspoon olive oil

1. Bring about 1 inch of water to a boil in large saucepan. Drop in spinach and cook for 30 seconds, or just until wilted. Drain, press out liquid, and chop coarsely. (Alternatively, place spinach in microwave-safe bowl, cover with vented plastic wrap, and microwave on high for 1 to 2 minutes.) Place spinach in small bowl. Stir in cheese and scallion.

2. Stir egg, egg whites, hot sauce, salt, and black pepper briskly with fork in medium bowl. Heat oil in 7- to 10-inch nonstick skillet over medium-high heat until hot. Tilt skillet to spread oil over surface. Pour in egg mixture. Immediately stir with heat-resistant rubber spatula or fork for a few seconds. Then use spatula to push cooked portions at edges toward the center, tilting skillet to allow uncooked egg mixture to fill in areas around edges. Sprinkle spinach mixture over omelet. Continue to cook until almost set and bottom is golden. The entire cooking process should take about 1 minute.

3. Use spatula to fold one-third of omelet over filling. Tip skillet and, using spatula as a guide, slide omelet onto plate so that it lands, folded in thirds, seam side down.

   Per serving: 235 calories, 20 g protein, 4 g carbohydrates, 1 g fiber, 15 g total fat, 6 g saturated fat

Summer Greens Scramble

Serves 4

Rich in protein, fiber, and a number of brain-boosting vitamins and antioxidants, kale is a true superfood that deserves a starring role during any meal, including breakfast.

2 cups shredded, stemmed fresh kale

5 large eggs

5 large egg whites

¼ teaspoon ground cumin

¼ teaspoon salt

¼ cup chopped lean deli ham

2 scallions, trimmed and thinly sliced

1. In large saucepan of boiling salted water, cook kale, 3 to 5 minutes, or until tender. Drain. Rinse under cold water. Drain well.

2. In large bowl, whisk together eggs, egg whites, cumin, and salt.

3. Coat large nonstick skillet with cooking spray. Heat over medium heat. Add egg mixture. Cook, stirring constantly, for 2 to 3 minutes, or until eggs start to thicken slightly. Stir in kale, ham, and scallions. Cook, stirring occasionally, for 2 to 3 minutes, or until eggs are soft-scrambled.

Per serving: 145 calories, 15 g protein, 5 g carbohydrates, 1 g fiber, 7 g total fat, 2 g saturated fat

Zucchini Frittata

Serves 6

To reduce fat and calories, only half the yolks are used. You can siphon off even more fat and calories by using no yolks at all.

4 eggs

4 egg whites

¼ cup grated Parmesan cheese

¼ teaspoon salt

2 tablespoons olive oil

1 clove garlic, minced

2 small zucchini, shredded

2 roasted red bell peppers, cut into thin strips

1. Preheat the oven to 400°F. In a medium bowl, whisk together the eggs, egg whites, cheese, and salt.

2. Heat the oil in a large ovenproof nonstick skillet over medium heat. Add the garlic and cook just until tender, 1 minute. Add the zucchini and peppers and cook 1 minute. Pour in the egg mixture and cook until the bottom of the frittata is set, 3 minutes. Bake until set, 10 minutes.

Per serving: 138 calories, 9 g protein, 5 g carbohydrates, 1 g fiber, 9 g total fat, 2 g saturated fat

LUNCHES

Broccoli Salad

Serves 6

Too often, we think lettuce is what makes a salad a salad. But that's just not true. In this version, you'll find a number of brain-healthy veggies, including broccoli and onions. The flaxseeds and almonds provide brain-boosting omega-3s.

- ¼ cup balsamic vinegar
- 2 tablespoons Dijon mustard
- 2 tablespoons honey
- ¼ teaspoon salt
- ¼ teaspoon black pepper
- 2 tablespoons flaxseed oil
- 2 tablespoons extra-virgin olive oil
- 2 heads broccoli
- 1 small red onion, cut into thin wedges
- ½ cup whole almonds, toasted and coarsely chopped
- ½ cup dried cranberries
- 4 ounces chèvre goat cheese, crumbled

1. In large bowl, whisk together the vinegar, mustard, honey, salt, and pepper. Whisk in the flaxseed and olive oils until well blended. Set aside.

2. Remove the florets from the broccoli and add to the vinaigrette. Trim the ends of the stalks and, with a vegetable peeler, peel off the thick outer layer. Shred the stalks with a food processor or by hand.

3. Add the shredded stalks, onion, almonds, and cranberries to the bowl and toss to coat well. Top with the cheese.

Per serving: 333 calories, 12 g protein, 33 g carbohydrates, 7 g fiber, 20 g total fat, 4 g saturated fat

Spinach Salad with Chickpeas

Serves 4

This salad includes a number of Brain Smart foods in just one dish. You'll reap a wealth of antioxidants from the spinach, onions, apples, and garlic. The chickpeas add a healthy dose of fiber, and the flaxseeds good-for-you fats that reduce inflammation.

- 2 medium onions, cut into ½-inch slices
- 15 ounces chickpeas, drained, rinsed, and patted dry
- ¼ cup lemon juice
- 2 tablespoons flaxseed oil
- 1 tablespoon olive oil
- 1 clove garlic, minced
- ½ teaspoon salt
- ½ cup crumbled feta cheese
- 5 ounces baby spinach
- 2 apples, cored and sliced
- 2 tablespoons ground flaxseeds

1. Preheat oven to 400°F. Coat baking sheet with olive oil cooking spray. Add onion slices and coat each with spray. Roast for 10 minutes. Add chickpeas and roast for 10 minutes, or until onions are tender and browned.

2. Meanwhile, in measuring cup, whisk together lemon juice, oils, garlic, and salt. Stir in cheese.

3. Place spinach in large bowl and toss with onions, chickpeas, apples, and flaxseeds. Drizzle with the vinaigrette.

Per serving: 292 calories, 9 g protein, 37 g carbohydrates, 10 g fiber, 14 g total fat, 3 g saturated fat

Spinach, Sweet Potato, and Shiitake Salad

Serves 4

This unusual combination of sweet potato, mushrooms, and spinach provides a good dose of antioxidants with appetite-suppressing fiber. To simplify lunch prep, bake a few sweet potatoes at the beginning of the week. Then just pull one or two from the fridge, as needed, to make this and other dishes.

- 1 pound sweet potatoes, peeled, halved lengthwise, and cut crosswise into ½-inch slices
- ⅓ cup walnuts
- 1 tablespoon plus 4 teaspoons olive oil
- 2 cloves garlic, slivered
- 12 ounces fresh shiitake mushrooms, stems discarded and caps thickly sliced
- ½ teaspoon salt
- 12 cups spinach leaves
- ½ cup red wine vinegar
- 1 tablespoon Dijon mustard

1. Preheat oven to 400°F. Place sweet potatoes on lightly oiled baking sheet and bake for 15 to 20 minutes, or until tender. Toast walnuts in separate pan in oven for 5 to 7 minutes, or until crisp. When cool enough to handle, coarsely chop nuts.

2. In large skillet, heat 1 tablespoon oil over medium heat. Add garlic and cook for 30 seconds, or until fragrant.

3. Add half the mushrooms, sprinkle with ¼ teaspoon salt, and cook for 4 minutes, or until they begin to soften. Add remaining mushrooms and ¼ teaspoon salt, and cook for 5 minutes, or until mushrooms are tender.

4. Place spinach in large bowl. Add sweet potatoes and walnuts. Remove mushrooms from skillet with slotted spoon and add to bowl.

5. Add vinegar, mustard, and remaining 4 teaspoons oil to the skillet, and whisk over high heat until warm. Pour dressing over salad and toss to combine.

Per serving: 283 calories, 9 g protein, 32 g carbohydrates, 8 g fiber, 15 g total fat, 2 g saturated fat

Mediterranean Salad with Edamame

Serves 8

The Mediterranean diet—rich in wholesome plant foods—has been shown to reduce risk for Alzheimer's disease, and this salad offers some of the best of what Mediterranean countries have to offer. You'll also see that this recipe includes its own dressing. Consider doubling or tripling the dressing ingredients, so you have dressing left over to use on salads throughout the week.

- 1 cup frozen shelled edamame beans
- ⅓ cup extra-virgin olive oil
- 3 tablespoons lemon juice
- 2 cloves garlic, minced
  Salt to taste
- ¼ teaspoon sugar
  Ground black pepper to taste
- 2 cups shredded romaine lettuce
- 2 cups cherry tomatoes, halved
- 1 cup sliced English cucumber
- ⅔ cup chopped scallions
- ½ cup pitted kalamata olives, halved
- ½ cup fresh mint leaves, washed, dried, and torn into ½-inch pieces
- ½ cup fresh flat-leaf parsley leaves, washed, dried, and torn into ½-inch pieces
- 1 cup crumbled feta cheese

1. Bring large saucepan of lightly salted water to a boil. Add edamame beans and cook, covered, over medium heat for 3 to 4 minutes, or until tender. Drain and rinse with cold running water.

2. In screw-top jar with tight-fitting lid, combine oil, lemon juice, garlic, salt, sugar, and pepper. Shake to blend.

3. In large bowl, combine lettuce, tomatoes, cucumber, scallions, olives, mint, parsley, and edamame beans. Just before serving, drizzle lemon dressing over salad and toss to coat well. Sprinkle each serving with cheese.

Per serving: 220 calories, 7 g protein, 10 g carbohydrates, 3 g fiber, 17 g total fat, 5 g saturated fat

Minted Mixed Grain Salad

Serves 4

This unusual summery salad is loaded with whole grains as well as veggies. You'll love the scent of parsley, mint, and lemon, too. Though it's low in calories, it's surprisingly filling.

⅓ cup bulgur
⅓ cup quinoa
1 small cucumber
2 large tomatoes
1 large green bell pepper
2 scallions
1 teaspoon sugar
   Grated zest and juice of 1 lemon
3 teaspoons olive oil
5 large mint sprigs, chopped
¼ cup chopped fresh parsley
1 head romaine lettuce, to serve

1. Place the bulgur and quinoa in a saucepan with 4 cups of boiling water. Return to a boil, reduce heat, cover and simmer for 15 minutes, or until the bulgur and quinoa are tender. Drain any water that was not absorbed. Finely dice the cucumber, tomatoes, and pepper, and thinly slice the scallions.

2. Mix the sugar, lemon zest, and juice in a large bowl, stirring until the sugar dissolves. Whisk in the oil and add the cucumber, tomatoes, pepper, and scallions. Stir in the cooked bulgur and quinoa, cover, and let cool for 15 minutes.

3. Stir the mint and parsley into the salad and season to taste just before serving. Divide the salad among four bowls and serve with a selection of lettuce leaves for wrapping and scooping.

Per serving: 267 calories, 7 g protein, 32 g carbohydrates, 3 g fiber, 13 g total fat, 2 g saturated fat

Grilled Salmon Salad

Serves 4

Salmon is rich in brain-healthy omega-3, fatty acids. To create a quick lunch on the go, modify this recipe by swapping canned wild salmon for the fillet and assembling the rest of the salad just before eating.

- 8 cardamom pods, crushed
- 1 teaspoon cumin seeds
  Finely grated zest and juice of 1 lime
  Juice of 1 large orange
- 1 tablespoon light soy sauce
- 1 tablespoon honey
  Salt and ground black pepper
- 4 pieces (4 ounces each) skinless salmon fillet
- 4 cups mixed salad leaves, such as oak leaf, red leaf lettuce, and baby chard, or use romaine
- 1 mango, peeled and cut into 1-inch cubes
- 1 papaya, peeled, seeded, and cut into 1-inch cubes
- 1 orange, peeled and segmented

1. Heat small nonstick skillet over medium heat. Scrape seeds from cardamom pods and add to hot pan with cumin seeds. Toast for a few seconds to release aromas and remove seeds to shallow nonmetallic dish.

2. Add lime zest and juice, orange juice, soy sauce, and honey to seeds. Season lightly with salt and pepper. Lay salmon pieces in dish and turn to coat both sides. Cover and let marinate for 30 minutes.

3. Preheat grill or oven broiler. Lift salmon out of marinade, place on grill rack or broiler pan, and grill or broil for 4 to 5 minutes on one side only. The fillets should still be slightly translucent in the center. Meanwhile, pour marinade into small saucepan and bring just to a boil.

4. Arrange salad leaves in middle of 4 plates. Scatter mango and papaya cubes and orange segments over salad. Place cooked salmon on top of salad and drizzle with warm marinade. Serve immediately.

Per serving: 313 calories, 26 g protein, 30 g carbohydrates, 4 g fiber, 10 g total fat, 2 g saturated fat

Curried Chicken Salad Sandwich

Serves 4

This version of the traditional chicken salad sandwich includes antioxidant-rich apples and is seasoned with curry powder, naturally rich in the spice turmeric. For optimal brain protection, stuff your sandwich with the darkest salad greens available. The darker the green, the more protective antioxidants it contains.

- ¼ cup low-fat plain yogurt
- 2 tablespoons low-fat canola mayonnaise
- 1½ teaspoons curry powder
- 1 teaspoon honey
- ¼ teaspoon salt
- 2 cups (8 ounces) chopped cooked chicken
- 1 apple, cored and chopped
- 2 celery stalks, chopped
- 4 lettuce leaves
- 2 whole grain pita breads (8 inches), halved

1. In a large bowl, whisk together the yogurt, mayonnaise, curry powder, honey, and salt. Add the chicken, apple, and celery.

2. Place a lettuce leaf in each pita half and fill with one-quarter of the chicken salad.

   Per serving: 253 calories, 23 g protein, 27 g carbohydrates, 4 g fiber, 6 g total fat, 1 g saturated fat

Tuna and Carrot Sandwich on Rye

Serves 2

Vegetables add an antioxidant-infused crunch to this healthier version of the typical tuna sandwich. If carrots aren't your thing, swap them for radishes or any other crunchy veggie. If you are trying to slim down, eat half a sandwich, and pair it with a salad.

- ⅔ cup shredded carrot (1 medium)
- 2 teaspoons lemon juice
- 2 teaspoons extra-virgin olive oil
- 1 tablespoon chopped scallions
- 1 tablespoon chopped fresh dill or parsley
- ⅛ teaspoon salt, or to taste
- 3 ounces water-packed chunk light tuna, drained and flaked
- ¼ cup finely chopped celery

2 tablespoons reduced-fat mayonnaise
4 slices rye or pumpernickel bread
4 lettuce leaves, rinsed and dried

1. In small bowl, combine carrot, lemon juice, oil, scallions, dill or parsley, and salt. Mix with fork.

2. In another small bowl, mix tuna, celery, and 1 tablespoon of mayonnaise.

3. Spread remaining 1 tablespoon mayonnaise over bread slices. Spread half of tuna mixture over 2 bread slices. Top with carrot salad and lettuce. Set remaining bread slices over filling. Cut each sandwich in half. One serving equals 2 sandwich halves. Sandwiches will keep, well wrapped, in refrigerator or cooler packed with ice packs for up to 1 day.

Per serving: 303 calories, 17 g protein, 38 g carbohydrates, 5 g fiber, 9 g total fat, 2 g saturated fat

Salmon and Fennel Lettuce Wraps

Serves 4

Canned salmon is one of the easiest ways to get in the habit of consuming more inflammation-lowering omega-3 fatty acids. Keep one or two cans of wild salmon in your pantry, and use it in salads, sandwiches, and wraps.

3 tablespoons reduced-fat mayonnaise
1 tablespoon reduced-fat sour cream
2 tablespoons fresh lemon juice
1 tablespoon chopped fresh dill
12 ounces canned Alaskan pink or sockeye salmon, drained
½ fennel bulb, trimmed and finely chopped
4 large Boston lettuce leaves

1. In medium bowl, whisk together mayonnaise, sour cream, lemon juice, and dill. Stir in salmon and fennel.

2. For each wrap, start about 1 inch up from bottom of lettuce leaf and mound one-fourth of salmon mixture in horizontal row along bottom third of lettuce.

3. Fold bottom of lettuce over filling, then fold in about 1 inch of sides. Roll firmly away from you.

4. Cut each wrap in half on a diagonal.

Per serving: 179 calories, 21 g protein, 5 g carbohydrates, 1 g fiber, 8 g total fat, 2 g saturated fat

Salmon Cake Sandwiches

Serves 4

Make all four of these salmon patties early in the week. That way, you've got four lunches ready to grab while you are on your way to work.

- ¼ cup mild salsa
- 2 egg whites
- ¼ cup low-fat canola mayonnaise
- ½ teaspoon ground cumin
- ¼–1 teaspoon hot red-pepper sauce
- 2 pouches (7 ounces each) salmon, patted dry
- 1 cup fresh whole wheat bread crumbs
- 4 lettuce leaves
- 4 whole wheat sandwich rolls
- 1 large tomato, cut into 4 slices

1. Drain salsa by placing it in a sieve over a bowl for about 10 minutes. Shake sieve to release any remaining liquid.

2. Line baking sheet with parchment paper. In medium bowl, whisk egg whites. Stir in salsa, mayonnaise, cumin, and red-pepper sauce. Add salmon and bread crumbs and gently fold in just until combined. Shape mixture into 4 cakes, place on baking sheet, and refrigerate for at least 30 minutes.

3. Coat nonstick skillet with cooking spray. Add cakes and cook over medium heat, turning once, for 6 minutes, or until browned and crisp.

4. Place lettuce leaf on each roll. Top with salmon cake and tomato slice.

Per serving: 367 calories, 30 g protein, 39 g carbohydrates, 6 g fiber, 11 g total fat, 1 g saturated fat

Open-Faced Sardine Sandwiches

Serves 2

Sardines offer a convenient way to get more brain-healthy omega-3s. By eating a sandwich open-faced with just one slice of bread, you halve blood-sugar-raising carbs and subtract about 100 calories, without sacrificing satisfaction.

- 1 tablespoon low-fat canola mayonnaise
- ½ teaspoon fresh lemon juice
- ¼ teaspoon grated lemon zest
- 2 slices (each ¾ inch thick) whole grain bread, such as 12-grain
- 1 small tomato, cut into 4 slices
- 3.75 ounces sardines in olive oil
- 2 slices (2 ounces) low-fat Jarlsberg cheese

1. Preheat the broiler. In a small bowl, combine the mayonnaise, lemon juice, and lemon zest. Spread half of the mixture onto each slice of bread.

2. Top each slice with half of the tomatoes, sardines, and cheese. Place on a broiler pan or baking sheet and broil until the cheese melts, about 3 minutes.

   Per serving: 228 calories, 20 g protein, 17 g carbohydrates, 5 g fiber, 9 g total fat, 1 g saturated fat

DINNERS

Chicken Curry Soup

Serves 6

Turmeric is one of the main spices in most curry mixes, making this soup especially good for your brain. Round out a bowl with a side salad and/or a slice of whole grain bread.

- 2 tablespoons olive oil
- 2 onions, chopped
- 4 large carrots, chopped
- 1 russet potato, peeled and finely chopped
- 1 tablespoon mild curry powder
- 1 carton (32 ounces) low-sodium chicken broth
- 1 cup water
- 1 pound boneless, skinless chicken breasts, cut into thin strips
- ½ small head cauliflower, cut into florets (2 cups)
- 1 cup frozen peas, thawed

1. Heat the oil in a large saucepan over medium heat. Add the onions and carrots and cook, stirring, until lightly browned, 5 minutes. Add the potato, curry powder, 1 cup of the broth, and 1 cup water. Cover and cook for 10 minutes or until the vegetables are tender.

2. Remove from the heat and let cool slightly, 5 minutes. Place in a food processor or blender and process until smooth.

3. Return the mixture to the saucepan and add the remaining broth and the chicken and cauliflower. Bring to a boil, reduce the heat to medium-low, and simmer until the chicken is cooked and the cauliflower is tender, 15 minutes. Add the peas and cook until heated through, 3 minutes.

   Per serving: 260 calories, 25 g protein, 26 g carbohydrates, 6 g fiber, 7 g total fat, 1 g saturated fat

Cock-a-Leekie Soup with Kale

Serves 4

Here, kale has been added to this traditional Scottish dish. This power green is good for your brain. Round it out with a side of whole grain bread and/or a salad.

 1 **pound boneless, skinless chicken breasts**
 ¾ **pound leeks**
 1 **tablespoon olive oil or canola oil**
 2 **large carrots**
 4¾ **cups hot chicken stock**
 1 **bunch kale (about ¾ pound)**
 ⅓ **cup pitted prunes, quartered**
    salt and ground black pepper

1. Cut the chicken breast fillets into 1½-inch cubes. Trim, slice, and rinse the leeks. Heat the oil in a large saucepan over high heat. Add the chicken and leeks, and cook for 5 minutes, reducing heat to medium after the first 1 to 2 minutes. Stir occasionally.

2. Slice the carrots. Pour the hot stock into the pan. Add the carrots and bring to a boil over high heat, stirring, and reduce heat to low. Cover and simmer for 10 minutes, or until the carrots are tender.

3. Finely shred the kale and stir into the pan. Return to a boil then reduce the heat, cover, and simmer for 4 minutes. Add the prunes and stir them into the soup. Simmer for 1 minute, season to taste with salt and pepper, and ladle into 4 bowls to serve.

 Per serving: 240 calories, 24 g protein, 15 g carbohydrates, 7 g fiber, 7 g total fat, 1 g saturated fat

Barbecued Flank Steak

Serves 4

Flank steak is lower in fat than other cuts of beef. In this recipe, you'll marinate it in a homemade, low-sodium barbecue sauce to help reduce the formation of harmful AGEs as it cooks on the grill.

 2 **cloves garlic, grated**
 1 **small onion, grated**
 ½ **cup tomato sauce**
 2 **tablespoons red wine vinegar**
 2 **tablespoons brown sugar**
 1 **tablespoon Worcestershire sauce**

¼ teaspoon salt
1 pound flank steak

1. In a large zipper-seal bag, combine the garlic, onion, tomato sauce, vinegar, brown sugar, Worcestershire, and salt. Add the steak, seal the bag, and turn to coat. Refrigerate for 6 hours or overnight.

2. Preheat the broiler or grill. Remove the steak from the marinade, reserving the marinade. Broil the steak 2 to 3 inches from the heat source or grill until a thermometer inserted in the center reaches 145°F for medium-rare, 13 minutes. Transfer to a cutting board.

3. Meanwhile, place the marinade in a small saucepan, bring to a boil, and cook for 4 minutes. Slice the steak and serve with the sauce.

Per serving: 219 calories, 25 g protein, 11 g carbohydrates, 1 g fiber, 8 g total fat, 3 g saturated fat

Beef in Lettuce Wraps

Serves 4

So often we create sandwiches by placing meat between two slices of bread or on a bun, but this can add up to a lot of calories. The bread is usually refined, too. In this version of a "sloppy Joe," you use lettuce to wrap the meat, reducing your calories by more than 100.

3 tablespoons hoisin sauce
2 tablespoons wine vinegar
1 tablespoon soy sauce
1 teaspoon toasted sesame oil
½ teaspoon ground ginger
1 pound lean ground beef
4 scallions, chopped
2 carrots, shredded
1 clove garlic, minced
12 Bibb or Boston lettuce leaves

1. In small bowl, whisk together hoisin sauce, vinegar, soy sauce, oil, and ginger.

2. In nonstick skillet over medium heat, cook beef for 5 minutes, or until browned. Add scallions, carrots, and garlic and cook for 3 minutes, or until tender. Stir in the hoisin mixture and cook for 3 minutes, or until thickened and flavors are blended.

3. Place 3 lettuce leaves on each of 4 plates and fill with beef mixture.

Per serving: 201 calories, 24 g protein, 13 g carbohydrates, 3 g fiber, 6 g total fat, 2 g saturated fat

Spinach-Stuffed Meat Loaf

Serves 8

Meatloaf is usually packed full of saturated fat, but this version artfully sneaks several different antioxidant-rich veggies into the meat, reducing fat and calories.

  1 teaspoon olive oil
  2 large onions, finely chopped
  6 cloves garlic, crushed, or to taste
 24 ounces chopped tomatoes
  ⅔ cup low-fat, reduced-sodium chicken broth
  1 teaspoon dried mixed herbs (try basil, oregano,
       and thyme)
Salt and ground black pepper
  1 pound fresh spinach leaves
  2 tablespoons low-fat plain yogurt
  ½ teaspoon freshly grated nutmeg
  1 pound lean (93%) ground beef
  1 pound lean ground pork
  1 celery stalk, finely chopped
  1 large carrot, grated
  ½ cup rolled oats
  2 teaspoons chopped fresh thyme
  5 tablespoons low-fat milk
  1 egg, beaten
  2 teaspoons Dijon mustard

1. Heat oil in saucepan over medium heat. Add onions and garlic and cook for 5 minutes, or until onions are soft.

2. Transfer half of onion mixture to large bowl and set aside. Stir tomatoes (with their juice), broth, and mixed herbs into onions in saucepan. Season lightly with salt and pepper. Bring to a boil, then cover, reduce heat, and simmer sauce very gently.

3. Preheat oven to 350°F. Put spinach in large saucepan, cover with tight-fitting lid, and cook over high heat for 2 to 3 minutes, or until the leaves are wilted. Drain spinach, squeeze it dry with your hands, then chop it coarsely and put into a bowl. Stir in yogurt and season with ¼ teaspoon of the nutmeg and salt and pepper to taste.

4. Put beef and pork into bowl with reserved onion mixture. Add celery, carrot, oats, thyme, milk, egg, mustard, and remaining ¼ teaspoon nutmeg. Season with salt and pepper. Mix ingredients together with your hands.

5. Lay large sheet of plastic wrap on work surface and place meat mixture in center. With a spatula, spread meat into a 9 x 7-inch rectangle. Spread

spinach mixture evenly over meat, leaving a ½-inch border. Starting at a short end, roll up meat and spinach. Pat sides and place on nonstick baking sheet, discarding plastic wrap.

6. Place meat loaf, uncovered, in the center of oven and cook for 45 minutes, then remove and brush lightly with a little tomato sauce. Return to oven and cook for 5 minutes to set glaze and brown slightly. To check if meat loaf is cooked through, insert a skewer into the center and remove after a few seconds. It should feel very hot when lightly placed on the back of your hand. When meat loaf is ready, remove from oven, cover loosely with foil, and leave to stand for 10 minutes. Serve with remaining tomato sauce.

Per serving: 250 calories, 30 g protein, 17 g carbohydrates, 5 g fiber, 7 g total fat, 2 g saturated fat

Lentil and Rice Paella with Clams

Serves 4

In this version of a traditional Mediterranean dish, lentils have been substituted for some of the rice, adding appetite-suppressing fiber.

  1   tablespoon olive oil
  2   large leeks, quartered lengthwise, thinly sliced crosswise, and well washed
  5   cloves garlic, minced
  3   large carrots, cut crosswise into ½-inch slices
  1   pickled jalapeño chile pepper, minced (wear gloves when handling)
  ⅔   cup lentils, picked over and rinsed
  3   cups water
  ½   teaspoon salt
  ⅔   cup rice
1⅓   cups frozen lima beans
  1   large tomato, coarsely chopped
  2   teaspoons finely slivered lemon zest
 18   littleneck clams, well scrubbed

1. In nonstick Dutch oven or flameproof casserole, heat oil over medium heat. Add leeks and garlic and cook, stirring frequently, for 7 minutes, or until leeks are tender.

2. Add carrots and chile pepper and cook for 5 minutes, or until carrots are crisp-tender.

3. Add lentils, stirring to coat. Add water and salt and bring to a boil over high heat. Reduce heat to a simmer, cover, and cook for 10 minutes.

4. Add rice, cover, and simmer for 10 minutes. Stir in lima beans, tomato, and lemon zest and cook for 2 minutes. Place clams on top of lentil-rice mixture. Cover and cook for 5 to 7 minutes, or until clams open (check after 3 minutes as some will open before others; discard any that do not open).

Per serving: 457 calories, 25 g protein, 79 g carbohydrates, 11 g fiber, 5 g total fat, 1 g saturated fat

Poached Salmon with Cucumber Dill Sauce

Serves 4

Poaching is one of the healthiest ways to cook meat and fish because the presence of water reduces the formation of harmful AGEs. It's also one of the tastiest. It seals juices into the meat, so the final result is moist rather than dry.

1½ cups water
 1 cup dry white wine or reduced-sodium chicken broth
 2 scallions, sliced
 8 black peppercorns
 4 salmon fillets (4 ounces each)
 ¾ cup nonfat sour cream
 ⅓ cup diced peeled cucumber
 2 tablespoons snipped fresh dill
 1 tablespoon fresh lemon juice
 ¼ teaspoon salt
 ⅛ teaspoon ground black pepper
    Fresh dill sprigs

1. Pour water into large nonstick skillet. Stir in wine or broth, scallions, and peppercorns. Put salmon in skillet in single layer and bring just to a boil over high heat.

2. Reduce heat to medium-low, cover, and simmer for 6 minutes, or until fish flakes when tested with a fork.

3. Meanwhile, in medium bowl, stir sour cream, cucumber, dill, lemon juice, salt, and pepper to make sauce. Refrigerate if not serving immediately.

4. Carefully transfer fillets with slotted spatula to large platter. Garnish with fresh dill sprigs. Serve hot or chilled with sauce.

Per serving: 229 calories, 27 g protein, 5 g carbohydrates, 0 g fiber, 10 g total fat, 2 g saturated fat

Curry-Seared Scallops

Serves 4

Low-fat yogurt gives this recipe a creamy texture without the saturated fat and calories of heavy cream. Serve over brown rice, quinoa, or another favorite whole grain.

½ cup low-fat plain yogurt
2 teaspoons cornstarch
1½ pounds sea scallops
1 tablespoon curry powder
½ teaspoon salt
3 tablespoons olive oil
1 package (10 ounces) grape or cherry tomatoes, halved
6 scallions, sliced

1. In a small bowl, combine the yogurt and cornstarch and set aside. Place the scallops in a medium bowl, sprinkle with the curry powder and salt, and toss to coat well.

2. Heat 2 tablespoons oil in a large nonstick skillet over medium-high heat. Add the scallops and cook, turning to brown all sides, until well browned and opaque, 3 to 6 minutes. With tongs or a slotted spoon, transfer to a plate.

3. Add the remaining 1 tablespoon oil to the skillet and reduce the heat to low. Add the tomatoes and scallions and cook until tender and lightly browned, about 4 minutes.

4. Return the scallops to the skillet along with the yogurt mixture. Cook until thickened and heated through, 2 minutes.

Per serving: 287 calories, 31 g protein, 12 g carbohydrates, 2 g fiber, 13 g total fat, 2 g saturated fat

Bok Choy, Tofu, and Mushroom Stir-Fry

Serves 4

A staple in Asian cuisines, bok choy is rich in several different antioxidants as well as inflammation-suppressing omega-3 fatty acids. You'll find it near other varieties of cabbage in the produce section of your grocery store.

- 15 ounces extra-firm tofu
- 3 tablespoons reduced-sodium soy sauce
- 4 teaspoons dark brown sugar
- 1½ teaspoons cornstarch
- 1 cup water
- 4 teaspoons olive oil
- 4 scallions, thinly sliced
- 2 tablespoons minced fresh ginger
- 3 cloves garlic, minced
- 8 ounces fresh shiitake mushrooms, stems removed and caps quartered
- 8 ounces button mushrooms, halved
- ¼ teaspoon salt
- 1 large head bok choy, sliced crosswise into 1-inch-wide strips

1. Halve tofu horizontally, then cut each piece into 12 squares or triangles. In small bowl, stir together soy sauce, brown sugar, cornstarch, and ½ cup water.

2. In large nonstick skillet, heat 2 teaspoons of the oil over medium heat. Add scallions, ginger, and garlic and cook for 1 minute, or until tender.

3. Stir in mushrooms. Add salt and remaining ½ cup water. Cover and cook, stirring occasionally, for 5 minutes, or until mushrooms are tender. Transfer to a bowl.

4. Add bok choy and remaining 2 teaspoons oil to skillet. Cook, stirring frequently, for 5 minutes, or until bok choy is tender.

5. Return mushroom-scallion mixture to skillet and add tofu. Stir soy sauce mixture to recombine and add to skillet. Cook for 2 minutes, or until tofu is heated through and vegetables are coated with sauce.

Per serving: 240 calories, 20 g protein, 20 g carbohydrates, 4 g fiber, 11 g total fat, 1 g saturated fat

Broccoli, Carrot, and Mushroom Stir-Fry

Serves 4

This quick vegetarian meal is loaded with brain-protecting antioxidants. It's also low in calories and rich in appetite-quelling fiber. It's a great meal to turn to when you're trying to lose weight.

- 2 tablespoons olive oil or canola oil
- 1 cup broccoli florets
- ⅔ cup carrots, julienned
- 8 scallions, sliced lengthwise
- ½ cup button mushrooms, sliced
- 2 cloves garlic, crushed
- 2 tablespoons light soy sauce
- 2 teaspoons honey
- 1 tablespoon rice vinegar
- 4 tablespoons cashew nuts

1. Heat 1 tablespoon olive oil or canola oil in a wok or nonstick frying pan. Add the broccoli florets and carrots, and stir-fry over high heat for 2 minutes.

2. Add the scallions and cook for another 2 minutes.

3. Stir in remaining olive oil or canola oil, plus the mushrooms and garlic. Stir-fry for 1 minute.

4. Pour in the soy sauce, honey, and rice vinegar. Heat through for 1 minute.

5. Remove from heat, sprinkle with the cashew nuts, and serve hot.

Per serving: 201 calories, 6 g protein, 15 g carbohydrates, 4 g fiber, 13 g total fat, 2 g saturated fat

Macaroni and Cheese with Spinach

Serves 6

In this version of this classic comfort food, we've added four whole cups of antioxidant-rich spinach, as well as fiber from wheat germ. Double the recipe and use the leftovers to accompany salads for lunch later in the week.

- 1¾ cups cold low-fat milk
- 3 tablespoons all-purpose flour
- 2 cups (6 ounces) grated extra-sharp Cheddar cheese
- 1 cup 1% cottage cheese
- ⅛ teaspoon ground nutmeg
- ½ teaspoon salt, or to taste
- Ground black pepper to taste
- 10 ounces frozen spinach or 4 cups individually quick-frozen spinach
- 8 ounces whole wheat macaroni
- ¼ cup toasted wheat germ

1. Preheat oven to 400°F. Coat 8-inch square baking dish (2-quart capacity) with cooking spray. Bring large pot of lightly salted water to a boil for cooking macaroni.

2. Whisk ¼ cup milk with flour in small bowl until smooth. Set aside. In heavy medium saucepan, heat remaining 1½ cups milk over medium heat until steaming. Add flour mixture and cook, whisking constantly, for 2 to 3 minutes, or until sauce boils and thickens. Remove from heat. Add Cheddar cheese, stirring until melted. Stir in cottage cheese, nutmeg, salt, and pepper.

3. Cook spinach according to package directions. Drain, refresh under cold water, and press out excess moisture.

4. Cook macaroni in boiling water, stirring often, for 4 to 5 minutes, or until not quite tender. (The macaroni will continue to cook during baking.) Drain, rinse with cold running water, then drain again.

5. In large bowl, mix macaroni with cheese sauce. Spread half of macaroni mixture in baking dish. Spoon spinach on top. Spread remaining macaroni mixture over spinach layer. Sprinkle with wheat germ.

6. Bake for 35 to 45 minutes, or until bubbly and golden.

Per serving: 357 calories, 22 g protein, 40 g carbohydrates, 6 g fiber, 12 g total fat, 7 g saturated fat

Thai Noodles with Cashews and Stir-Fried Vegetables

Serves 4

This Asian-inspired dish is packed with brain-protecting antioxidants and is super easy to toss together. You'll find Thai curry paste in the international section of your grocery store or at a specialty Asian market.

- 1 onion
- ⅓ cup mushrooms
- 1 red bell pepper
- ½ pound bok choy
- ⅔ cup bean sprouts
- 2 tablespoons olive oil or canola oil
- 2 cloves garlic, crushed
- ⅓ cup unsalted cashew nuts
- ½ cup frozen soybeans
- 1 tablespoon Thai green curry paste
- 14 ounces fresh egg noodles

1. Finely slice the onion and mushrooms and dice the pepper. Wash and shred the bok choy and thoroughly wash the bean sprouts. Heat the oil in a large frying pan or wok over high heat. Add the garlic, onion, mushrooms, and pepper.

2. Stir-fry the vegetables for 2 minutes, then add the cashew nuts and continue to cook for another 3 minutes. Add the frozen soybeans and Thai green curry paste. Stir in the noodles, breaking them up with a spoon, then add the bok choy.

3. Stir-fry the mixture for 2 minutes, adding 1 to 2 tablespoons of cold water if it becomes too dry and the bok choy doesn't wilt. Add the bean sprouts and cook for a final minute before serving.

Per serving: 649 calories , 22 g protein, 82 g carbohydrates, 8 g fiber, 28 g total fat, 5 g saturated fat

SIDES

Fruity Brussels Sprouts

Serves 4

Many people avoid this antioxidant powerhouse veggie because they remember eating overcooked, mushy sprouts when they were children. This recipe chops the sprouts so finely and mixes them with so many other tasty foods that you and your family won't realize what you are eating. Serve it for dinner as a side dish to fish or chicken or as the main course for lunch.

- 3 teaspoons crème fraîche
- 1½ tablespoons low-fat mayonnaise
- 2 teaspoons olive oil
  Grated zest and juice of 1 orange
- 2 teaspoons white wine vinegar
  Salt and ground black pepper
- 8 ounces Brussels sprouts
- 1 apple
- 1 carrot, grated
- 3 celery stalks, chopped
- 2 tablespoons chopped fresh cilantro
- 1 ounce fresh dates, stoned and chopped

1. In a small bowl, whisk together crème fraîche, mayonnaise, oil, orange zest and juice, and vinegar. Season to taste with salt and pepper. Set dressing aside.

2. Trim off and discard bases and outer leaves of sprouts, then shred finely and put into a large bowl. Cut unpeeled apple into quarters, remove core, and chop into small chunks. Add to bowl along with carrot and celery.

3. Stir in enough dressing to coat salad, saving any left over to serve on the side. Scatter cilantro and dates over salad and serve.

   Per serving: 122 calories, 2 g protein, 18 g carbohydrates, 4 g fiber, 5 g total fat, 1 g saturated fat

Warm Potato and Lima Bean Salad

Serves 4

Lima beans add fiber to this traditional picnic offering, helping to slow the release of sugar into the bloodstream. Serve it as a side dish to fish or chicken.

- 1 pound baby new potatoes
- 4 cups fresh lima beans or
- 1²⁄₃ cups frozen baby lima beans
- 1 teaspoon sugar
- 1 teaspoon English mustard
- 1 teaspoon cider vinegar
- 3 tablespoons olive oil
- 3 large sprigs thyme
     Salt and ground black pepper
- 4 ounces beet leaves or mixed
     salad leaves
- 4 tablespoons snipped fresh chives

1. Put the potatoes in a large saucepan and add boiling water to cover. Return to a boil, reduce heat, cover, and cook for 10 minutes. Meanwhile, shell the lima beans, if using fresh ones. Soak the shelled beans in a bowl of hot water for 3 to 4 minutes before peeling off the pale green outer skins. Add the beans to the potatoes, return to a boil, cover, and cook for 4 minutes or until tender.

2. Make a vinaigrette by whisking the sugar, mustard, and vinegar in a large bowl until the sugar has dissolved. Whisk in the oil and rub the thyme leaves off the stalks and into the bowl. Season to taste with salt and pepper.

3. Make a bed of salad greens on 4 plates. Drain the potatoes and beans and stir them into the vinaigrette. Sprinkle with chives and mix again. Top the greens with the potato and bean salad.

Per serving: 247 calories, 7 g protein, 28 g carbohydrates, 6 g fiber, 13 g total fat, 2 g saturated fat

Napa Cabbage Slaw with Peanut Dressing

Serves 6

Regular coleslaw is full of fat and calories, but this version uses vinegar, soy sauce, and hot sauce to give this picnic favorite an Asian feel. A rich variety of brain-protecting antioxidants comes from the cabbage, carrots, tea, and hot sauce. Serve it as a side dish for lunch or dinner.

- ⅓ cup natural peanut butter
- ¼ cup hot brewed black or green tea
- 4 teaspoons reduced-sodium soy sauce
- 4 teaspoons rice vinegar
- 1½ teaspoons brown sugar
- 1 teaspoon hot sauce, such as sriracha, chile-garlic sauce, or Tabasco
- 1 clove garlic, minced
- 4 cups thinly sliced napa cabbage
- 1 cup shredded carrots
- ½ cup chopped scallions
- ⅓ cup unsalted roasted peanuts

1. Place peanut butter in large bowl and gradually whisk in hot tea. Add soy sauce, vinegar, brown sugar, hot sauce, and garlic and whisk until smooth.

2. Add cabbage, carrots, and scallions and toss to coat well. Sprinkle with peanuts.

Per serving: 158 calories, 7 g protein, 11 g carbohydrates, 3 g fiber, 11 g total fat, 2 g saturated fat

Braised Mixed Greens with Dried Currants

Serves 4 to 6

Here's a quick and easy way to cook up a serving of delicious brain-protective greens. Make this side dish over and over again until you've got it stored in your brain as a habit loop.

- 1 tablespoon extra-virgin olive oil
- 3 cloves garlic, thinly sliced
- 1 pound mixed cooking greens (collards, kale, turnip greens, and mustard), rinsed and slightly drained
- 1 tablespoon dried currants

1. In small skillet, heat oil and garlic over low heat, stirring, until garlic begins to sizzle. Watch carefully and remove from heat when garlic begins to turn golden, after about 5 minutes. Set aside.

2. In large wide pan, cook greens and currants over medium heat, covered, turning once or twice with tongs, for 10 minutes, or until wilted and tender. Raise heat to high. Cook, uncovered, to evaporate any excess moisture.

3. Add garlic and reheat, stirring, for 1 minute.

Per serving: 81 calories, 3 g protein, 10 g carbohydrates, 4 g fiber, 4 g total fat, 1 g saturated fat

New Potatoes with Nori

Serves 4

By boiling the potatoes instead of roasting them, you reduce the formation of harmful acrylamide. Serve them as a side dish.

- 1 **pound unpeeled small new potatoes**
- 1 **ounce butter**
  Grated zest and juice of ½ small lemon
- 1 **sheet toasted sushi nori, about 8 x 7 inches**
  Salt and ground black pepper
- 2 **tablespoons snipped fresh chives**

1. Cook potatoes in saucepan of boiling water for 12 minutes, or until just tender.

2. Reserve 3 tablespoons of cooking water, then drain potatoes and return them to saucepan with reserved water. Add butter and lemon zest and juice, and toss potatoes to coat with liquid.

3. Use scissors to snip sushi nori into fine strips. Sprinkle nori over potatoes and cover pan. Cook over low heat for 1 to 2 minutes, or until nori has softened. Add salt and pepper to taste, sprinkle with chives, and serve.

Per serving: 134 calories, 2 g protein, 19 g carbohydrates, 2 g fiber, 6 g total fat, 4 g saturated fat

DESSERTS

Chock-Full Chocolate Chip Cookies

Makes 5 Dozen

Dark chocolate provides plenty of brain-boosting antioxidants. And at just 97 calories per cookie, these dark chocolate–rich treats come in the perfect portion size to enjoy.

- 1½ cups whole wheat pastry flour
- 1 cup whole oats, ground
- ⅓ cup cocoa powder
- 1 teaspoon baking soda
- ½ teaspoon salt
- 1 cup nonhydrogenated butter-replacement stick margarine
- ½ cup granulated sugar
- 1 cup packed light brown sugar
- 2 eggs
- 1 tablespoon vanilla extract
- 1 cup bittersweet chocolate chips (60% or higher cocoa content)
- 1 cup raisins
- 1 cup walnuts, coarsely chopped

1. Preheat the oven to 350°F. In a medium bowl, whisk together the flour, oats, cocoa, baking soda, and salt.

2. In a large bowl, with an electric mixer at medium speed, beat the margarine with the granulated and brown sugar until light and fluffy, 2 minutes. Add the eggs and vanilla and beat until smooth. Beat in the flour mixture until combined. Stir in the chocolate chips, raisins, and walnuts. Drop by teaspoons onto a baking sheet.

3. Bake until browned, 10 minutes. Let cool on the baking sheet for 2 minutes, then transfer to a rack and let cool completely.

Per serving: 97 calories, 1 g protein, 12 g carbohydrates, 1 g fiber, 5 g total fat, 2 g saturated fat

Chocolate Fondue

Serves 10

Fondue offers a wonderful way to turn any healthy food into a sweet dessert. Use it as a dip for apples, figs, oranges, pears, strawberries, and every other variety of fruit that you love.

- 1 **cup low-fat evaporated milk**
- ¼ **cup sugar**
- ¼ **cup cocoa powder**
- 1 **tablespoon vanilla extract**
- ½ **package (6 ounces) bittersweet chocolate chips (60% or higher cocoa content)**

1. In a small saucepan, whisk together the milk, sugar, cocoa, and vanilla until well blended. Add the chocolate chips.

2. Place over low heat and cook, stirring occasionally, until melted, 10 minutes. Pour into a fondue pot or small slow cooker set on low.

   Per serving: 128 calories, 3 g protein, 20 g carbohydrates, 1 g fiber, 5 g total fat, 3 g saturated fat

Fig, Apple, and Cinnamon Compote

Serves 4

This delicious, antioxidant-rich snack uses cinnamon as a sweetener instead of sugar, bringing the calories down to just 143 per serving.

- 2 **eating apples (such as McIntosh or Red Delicious)**
- 1 **baking apple (such as Granny Smith)**
- ½ **cup orange juice**
- 4 **dried figs, chopped**
- 1 **teaspoon ground cinnamon**
- 2 **tablespoons toasted pine nuts**

1. Slice apples and place in a saucepan with orange juice, figs, and cinnamon.

2. Bring to a boil, then reduce the heat and simmer, uncovered, for 20 minutes, or until the apples are tender when gently pressed with the back of a spoon.

3. Sprinkle with pine nuts, divide among 4 bowls, and serve hot.

   Per serving: 143 calories, 2 g protein, 22 g carbohydrates, 4 g fiber, 6 g total fat, 0 g saturated fat

Fresh Figs with Raspberries and Rose Cream

Serves 4

Figs are a delicious treat that happen to be loaded with antioxidant goodness.

3½ ounces crème fraîche, or sour cream mixed with a little confectioners' sugar
2 teaspoons raspberry jam
Finely grated zest of 1 lime
1–2 tablespoons rosewater, or to taste
8 small ripe, juicy figs
4 large fresh fig leaves (optional)
7 ouncees fresh raspberries
Fresh mint leaves

1. Place crème fraîche in a bowl and beat in raspberry jam and lime zest until jam is well distributed. Add rosewater and stir to mix. Transfer rose cream to a serving bowl.

2. Cut each fig vertically into quarters without cutting all the way through, so they remain whole. Arrange fig leaves, if using, on 4 plates and place 2 figs on each plate.

3. Spoon a dollop of rose cream into center of each fig. Serve remaining cream separately. Scatter raspberries over plates, garnish with mint leaves, and serve.

Per serving: 162 calories, 2 g protein, 20 g carbohydrates, 5 g fiber, 10 g total fat, 6 g saturated fat

Pineapple and Kiwifruit with Gingersnap Cream

Serves 4

This light dessert helps you get in a serving of kiwifruit, known to improve sleep.

½ pineapple
4 kiwifruit
4 pieces preserved ginger stem
6 large fresh mint leaves
4 gingersnaps
1 cup low-fat cream cheese, softened
4 sprigs fresh mint, to garnish

1. Peel, core, and slice the pineapple into wedges. Peel, thickly slice the kiwifruit, and cut each slice in half. Thinly slice the preserved ginger stem. Shred the mint leaves and toss with the pineapple and kiwifruit.

2. In a plastic bag, crush the gingersnaps with a rolling pin to make fine crumbs. Stir the gingersnap crumbs into the cream cheese.

3. Arrange the pineapple and kiwifruit on 4 plates with a large spoonful of gingersnap cream cheese on the side. Top the cream cheese with sliced ginger and garnish each portion with a mint sprig.

Per serving: 217 calories, 9 g protein, 33 g carbohydrates, 4 g fiber, 5 g total fat, 2 g saturated fat

Pomegranate Ice

Serves 4

Pomegranates are loaded with brain-protecting antioxidants. Commercially prepared Italian ice is often heavy on the sugar and light on the fruit. Though this version requires you to plan ahead, it tastes just as delicious as anything you could buy at a store.

    2 cups pomegranate-blueberry juice (100% juice)
    ¼ cup lime juice
    2 tablespoons sugar

In a 9-inch square metal baking pan, whisk together the pomegranate juice, lime juice, and sugar until the sugar dissolves. Freeze for 1 hour, then stir to blend in any frozen portions. Freeze, stirring every 45 minutes to incorporate frozen portions, until the mixture has a uniform slushy consistency and ice crystals form, about 4 hours.

Per serving: 98 calories, 1 g protein, 25 g carbohydrates, 0 g fiber, 0 g total fat, 0 g saturated fat

CHAPTER 11

....

Brain Smart Fitness Routines

In this chapter you'll find two fitness routines. The first is a more intense circuit that's appropriate for people without joint or mobility issues. The second is a lower-impact routine designed for people who are frail, out of shape, or who have joint pain. Choose the routine that is right for you.

The 7-Minute Circuit

Designed by Chris Jordan, Director of Exercise Physiology at the Johnson & Johnson Human Performance Institute, the workout has helped over 1.3 million people get the most out of every minute. Depending on your fitness and available time, you can do this routine just once or you can cycle through it two or three times to create a 14- to 21-minute session. Move swiftly from one exercise to another, trying to rest as little as possible between movements. Visit *https://7minuteworkout.jnj.com/* for more information about the free app that guides you through the workout.

Jumping jacks: Stand with your feet shoulder-width apart, knees slightly bent, arms at your sides. Jump your feet out to either side and extend your arms overhead. Return to the starting position and repeat for 30 seconds.

TIPS Stay on your toes. Keep your knees slightly bent.

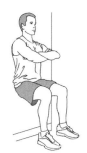

Wall sit: Stand with your feet shoulder-width apart, knees bent at 90 degrees, and back straight and supported against a wall. Fold your arms across your chest and hold this position for 30 seconds.

TIPS Make sure your knees are directly above your ankles. Keep your back flat against the wall. Don't forget to breathe!

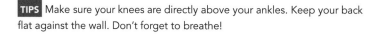

Push-ups: Start in the plank position, supporting your body with your hands and feet. Your hands should be just wider than shoulder-width apart, your body straight from head to heels, arms fully extended but not locked. Lower your body until your elbows are bent at 90 degrees, keeping your core muscles engaged. Return to the starting position and repeat for 30 seconds.

TIPS Keep your hips up and body straight. Don't sag! Breathe out as you push up. If you lack the strength for a regular push-up, start with a wall push-up. Stand with your feet a foot or two away from the wall. Then, keeping your back straight, bend your arms as you bring your chest closer to the wall. Straighten your arms to push away. Once wall push-ups feel easy, progress to regular push-ups but with your knees on the floor. Then, progress to doing some and eventually all of your push-ups with your legs extended.

Abdominal crunches: Lie on your back with your feet flat on the floor, knees bent. With arms extended over your thighs, engage your abs and raise your upper body slightly off the floor, keeping your chin off your chest. Return to the starting position and repeat for 30 seconds.

TIPS Look upwards and don't tuck your chin into your chest. Focus on squeezing your abs, not crunching up as high as you can. Don't pull on your head with your hands. Keep your head and neck in a neutral position.

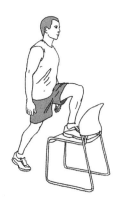

Step-ups: Stand in front of a chair, step, or bench with your feet shoulder-width apart, knees slightly bent, arms at your sides. Step up onto the chair with your left foot, then bring your right foot up so that you are standing with both feet on the chair. Step back down to the floor with your left foot, then your right. Repeat with your right foot leading. Switch back and forth for 30 seconds.

TIPS Make sure your entire foot is on the chair before you step up. Use a wall to help you balance, if necessary.

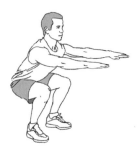

Squats: Stand with your feet shoulder-width apart, knees slightly bent, arms at your sides. Squat down by bending your knees, keeping your back straight and raising your arms in front of you until they are at shoulder level. Return to the starting position and repeat for 30 seconds.

TIPS When you bend down, don't let your knees stick out in front of your toes. And don't let your heels come off the floor. Use your arms to counterbalance you.

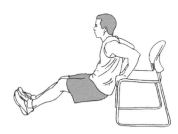

Triceps dips: Sit on a sturdy chair with your legs extended in front, feet on the floor. Hold on to the chair, arms fully extended but not locked. Slowly lower your body off the chair by bending your elbows to 90 degrees. Return to the starting position and repeat for 30 seconds.

TIPS Keep your knees slightly bent and your core engaged. Focus on bending your elbows and lowering yourself directly down towards the floor. Avoid going so deep that you feel pain in your shoulders.

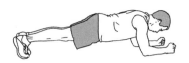

Forearm plank: Start facing the floor, supporting yourself on your elbows and forearms and the balls of your feet. Your body should be straight from head to heels. Hold for 30 seconds.

TIPS Keep your hips up and body straight. Don't sag, and don't forget to breathe.

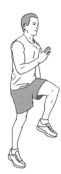

High knees: Run in place for 30 seconds, lifting your knees high, swinging your arms, and keeping your back straight.

TIPS Stay on your toes and keep your core engaged. Lift your knees as high as you can and swing your arms forcefully.

Lunges: Stand with your feet together, knees slightly bent, hands on hips. Step one foot forward and squat down by bending your knees, keeping your back straight and your front knee behind your toes. Return to the starting position and repeat with the other foot. Switch back and forth for 30 seconds.

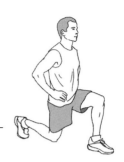

TIPS Lunge slowly at first and make sure you are stable. Focus on squatting down, not lunging forward, while maintaining an upright posture.

Push-ups with rotation: Start with your hands and feet on the floor, hands just wider than shoulder-width apart, body straight from head to heels, and arms fully extended but not locked. Lower your body until your elbows are bent at 90 degrees, keeping your core muscles engaged. Push up, rotate your upper body, and extend your right arm upwards. Return to the starting position and repeat, rotating to the other side. Switch back and forth for 30 seconds.

TIPS Keep your hips up and body straight. Don't sag! Rotate slowly at first and make sure you are stable. Use a wider foot stance to help maintain your balance, if necessary. Breathe out as you push up.

Side planks: Start on your right side, supporting yourself on your right elbow and forearm, legs extended, with the side of your right foot on the floor and your body straight from head to heels. Hold for 30 seconds. Repeat on the left side.

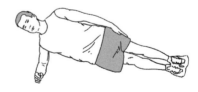

TIPS Keep your hips up and body straight. Don't sag, and don't forget to breathe.

Low-Impact Routine for People with Alzheimer's and/or Mobility Issues

Start by doing the routine just once. As fitness improves, restart at the beginning and do it one more time. You can also increase the challenge by holding hand weights or by using ankle weights. Start with 1-, 3-, or 5-pound weights and progress from there.

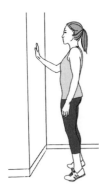

Toe and heel lifts: Stand with your feet hip distance apart. Place one or both hands against a wall or chair for balance. Lift onto the balls of your feet. Hold for a count of five. Lower and repeat 12 times.

Alternate each heel lift with a toe lift: Rock back onto your heels, lifting your toes off the ground. Hold for a count of five. Repeat 12 times.

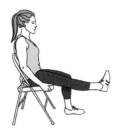

Knee straightening: Sit in a chair or on a bench. Raise and straighten one leg. Hold for a count of two, lower, and repeat 12 times. Then do the same with the other leg.

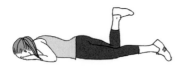

Back knee bends: Lie on your stomach. Bend one knee, moving your lower leg toward your thigh. Lower and repeat 12 times. Then switch and repeat with the other leg.

Marching: Stand with your feet hip distance apart. Slowly lift one knee, bringing your thigh toward your stomach. Lower and repeat with the other leg. Continue to switch back and forth until you've completed a total of 12 repetitions with each leg.

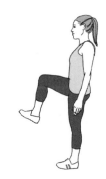

Side leg lifts: Stand with your feet hip distance apart. Slowly lift one extended leg out to the side. Lower and repeat 12 times. Then switch legs.

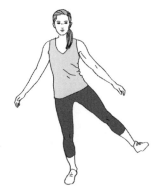

Back leg lifts: Stand with your feet hip distance apart. Slowly lift one extended leg behind you, as if you were trying to wipe mud off your shoes. Hold for a count of two. Repeat 12 times. Then switch to the other leg.

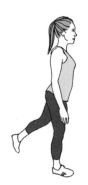

Chair squats: Stand just in front of a chair and with your feet hip distance apart. Slowly bend your knees as you lower your buttocks toward the seat of the chair. Just as your buttocks touch the seat, press into your feet as you raise back up. Repeat 12 times.

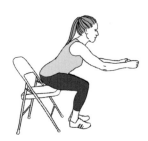

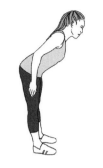

Forward lean: Stand with your feet hip distance apart. Keeping your back straight, slowly bend forward from your hips, just until you feel your abdominals tighten. Hold for a count of five. Raise and repeat 12 times.

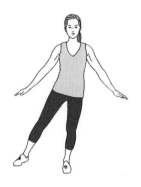

Balancing on one foot: Stand with your feet hip distance apart. Shift your body weight into one foot, lifting the other off the ground. Hold for as long as you can maintain your balance, placing a hand against a wall as needed. Lower and repeat with the other foot.

If this exercise becomes easy, you can increase the challenge by lifting your leg higher and then lowering and repeating, never allowing your foot to touch the ground. You can also try it while moving your arms into various positions—at your hips, out to the sides, out in front, extended overhead. Try turning your head back and forth or standing with your eyes closed.

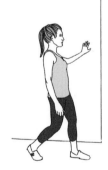

Backward walking: Walk backward, using your hand against a wall for balance. If backward walking is easy, try doing it with your eyes closed. And know the path so you don't fall.

CHAPTER 12

Brain Smart Games

You'll find almost 30 puzzles, games, and memory builders in the following pages. Make a habit of trying a few a day to challenge your mind. Once you run out of options here, keep up the habit by signing up for apps such as Clockwork Brain, What's the Word?, and Unblock Me, by doing the puzzles and jumbles that come in your newspaper, or by buying puzzle books.

Brain-Teasing Puzzles and Problems

These challenging, but fun, exercises help to strengthen your spatial and problem-solving skills.

SEATING PLAN

People to seat:

Kate's Aunt Alice and Uncle Bob (married couple)

Larry's Cousin Carl

Kate's Cousin Dave

Larry's Aunt Ella and Uncle Frank (married couple)

Kate's Uncle George

Larry's Aunt Harriet

Kate's Cousin Ida

Larry's Uncle Jack

Seating restrictions (in order of importance)

1. All of Kate's relatives sit together, and all of Larry's relatives sit together

2. Married couples must sit together

3. Cousin Dave plays in a rock band and wants to sit as close to the band as possible

4. You're trying to get Cousin Carl to date Cousin Ida, so seat them together

5. Uncle Frank isn't talking to Uncle Jack, so they can't sit next to each other

6. Uncle George owes money to Cousin Dave, so he wants to sit as far from Dave as possible

7. Uncle Bob hasn't seen Uncle George for 20 years, and they have a lot to catch up on

Answers on page 254

ROCK BAND

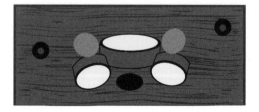

DINING WITH FRIENDS

	Vincent	Laura	Paul	Sophie	Matthew	Charlotte	
2	chocolate eclairs	roast beef	salad	apple tart	soufflé	courgette gratin	0
2	lamb stew	ratatouille	roast beef	asparagus	apple tart	grilled cheese	0
1	apple tart	bruschetta	soufflé	meat pie	courgette gratin	roast beef	1
2	courgette gratin	couscous	soufflé	roast beef	chocolate eclairs	apple tart	2
0	cake	soup	mashed potatoes	meat pie	macaroni and cheese	ratatouille	0
2	asparagus	apple tart	salad	couscous	courgette gratin	sweets	2
1	soup	cake	macaroni and cheese	grilled cheese	mashed potatoes	ratatouille	1
3	couscous	lamb stew	sweets	asparagus	chicken	mashed potatoes	0

Dining with friends

Three couples get together to organize an evening with friends. As there will be many guests, they have decided to share the work of preparing or buying the various items for the meal. You have to determine who will be preparing what.

In each horizontal row, the number on the left indicates how many of the dishes will be prepared by the cooks, and the figure on the right tells you how many of these dishes are recorded under the name of the right person.

Don't do this logigram if you are tired, because it needs sustained concentration. Choose a time when you feel relaxed and can think clearly. And, most especially, take time to understand, analyze, and organize your ideas. You might want to note them down on a piece of paper.

Answers on page 254

STACK TRACKING

For this exercise you'll need:
- **A pen or pencil**
- **A watch or clock with a second hand**

Below you'll see a grid containing geometric shapes with the names of the shapes underneath. Your goal is to ensure that the shapes and names match, so that each shape has a correct name in the corresponding position on the grid. If you run across a mistake, circle the incorrect word and continue on.

For example:

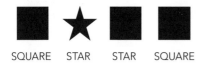

SQUARE   STAR   STAR   SQUARE

Third word ("star") should be circled.

These exercises will be scored for accuracy. But time is also important, so work as quickly as possible. When you have completed each page, write down the amount of time you needed to finish in the space provided at the bottom. Score the exercise before moving on to the next one. When you are ready, set the timer and begin!

Stack Tracking #1

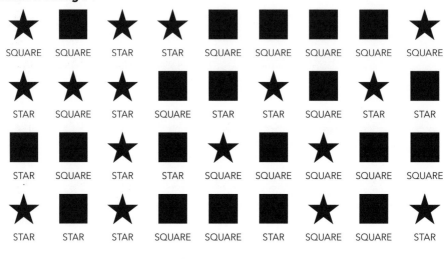

TIME _____ ITEMS CIRCLED INCORRECTLY _____ MISSED MISTAKES _____

STACK TRACKING (CONTINUED)

Stack Tracking #2

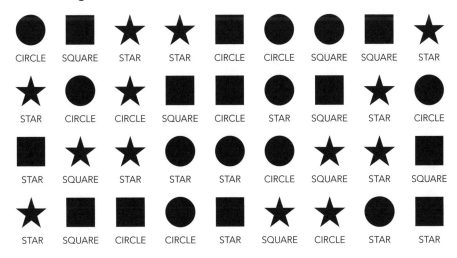

CIRCLE	SQUARE	STAR	STAR	CIRCLE	CIRCLE	SQUARE	SQUARE	STAR
STAR	CIRCLE	CIRCLE	SQUARE	CIRCLE	STAR	SQUARE	STAR	CIRCLE
STAR	SQUARE	STAR	STAR	STAR	CIRCLE	SQUARE	STAR	SQUARE
STAR	SQUARE	CIRCLE	CIRCLE	STAR	SQUARE	CIRCLE	STAR	STAR

TIME _____ ITEMS CIRCLED INCORRECTLY _____ MISSED MISTAKES _____

Stack Tracking #3

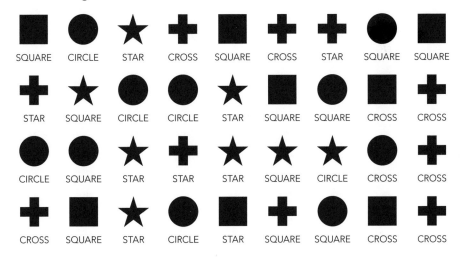

SQUARE	CIRCLE	STAR	CROSS	SQUARE	CROSS	STAR	SQUARE	SQUARE
STAR	SQUARE	CIRCLE	CIRCLE	STAR	SQUARE	SQUARE	CROSS	CROSS
CIRCLE	SQUARE	STAR	STAR	STAR	SQUARE	CIRCLE	CROSS	CROSS
CROSS	SQUARE	STAR	CIRCLE	STAR	SQUARE	SQUARE	CROSS	CROSS

TIME _____ ITEMS CIRCLED INCORRECTLY _____ MISSED MISTAKES _____

STACK TRACKING (CONTINUED)

Stack Tracking #4

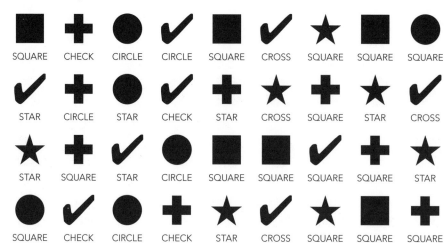

TIME _____ ITEMS CIRCLED INCORRECTLY _____ MISSED MISTAKES _____

Stack Tracking #5

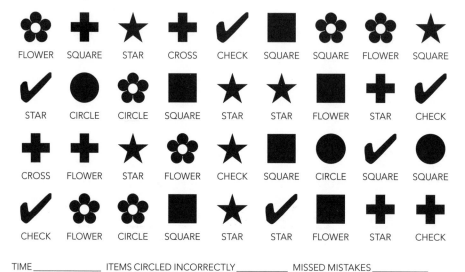

TIME _____ ITEMS CIRCLED INCORRECTLY _____ MISSED MISTAKES _____

Answers on page 254

WORDS AND NUMBERS

These exercises will help you solve everyday problems involving numbers.

Words and Numbers #1

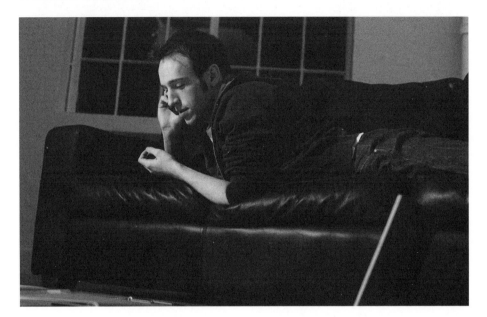

Dan is a full-time college student who has a part-time job. His girlfriend lives hundreds of miles away. On a particular day, his classes end at 4 p.m., after which he immediately drives to his job, arrives at 4:15 p.m., and works for 3½ hours, plus a 45-minute break for dinner. After work, he drives straight home, immediately starts studying, and continues studying for 2 hours and 10 minutes, and then telephones his girlfriend at 11 p.m. How long was Dan's drive from work to his home?

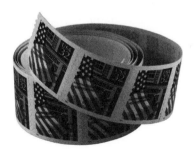

Words and Numbers #2

Dorothy loves entering contests by mail. She had an old roll of 100 42-cent stamps and used 55 of them before the rate went up to 44 cents per letter. If she already has 7 1-cent stamps and 8 2-cent stamps, how much does she have to spend on additional postage so she can use her remaining 42-cent stamps to mail her contest entries?

WORDS AND NUMBERS (CONTINUED)

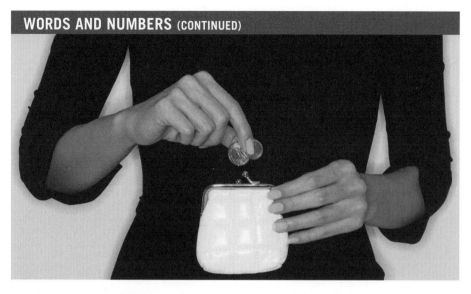

Words and Numbers #3

Jacqueline has 11 coins in her purse, all pennies, dimes, or quarters, and doesn't have any combination of coins that adds up to exactly $1.00. If the total value of her coins is more than $1.00, how many each of pennies, dimes, and quarters does she have?

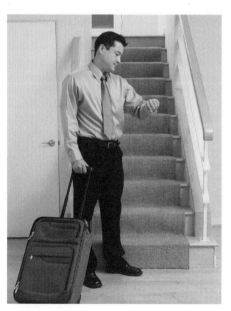

Words and Numbers #4

A certain airline has a weight limit of 20 pounds for a piece of carry-on baggage. Marc's empty suitcase weighs 1 pound, and he has these items that he'd like to put in it for his flight:

Jar of snacks: 2 pounds

Travel iron: 3 pounds

Crossword dictionary: 4 pounds

Gift for his mother: 7 pounds

Laptop computer: 9 pounds

Which of these items should he take, if he'd like to take as much (by weight) as possible?

Answers on page 255

OVERLAPPING SHAPES

How many squares can you see?

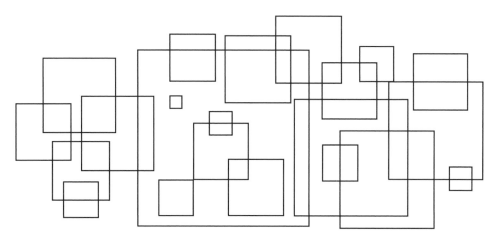

Answers on page 255

THE RIGHT TIME

1. Find the clock giving the right time, taking into account that one of the clocks is 7 hours fast while another is 7 hours slow.

2. Same question, but this time one of the clocks is 5 hours slow and another 5 hours fast.

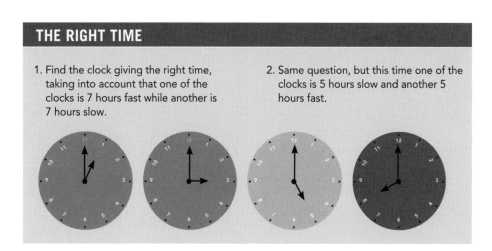

Answers on page 255

NUMBER SEQUENCES

Complete the logical sequence of the following numbers, taking due note of the geometric shapes associated with them.

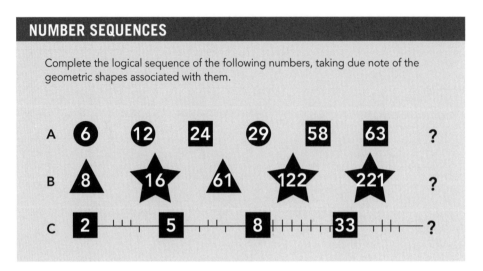

Answers on page 255

MATCHES

Move only one match to change the five squares into six squares.

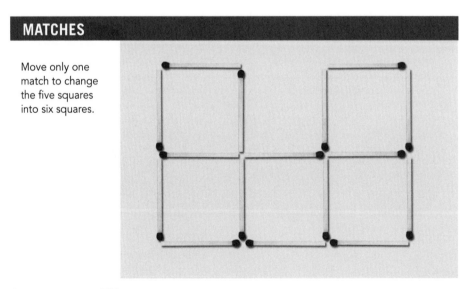

Answers on page 255

MAGIC SQUARE

On this box are superimposed three rows of three circles, the central one of which contains the number 5. Using a range of numbers from 1 to 9 fill in the circles in such a way that each line of three circles, vertical, diagonal, and horizontal, adds up to the number 15. You will have to feel your way through this puzzle.

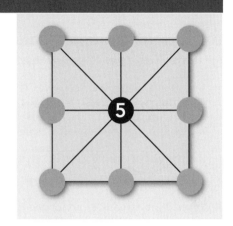

Answers on page 255

NUMBER PYRAMID

Each brick in the number pyramid is the sum of the two bricks immediately below it. Fill in all the numbers by making use of those already in place.

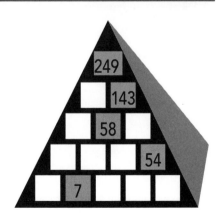

Answers on page 256

Memory Joggers

These exercises and games will take you or the person you are caring for on a trip down memory lane. Each one helps you to uncover memories of the past with the help of your senses (sight, touch, sound, sensation).

YOU MUST REMEMBER THIS

For this exercise, you'll need a timer.

Set the timer for 5 minutes. Read one of the questions, then close your eyes and remember all the details you can. Try to think on all sensory fronts: sight, sound, smell, taste, and touch. Don't rush the process; take the full 5 minutes. After the timer goes off, open your eyes. Did you remember more than you thought you would?

1. How did you celebrate your 13th birthday?

2. How did you get to school in the 5th grade?

3. What do you remember about your best friend's wedding?

4. What do you remember about your most recent vacation?

5. Where and with whom was your first kiss?

6. What was the best birthday present you ever got?

7. What do you remember most about your grandparents?

8. How did you spend summers as a child?

9. Which dance steps or music groups were popular when you were in high school?

10. What do you remember about the first job you ever held?

11. What books did you read in the past year?

12. What movies did you see in the past year?

13. How did you and your friends spend your time after school when you were 10?

14. What was your first pet?

15. What was your most intimidating moment?

16. When did you get your first bicycle?

17. What was your favorite book as a kid?

18. Who was your favorite grade-school teacher?

19. What did the first house you lived in look like?

20. Who was your first crush?

ASSOCIATE THE SMELLS

Dig deep into your memory to find links between these kinds of smells and events or emotions you have experienced.

Burning Body odor Chlorine Musk **Fruit**

Iodine *Sulphur*

Cleanliness **Ammonia** Flowers

Caramel Mold

Rotting fish

▶ Smells stimulate all the senses. The more highly developed your sense of smell, the more alert your senses will be. Try to copy animals—they make full use of an excellent sense of smell—by going beyond merely visual and/or auditory perception to enable your brain to respond to all aspects of the information reaching it. When choosing a melon, for example, don't just look at it—smell it and touch it as well.

HOLIDAY MEMORIES

Give examples of holiday memories relating to each of your five senses.

Example: the sound of waves crashing on a beach outside your window at night, the taste of a local cheese in a cheese factory, the sights of a souk in Marrakesh with its colorful display of exotic goods, the smell and vivid colors of a spice market.

Sights ....

....

Sounds ....

....

Tastes ....

....

Smells ....

....

Touch ....

....

SCENTS AND SENSIBILITY

For this exercise, you'll need:
- **A pen or pencil**
- **A timer**

Certain scents have the amazing ability to bring you right back to a particular time, place, or moment in your life. The olfactory bulb, the area of the brain that perceives smells, is part of the brain's limbic system, which plays a major role in long-term memory, especially emotional memories.

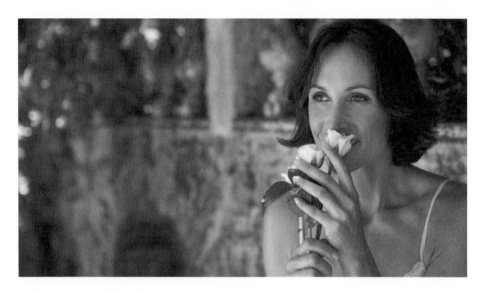

Scents and Sensibility #1

Set the timer for 5 minutes. Look at the list below and choose one of the scents. If you happen to have access to the scent, take a good whiff. Then, sit down without any distractions and imagine the smell as best you can. Let your mind recall every detail of the memories it evokes. Don't rush the process; take the full 5 minutes. Later, come back and do this exercise with other scents from the list.

Cinnamon	Floral perfume	Rubbing alcohol
Warm apple pie	Baby powder	Aftershave
Warm chocolate chip cookies	Cut grass	Nutmeg
Freshly sharpened lead pencil	Worms after a rainstorm	Shoe polish
Fresh pine (or a pine-scented candle)	Manure	Baking bread
	Homemade chicken soup	Burning leaves
Roses	Mulled wine	Stinky cheese
Musk	Musty books	Strawberry lip gloss
Skunk	Wood smoke	Lake water
	Hay	Chlorine
	Tobacco	

Scents and Sensibility #2

Think of a scent that has special meaning for you. Maybe it's the perfume your mother wore to church on Sundays, an old lover's aftershave, chicken fat from your grandmother's kitchen, a sycamore tree from your childhood backyard, a leather chair from your father's study, machine oil or melting solder or sawdust from your uncle's workshop, or burnt marshmallows from summer camp. The possibilities are endless. For each scent you think of, write down the memory you associate with it.

Scent: _____

Memory: _____

_____

_____

_____

Scent: _____

Memory: _____

_____

_____

_____

Scent: _____

Memory: _____

_____

_____

_____

Scent: _____

Memory: _____

_____

_____

_____

Memory Skills

Do you have trouble remembering your PIN number? Passwords to the computer? These exercises will help you to learn and practice skills like "chunking" and "repeating" to make remembering a series of numbers, letters, or shapes come more easily.

PIN MANIA

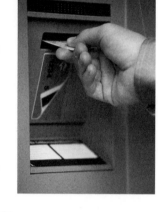

These days, most of us have far too many PINs (personal identification numbers) to remember. Take a look at each of the four PINs below, and try to make an association with the number to help you remember it. Once you've thought of something solid, move on to another puzzle, then turn to page 256 to see if you can write in the PIN numbers you memorized.

For example: 7613

A person familiar with the song "Seventy-Six Trombones" from The Music Man might think of that song for the first two digits. Someone with a 13-year-old child might use the child's age to remember the second two.

PIN Mania #1
Richard's ATM PIN: 4923

PIN Mania #2
Edwin's email PIN: 403214

PIN Mania #3
Michelle's online banking PIN: 120489

PIN Mania #4
Eric's online travel site PIN: 52547

CALLER ID

Who's calling? Look at the names and phone numbers below. Try to remember which phone numbers are whose. Then turn to page 246 and see how well you do.

Caller ID #1

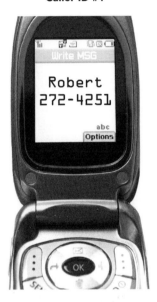

Robert
272-4251

Caller ID #2

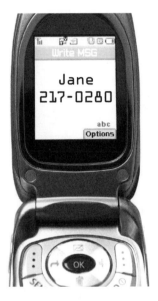

Jane
217-0280

Caller ID #3

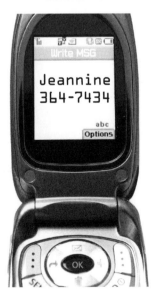

Jeannine
364-7434

Caller ID #4

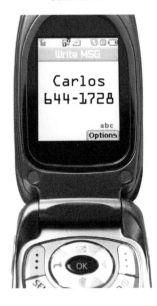

Carlos
644-1728

CALLER ID (CONTINUED)

Circle the correct name for each of the numbers, then turn back to page 245 to see how you did.

Caller ID #1
272-4251

A. Jane
B. Carlos
C. Robert
D. Jeannine

Caller ID #2
217-0280

A. Jane
B. Carlos
C. Robert
D. Jeannine

Caller ID #3
364-7434

A. Jane
B. Carlos
C. Robert
D. Jeannine

Caller ID #4
644-1728

A. Jane
B. Carlos
C. Robert
D. Jeannine

DRAWING FROM MEMORY

Look carefully at these drawings. Close your eyes and try to visualize them in relation to each other. If you forget one of them, look at it again to consolidate the image.

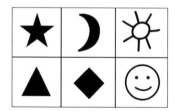

Cover the pictures and try to
draw them all from memory.

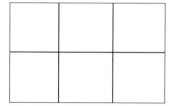

TEST YOUR NUMBER SPAN

5 4 2   ....

0 3 6   ....

6 0 9 2   ....

9 5 1 8   ....

6 4 2 9 6   ....

7 4 2 8 1   ....

5 4 8 2 6 3   ....

3 9 5 7 6 2   ....

0 1 5 1 2 3 7   ....

1 9 6 3 7 5 1   ....

7 5 8 2 6 3 6 4   ....

6 5 2 9 3 7 6 0   ....

5 6 3 2 1 4 8 7 0   ....

2 8 4 6 1 0 3 5 9   ....

5 6 3 2 8 9 7 4 0 1   ....

8 5 9 3 2 6 4 0 1 7 ....

Before starting this exercise, make sure you have something with which you can cover up the lines of numbers. Uncover the first line and read the digits one at a time. Cover them again and in the space opposite write down those you remember. When you've done that, move to the following line and repeat the exercise to the end.

Now check your answers. The last line of digits that you have correctly noted down will give you your number span. For example, if your mistakes start at line 13, then you have a number span of 8 (line 12 has 8 digits).

▶We tend to remember numbers only if they interest us for a special reason, if they have an emotional connotation, or if we can associate them with something familiar to us. Such a figure would be the age of someone close to you, your graduation day, the birth of a child, your zip code, etc. If they don't evoke anything in particular and remain abstract entities, without associations that make them easy to remember, it would be difficult, if not impossible, to recall them. This could explain why the number span is lower in some people than in others and, more generally, why a fair number of people feel a certain resistance, if not blockage, when it comes to numbers.

Vocabulary Builders

These fun exercises will all help you boost and strengthen your vocabulary, bolstering your cognitive reserve.

IRREGULAR WORDS

Below are groups of words. Within each group, one of the words does not fit in the same category as the others. Circle the irregular word.

1. Broccoli, Carrots, Spinach, Peas

2. Wristwatch, Bubble, Baseball, Globe

3. Eagle, Sparrow, Ostrich, Swan

4. Tennis, Ping-Pong, Polo, Volleyball

5. Antagonize, Anger, Inspire, Infuriate

6. Braille, Morse Code, Dominoes, Zebras

7. Duck, Badger, Camel, Hog

8. Tree, Ball, Watch, Mitt

9. Plant, Car, Money, Cash

10. Television, Magazine, Baseball Game, Movie

11. Tea Kettle, Whistle, Bathtub, Bird

12. Plant, Pipe, Brain, Toenail

13. Ice Skates, Roller Skates, Knife, Razor

14. Boat, Kickboard, Sunglasses, Wine Cork

OPPOSITES ATTRACT

Match each word with its antonym by writing a number next to each letter.

Opposites Attract #1

1. Elated   ____ **a.** Ally

2. Inspired   ____ **b.** Support

3. Lazy   ____ **c.** Beneficial

4. Obscure   ____ **d.** Acknowledge

5. Adversary   ____ **e.** Dejected

6. Pernicious   ____ **f.** Industrious

7. Oppose   ____ **g.** Ornery

8. Deny   ____ **h.** Ignore

9. Address   ____ **i.** Evident

10. Affable   ____ **j.** Unmotivated

Opposites Attract #2

1. Futile   ____ **a.** Yield

2. Penitent   ____ **b.** Disparaging

3. Boldness   ____ **c.** Unseemly

4. Agreeable   ____ **d.** Contrary

5. Defy   ____ **e.** Remorseless

6. Incessant   ____ **f.** Loquacious

7. Taciturn   ____ **g.** Useful

8. Careless   ____ **h.** Cowardice

9. Elegant   ____ **i.** Thoughtful

10. Fawning   ____ **j.** Intermittent

LINKUP

Below is a series of analogies. It's up to you to fill in the blanks. We've helped by providing the correct number of spaces needed.

1. DOWNPOUR is to RAIN as BLIZZARD is to: ___ ___ ___ ___

2. DOLLAR is to CENT as CENTURY is to: ___ ___ ___ ___

3. RECIPES is to COOKBOOK as MAPS is to: ___ ___ ___ ___ ___

4. BASEBALL is to BAT as TENNIS is to: ___ ___ ___ ___ ___ ___

5. BLUE is to SAPPHIRE as RED is to: ___ ___ ___ ___

6. COUGAR is to LEAP as WHALE is to: ___ ___ ___ ___ ___ ___

7. HEN is to ROOSTER as FILLY is to: ___ ___ ___ ___

8. MOON is to CRATER as PAVEMENT is to: ___ ___ ___ ___ ___ ___ ___

9. SPIDER is to CRAWL as SNAKE is to: ___ ___ ___ ___ ___ ___ ___

10. CANDY is to SUGAR as TIRE is to: ___ ___ ___ ___ ___ ___

11. AIRPLANE is to PILOT as LIMOUSINE is to: ___ ___ ___ ___ ___ ___ ___ ___ ___

12. HERD is to BUFFALO as GAGGLE is to: ___ ___ ___ ___ ___

13. SOLAR SYSTEM is to SUN as ATOM is to ___ ___ ___ ___ ___ ___ ___

14. ACROPHOBIA is to HEIGHTS as PYROPHOBIA is to: ___ ___ ___ ___

15. DOUGHNUT is to HOLE as IRIS is to: ___ ___ ___ ___ ___

16. EQUINE is to HORSE as AQUILINE is to: ___ ___ ___ ___ ___

17. TETHER is to BALL as CORD is to ___ ___ ___ ___ ___

Answers on page 256

KISSING COUSINS

Match each word with its synonym by writing a number next to each letter.

Kissing Cousins #1

1. Settle	____**a.** Resist
2. Entreat	____**b.** Compromise
3. Acquiesce	____**c.** Grave
4. Dismiss	____**d.** Coarse
5. Peevish	____**e.** Wander
6. Vulgar	____**f.** Enlarge
7. Roam	____**g.** Petulant
8. Oppose	____**h.** Implore
9. Amplify	____**i.** Ignore
10. Solemn	____**j.** Comply

Kissing Cousins #2

1. Egotism	____**a.** Evasiveness
2. Grateful	____**b.** Rugged
3. Approach	____**c.** Fixed
4. Rough	____**d.** Overstate
5. Immobile	____**e.** Unwavering
6. Imitate	____**f.** Vainglory
7. Secrecy	____**g.** Vanquished
8. Exaggerate	____**h.** Advance
9. Persistent	____**i.** Mirror
10. Conquered	____**j.** Appreciative

Answers on page 257

MOCK EXAM

You have 10 minutes to find 30 words beginning with the letter **A:** 5 first names, 5 plants, 5 animals, 5 countries, 5 cities in the world and, finally, 5 celebrities. Do the same with the letters **E, M,** and **P**.

Be methodical—think of the letters of the alphabet that could follow the first letter—and don't be put off by the stress imposed by the time limit. You could play this game alone or with several others, and further extend the game to include any other letters, or groups of letters (Pi, Mo, Dr…).

	Name	Plant	Animal	Country	City	Celebrity
A	....	....	....	....	....	....
	....	....	....	....	....	....
	....	....	....	....	....	....
	....	....	....	....	....	....
	....	....	....	....	....	....
E	....	....	....	....	....	....
	....	....	....	....	....	....
	....	....	....	....	....	....
	....	....	....	....	....	....
	....	....	....	....	....	....
M	....	....	....	....	....	....
	....	....	....	....	....	....
	....	....	....	....	....	....
	....	....	....	....	....	....
	....	....	....	....	....	....
P	....	....	....	....	....	....
	....	....	....	....	....	....
	....	....	....	....	....	....
	....	....	....	....	....	....
	....	....	....	....	....	....

▶ This mini-test is a good way to put your memory to work and stimulate verbal fluency. The unimpeded flow of words in the brain is an indication of rapid association. Remembering then becomes much easier.

THE LETTER CHASE

Change one letter in each of these words so that each new vertical column has a group of words on a single theme (one theme per set).

Set 1

CARE ....

DISH ....

SOCKS ....

LATER ....

BENCH ....

Set 2

BIND ....

ALOUD ....

PLANT ....

GUN ....

MOAN ....

Answers on page 257

CATERPILLAR

Move from one word to the next by replacing the letters indicated and changing the order of the letters.

CAPABLE

−B + S ....

−A + U ....

−P + S ....

−L + R ....

−C + D ....

−R + M ....

−U + A ....

−D + G ....

−A + E **MESSAGE**

Answers on page 257

ANAGRAMS

Find the animals hiding within the following anagrams.

1. SHORE ....

2. BRAZE ....

3. FLOW ....

4. DOING ....

5. PAROLED ....

6. TOAST ....

7. CORONA ....

8. TORTE ....

9. LOOPED ....

10. BARGED ....

Answers on page 257

WORD HOLES #1

Find the consonants that will enable you to complete the following words.

1. _ E _ E _ _ I _ I _ _

2. _ A _ A _ A _ I A

3. _ O _ O _ E _ O U _

4. _ I _ _ I _ _ I _ E

5. _ A I _ _ _ A _ E

6. _ _ I _ E _ I O _

Answers on page 257

WORD HOLES #2

By replacing each space with a letter, find six words that start with I, keeping to the same structure.

1. I _ _ _ _ _ G   4. I _ _ E _ _ M

2. I _ _ Q _ _ L _ _ Y   5. I _ L _ M

3. I _ S _ L _ _   6. I _ Y _ _

Answers on page 257

ANSWER KEY

SEATING PLAN

Clockwise from bottom center: Dave, Alice, Bob, George, Ida, Carl, Jack, Harriet, Frank, Ella

DINING WITH FRIENDS

Vincent: asparagus – **Laura:** chicken – **Paul:** soufflé – **Sophie:** grilled cheese – **Matthew:** chocolate eclairs – **Charlotte:** sweets.

STACK TRACKING

Stack Tracking #1

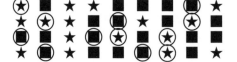

Stack Tracking #2

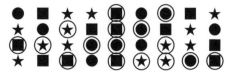

Stack Tracking #3

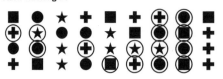

Stack Tracking #4

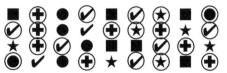

Stack Tracking #5

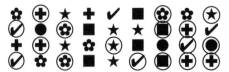

WORDS AND NUMBERS

Words and Numbers #1

20 minutes

Words and Numbers #2

67 cents

Words and Numbers #3

4 pennies, 4 dimes,
3 quarters

Words and Numbers #4

Travel iron, gift for mother, and laptop computer.
Total weight: 19 pounds.

OVERLAPPING SHAPES

There are 32 overlapping shapes.

THE RIGHT TIME

1. The clock registering 8 o'clock matches all the conditions. The one reading 1 o'clock is 7 hours behind, and the one reading 3 o'clock (pm) is 7 hours fast.

2. The answer is once again the clock showing 8 o'clock. The clock that reads 1 o'clock (pm) is 5 hours fast and the one reading 3 o'clock is 5 hours slow.

NUMBER SEQUENCES

A. 68: In a circle, you multiply by 2; in a square, you add 5. The next one is 63 + 5.

B. 122: a triangle multiplies by 2, a star reverses the meaning of what is written. So 221 is written from right to left and you get back to 122.

C. 62: multiply by the number of sticks above the line, and subtract the number of sticks below. The next is 33 x 2 – 4.

MATCHES

Four of the original squares are still in place, but two new squares have been created, four times larger than the original ones, made up of the two tiers on the left or the two tiers on the right of the figure. So the total is now 6 squares.

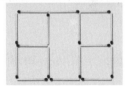

MAGIC SQUARE

This solution is one example, but there are several other possible solutions.

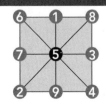

NUMBER PYRAMID

Start with 143. 143 – 58 = 85 to the right of 58. Then 85 – 54 = 31 to the left of 54, 58 – 31 = 27 to the left of 31. The numbers at the base are thus, to the right of the 7: 27 – 7 = 20, then 31 – 20 = 11 and 54 – 11 = 43 at the end on the right. Start at the top to finish the puzzle; on the fourth line up from the base, you have 249 – 143 = 106, on the third 106 – 58 = 48, on the second 48 – 27 = 21.

The first number at the left of the base is thus 21 – 7 = 14.

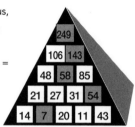

PIN MANIA

Write down the numbers you remember, then turn back to page 245 to see how you did.

PIN Mania #1
Richard's ATM PIN: _____

PIN Mania #3
Michelle's online banking PIN: _____

PIN Mania #2
Edwin's email PIN: _____

PIN Mania #4
Eric's online travel site PIN: _____

CALLER ID

Caller ID #1	**Caller ID #2**	**Caller ID #3**	**Caller ID #4**
272-4251	217-0280	364-7434	644-1728
A. Jane	**A.** Jane (circled)	**A.** Jane	**A.** Jane
B. Carlos	**B.** Carlos	**B.** Carlos	**B.** Carlos (circled)
C. Robert (circled)	**C.** Robert	**C.** Robert	**C.** Robert
D. Jeannine	**D.** Jeannine	**D.** Jeannine (circled)	**D.** Jeannine

IRREGULAR WORDS

1. Carrots (not green)
2. Wristwatch (not spherical)
3. Ostrich (can't fly)
4. Polo (not played with a net)
5. Inspire (not negative)
6. Zebras (don't have dots)
7. Camel (not a verb)
8. Watch (not four letters)
9. Money (the only word without the vowel "a")
10. Magazine (not something you watch)
11. Bathtub (doesn't make noise)
12. Pipe (doesn't grow)
13. Roller skates (aren't sharp)
14. Sunglasses (don't float)

LINKUP

1. snow **2.** year **3.** atlas **4.** racket **5.** ruby **6.** breach **7.** colt **8.** pothole **9.** slither **10.** rubber **11.** chauffeur **12.** geese **13.** nucleus **14.** fire **15.** pupil **16.** eagle **17.** phone

KISSING COUSINS

Kissing Cousins #1

1. b **2.** h **3.** j **4.** i **5.** g **6.** d
7. e **8.** a **9.** f **10.** c

Kissing Cousins #2

1. f **2.** j **3.** h **4.** b **5.** c **6.** i
7. a **8.** d **9.** e **10.** g

OPPOSITES ATTRACT

Opposites Attract #1
1. e **2.** j **3.** f **4.** i **5.** a **6.** c **7.** b **8.** d **9.** h **10.** g

Opposites Attract #2
1. g **2.** e **3.** h **4.** d **5.** a **6.** j **7.** f **8.** i **9.** c **10.** b

THE LETTER CHASE

CARE	CAPE	BIND	BIRD
DISH	FISH	ALOUD	CLOUD
SOCKS	ROCKS	PLANT	PLANE
LATER	WATER	GUN	SUN
BENCH	BEACH	MOAN	MOON

CATERPILLAR

CAPABLE

−B + S PALACES
− A + U CAPSULE
− P + S CLAUSES
− L + R SAUCERS
− C + D ASSURED
− R + M ASSUMED
− U + A AMASSED
− D + G MASSAGE
− A + E **MESSAGE**

ANAGRAMS

1. Horse
2. Zebra
3. Wolf
4. Dingo
5. Leopard
6. Stoat
7. Raccoon
8. Otter
9. Poodle
10. Badger

WORD HOLES #1

1. Serendipity
2. Macadamia
3. Homogenous
4. Discipline
5. Fairytale
6. Criterion

WORD HOLES #2

1. Iceberg
2. Inequality
3. Insular
4. Interim
5. Islam
6. Idyll

Brain Smarts Resources

A wide range of tools—ranging from the simple to the complex—can complement your efforts to outsmart Alzheimer's. In the following pages, you will find resources to help you incorporate Brain Smarts into your life and help support someone who is living with the disease.

Social Smarts Resources

As Alzheimer's progresses, it can become more difficult to remain socially connected. The following tech resources offer ways to stay socially connected, even when your memory is failing or your mobility is limited.

Tablets: The iPad and other handheld tablets (price range $50 to $400) can connect you with others without you ever leaving your home. Social media like Facebook allow you to see what friends and family are up to. Email and text messages can also help you to stay in touch, and FaceTime, Skype, and other video-messaging programs allow you to see the person you are talking to, and many of them are free.

Picture Phones: It's not always easy to remember a phone number or where to find it in an address book. Because of this, various landline phones come with auto-dial features, and some allow you to affix photos of the people you call most often. One of these phones, made by ClearSounds ($60 to $80), allows you to affix up to eight photos onto eight programmable buttons for easy speed dialing. The Big Button Phone Dialer from Sharper Image ($50) allows up to 12 photos to accompany frequently dialed numbers, and it can be connected to your existing phone. Many other brands and styles are also available.

POV Cameras: The same wearable technology that has provided us all with stunning adventure footage can also be used to help you remember your day, complementing your *autobiographical memory*.[414] These tiny, wearable cameras include wide angles and are nearly indestructible. You can set them to take a photo every few seconds throughout your day. Then you can download and review the photos each evening to remind yourself of what you did and, if possible, have a conversation with a friend, spouse, or other family member about your day.

The Narrative Clip camera is tiny and lightweight and can be affixed to your collar or lapel. It transmits images wirelessly to a smartphone app. Google Glass is similar in concept, but comes as a pair of eyeglasses that take photos, offer directions, translate languages, and perform other functions.

Another wearable camera, Looxcie is worn over your ear, and GoPro offers a wide variety of POV cameras that can be strapped to your body. The cameras vary in prices, from around $129 to well over $400. Some are waterproof and shock resistant, too.

Meal Smarts Resources

Other than a good knife, cutting board, measuring cups and spoons, and various pans and pots, you don't need much to cook a healthy meal. There are a few optional items, however, that can help you to accomplish your goal of eating more fruits and veggies as well as filling up on fewer calories.

Blender

These range in price from just $19.99 for the simplest, least powerful types, all the way up to $400 or even more for heavy-duty blending action. If you plan to make "green" smoothies with kale, you may want one of the more expensive ones, because their powerful motors help to emulsify greens so your drink is smooth and creamy rather than gritty and chunky. If you plan to mostly use fruit, an inexpensive, standard blender will probably work just fine.

Appetizer Plates

To fill up on fewer calories, you may also wish to invest in a set of multi-colored appetizer plates and matching tablecloths. Research done at the Cornell Food and Brand lab found that we perceive food portions as larger—and consequently feel more satisfied—when they appear on small plates. For example, the exact same size serving of pasta appears larger on a small appetizer plate than it does on a large dinner plate. Here's more: If the plate is the same color as the food, we tend to eat more. But if the plate is a different color, we eat less because, again, a serving of pasta with red sauce appears larger on a white plate than it does on a red plate. Finally, if we put our plate on a tablecloth that's the same color as the plate, our serving appears larger still—making it easier to fill up on fewer calories.[415]

Aerobic Smarts Resources

7 Minute Workout App

The 7-minute workout we included in Chapter 11 has a companion app, which includes additional exercises, videos, tracking capabilities, and more. Visit *https://7minuteworkout.jnj.com/* for more information.

Fitness trackers

Wearable technology—whether in the form of a wristband, watch, clip, or phone app—can keep track of your fitness efforts by counting your steps, distance, speed, calorie burn, and/or sleep time. Some, like Garmin's Vivosmart, will vibrate and alert you when you've been inactive for more than an hour. The Epix, originally designed for hikers and backpackers, offers detailed maps of your location and includes a TracBack feature that may help you find your way back home if you or the person you are caring for becomes disoriented.

Indoor gaming systems

For indoor exercise, gaming systems such as Nintendo's Wii Fit and Xbox Fitness can also help you stay fit. Try tennis for multitasking, bowling and shooting for hand-eye coordination, or boxing for an aerobic workout. Some gaming systems allow you to link up with, and play against, others virtually, so you can strengthen Social Smarts while you improve your Aerobic Smarts.

Vibrating shoes

Finally, if you are unsteady on your feet, it can make fitness difficult and increase your risk of falls. In the spring of 2015, Good Vibrations Shoes unveiled a line of state-of-the-art vibrating shoe wear. The shoes use sound waves to stimulate the bottom of the feet, warming them and increasing circulation. A small study done by researchers at Harvard and several other institutions found that the shoes improved balance in seniors.[416] They come with a remote control to turn the vibrating feature on and off. You can charge the shoes in much the same way you'd charge a phone—by using a USB adaptor to connect the sole of the shoe with a wall outlet.

Resilience Smarts Resources to Prevent Alzheimer's Disease

Biofeedback devices

How do you relax if you don't know what relaxation feels like? Years ago, to help people learn the sensations around relaxation, they were wired to a machine that measured their heart rates, skin temperature, and blood pressure. As you relaxed certain muscles, the machine would encourage you with sounds or light. Called *biofeedback*, the treatment required a lengthy office visit.

Now, with the use of smart technology, you can gain some of the benefits of biofeedback at home.

HeartMath, for example, sells a pulse sensor ($129 to $299) that can be fitted to a finger or to your ear, and it communicates with a smartphone, tablet, or computer. Various relaxation techniques are offered, and your pulse data is stored long term. Graphs can show you how your heart rate changes when you relax, sleep, dream, meditate, and deal with everyday work hassles.

A different biofeedback device called Muse ($299) comes as a headband that slips on like a pair of glasses. It contains seven sensors that record the brain's electrical activity, along with relaxation programs to try. Like HeartMath, the readings are recorded, stored in a cloud, and turned into easy-to-understand graphs that show you how you are doing and offer you tips for improvement.

Apps

A variety of apps can also help you follow through on your resilience goals. Happify, for example, is a free app that helps you remember to stay in the moment, practice gratitude, set and meet goals. ReliefLink, also free, can help you track your mood, and it offers coping suggestions for when life becomes stressful.

Train-Your-Brain Smarts Resources

Brain-training systems

Lumosity (*lumosity.com*), Brain HQ (*brainhq.com*), Dakim (*dakim.com*), and others offer personalized courses that prompt you to do their brain-training exercises on a set schedule.

Apps

In addition to those comprehensive subscription-based services, you'll find multitudes of individual technological resources that may help you sharpen your attention, reaction speed, and more. Apps for smartphones and tablets include puzzles and games such as Threes!, Sudoku, and Words with Friends. They can support your efforts to learn a language (Duolingo) and even learn to dance (Tap App, Salsa, Learn to Dance). Other great brain-racking puzzle apps include: Puzzle Juice, Bonza, Bicolor, Quento, Trainyard Express, Blek, The Heist, and Monument Valley.

Anki (*ankisrs.net*) offers free electronic flash cards that can help you learn everything from the periodic table to advanced math to foreign languages. The open-source system contains many different decks that have already been created by others. You can use the ones that are already there or create your own. It's up to you whether you use the cards you create only for your own purposes or whether you share them so others can benefit from them as well. It can handle decks up to more than 100,000 cards, and you can review them anywhere to help you remember important information. SuperMemo (*supermemo.net*) offers something similar, but the flash cards are already pre-made to help you learn a variety of languages.

Finally GE Healthcare offers a free app for people with neurological disorders, including Alzheimer's disease. Called GE MIND app (Make an Impact on Neurological Disorders), it features art, music, and dance activities. You can create your own music, watch dance and exercise videos, and enjoy music from different countries.

Sleep Smarts Resources

Other than a comfortable mattress and pillow, you really don't need much in the way of technology to get a good night's sleep. That said, if you tend to toss and turn at night, you may wish to look into any number of options.

White noise machine
A white noise machine or a fan may help to drown out street noise that may disturb your sleep. These machines come in various shapes and sizes and range in price from $20 to $50.

Blinds
If you don't have them already, you may also want to invest in a set of blinds to block out light from streetlights, car headlights, the moon, and so on.

Natural light alarm clock
Made by Verilux, BlueMax, and other companies, these clocks slowly begin to illuminate your bedroom as it nears your waking time. Some of them, like Body-Clock ACTIVE 250 ($153), double as white noise machines. And the BlueMax Sunrise System ($165) uses the stimulating LED "blue" light to simulate dawn.

Sleep-monitoring apps and devices
If you suffer from insomnia or just feel chronically unrested, you might want to look into sleep-monitoring apps and devices to help you and your health care provider discover what's leading to your tossing and turning. Beddit ($149), for example, is a smartphone app and monitoring device that measures your bodily movements as you sleep and uses them to estimate your heart rate, respiration,

sleep cycle, and sleep time. ResMed's S+ (also $149) is a similar device and app, and many of the wearable trackers—including Jawbone® and Fitbit—are capable of monitoring your sleep cycle, too.

CPAP

Finally, as I mentioned earlier, if you've been told you snore or have any other symptoms of sleep apnea, it's worth undergoing an evaluation by a sleep specialist to see if a CPAP machine could help you sleep more restfully.

Security Resources for Caregivers

As Alzheimer's progresses, the risk of falls, wandering, disorientation, and getting lost may increase. The person you are caring for may leave but forget to lock the door; may wander into the neighborhood and get lost; or may walk too far and not have the endurance to get back home.

This is where security sensors and other related technology can help. Sensors can be attached to key chains, inserted into shoes, slipped under a mattress, and installed at strategic locations around the house, allowing you to tell if the person you are caring for:

- has left the door unlocked or the water running;

- is still in bed in the middle of the day;

- has left the house at an unusual hour (such as the middle of the night) or gone out and not returned by a specified time;

- has wandered beyond an established comfort zone;

- has taken their medication;

- has fallen

On the simplest end of the spectrum are stand-alone GPS tracking devices. Think of these as "find my iPhone," but they help you find your loved one, instead. These come as ankle bracelets, pendants, shoes, soles inserts, and watches, and they can be set up with or without a trained response team. For example, Vision Localization Systems Keruve 2010 is a GPS tracking system that includes a waterproof GPS watch, and it allows you to determine the location of the watch at any time. The watch is paired with a touchscreen portable receiver, which pinpoints the wearer's location on a map.

In addition to sensors that track someone's movements, technology can also allow you to lock or unlock a door remotely, flip lights on or off, and control the thermostat. You can increase safety by installing lighting that is triggered by motion sensors, especially if the person you are caring for tends to wander or get up in the middle of the night. Automatic shut-off features on irons and similar devices are also a good idea.

Security companies like Alarm.com and ADT offer this technology, though not specifically designed for people with Alzheimer's. And Staples, Home Depot, Best Buy, and AT&T all offer home-monitoring systems and starter kits. What follows is a rundown on specific home-monitoring companies and the security programs they offer that are designed specifically for seniors and people with Alzheimer's and other forms of dementia.

GrandCare Systems

This home-monitoring system includes a large touchscreen that someone with Alzheimer's can use to communicate with others. The menu screen includes large buttons that can be pressed to obtain news, photos, letters, games, wellness information, a calendar, and more. The screen allows someone with Alzheimer's to video chat with family members and caregivers, and it is designed to sync with telehealth technology such as digital scales, glucose monitors, and blood-pressure cuffs. It also can give instructions and reminders regarding appointments, medication, and more.

You can add motion detectors, contact sensors, and pressure sensors (for example, on a bed to show if someone is sleeping) to the monitoring package. Learn more at grandcare.com.

The Alzheimer's Association's "Comfort Zone"

The Alzheimer's Association is a worldwide nonprofit that works to enhance the care and support for people with Alzheimer's disease. Comfort Zone is the association's web-based GPS location management service. The person with Alzheimer's wears a location device (such as a pager or watch) that communicates his location to a web-based portal that caregivers and family members can monitor. If the person with Alzheimer's goes outside of a pre-set zone, the family member receives an alert. If needed, an emergency response service can be called to retrieve someone with Alzheimer's who may have gotten lost. Learn more at *alz.org/comfortzone.*

Healthsense's eNeighbor

This is another remote monitoring system specifically designed to support caregivers. Depending on which sensors you install, you can monitor someone's location, tell if doors are opened or closed, and even know if the person you are caring for is asleep or sitting in his or her favorite chair. A toilet sensor alerts you to overflows. Learn more at *healthsense.com.*

Live!y

This system includes a watch, pillbox sensor, refrigerator sensor, and assorted other activity sensors that can be placed around the house in strategic locations. The devices communicate with an online hub, and the waterproof watch is capable of sending and receiving calls from a professional care team. The trained operators communicate with the watch wearer and can call emergency services, if needed. The watch also can issue reminders to take medications. Learn more at *mylively.com*.

Be Close

This home-monitoring system also includes a variety of sensors, relaying information to caregivers by text, email, or phone when something is out of the ordinary. Family members can go to a website to see what the person they are caring for is doing: sleeping, sitting, and so on. They can tell whether someone has taken medication, is sitting in a favorite chair, and where in the house she's gone and when.

Medical Resources for People with Alzheimer's Disease and Caregivers

About 42 percent of Alzheimer's patients do not take their medicines as prescribed,[417] and of all medication-related hospitalizations, between one-third and two-thirds are the result of poor medication adherence.[418]

There are many reasons a patient may not take medications as prescribed, but, for patients with Alzheimer's, a leading one is this: they forget. Even for those of us without diagnosed memory problems, it can be difficult, during the pre-caffeine morning haze, to remember: *Did I take my pills? If I take one now, will I accidentally double-dose myself?*

We've done it so many times that downing a pill with a gulp of water can become an automatic behavior, right up there with locking your front door. Do you remember locking your door as you left your home today or yesterday? Because we often do these tasks while on autopilot, it's hard to remember whether we've done them.

Thankfully, when it comes to medicine, technology can help. Some medicines come as transdermal patches that you can wear on your body for a few months at a time. The medicine slowly seeps through your skin and into your bloodstream over time. Rather than remembering to take it every day, you only have to remember to change the patch once every month or every three months, depending on the medication, and some research shows this can improve adherence.[419]

For medicines that are not available as patches, it may help to schedule reminders for yourself, treating medications in much the same way you would any other important appointment. By scheduling them into a computerized calendar, you can set the calendar to remind you to take them. The following technological resources may also help.

Pill organizers

These simple organizational tools allow you to sort pills into separate compartments for different times of the day and/or days of the week or month. They're available in many different styles and colors and can be purchased from your local pharmacy or convenience store.

Electronic pill organizers

These higher-tech pill organizers will sound an alarm to remind you to take pills at programmed times and days. For example, the MedFolio pill box ($248) beeps when it's time for you to take a scheduled medication dose, and a green circle on the box also lights up. MedCenter System's electronic monthly pill organizer allows you to program your doses up to a month in advance and talks to you to remind you to take the pills for that time and day. (It comes with various options that range in price from $37.95 to $64.95). Learn more about these tools at *medcentersystems.com* and *medfoliopillbox.com*.

Electronic pill bottles

These high-tech caps ($59 to $79) fit over most prescription pill containers. Inside the lid of the cap is a microchip that monitors when the bottle has been opened. The GlowCap brand will flash orange when it's time for you to take your medicine. If you don't respond by opening the bottle, then an audible alarm begins to beep. If you still don't respond, the cap wirelessly sends an email, text, or call to remind you or a caregiver that the medication has not been taken. To refill, you just push the button at the base of the lid, and it sends the refill request to the pharmacy. Learn more at *glowcaps.com*.

Similar to GlowCap, the e-Pill Multi-Alarm TimeCap ($29.95) can be programmed with up to 24 daily alarms. Its display will also tell you when the bottle was last opened. Learn more at *epill.com/timecap*.

Medication apps

The MedCoach (free) and Pill Monitor (99 cents) apps are just two of many apps available for smartphones and tablets that will remind you to take your pills. Many of them will prompt you to input data about dosage, refills, and specific instructions such as whether to take the medicine with or without food.

Glossary

Acetylcholine: One of the most common chemicals (called a *neurotransmitter*) in the brain. It is believed to be important for memory and thinking. It's sometimes abbreviated as ACh.

Advanced glycation end products: Usually abbreviated as AGEs, these harmful substances are created when proteins and fats react with sugars under high heat and pressure. They are found in particularly high levels in bacon, sausages, processed meats, and fried and grilled foods.

Autobiographical memory: What you remember based on your knowledge and life experiences.

Axons: These long, slender fingers extend from a nerve cell (called a *neuron*), allowing it to communicate with other cells.

Beta-amyloid plaque: A dangerous protein fragment that can accumulate and clump together, damaging brain cells and impairing the communication between them.

Biofeedback: A mind-body technique that helps you influence your heartbeat, blood pressure, and other automatic bodily processes. During a biofeedback session, you are connected to electrical sensors that measure information (*feedback*) from your body (*bio*), showing you that information as a graph or lights on a screen.

Body mass index (BMI): This is a number that is calculated based on your weight and height. A BMI less than 18.5 is considered underweight, 18.5 to 24.9 is normal weight, and above 25 is overweight.

Brain reserve: Also called *cognitive reserve,* this term refers to your brain's ability to compensate for damage by building connections to or leaning more heavily on nondamaged areas.

Dementia with Lewy bodies: Named after Frederick H. Lewy, MD, Lewy bodies are microscopic abnormal clumps of protein that form throughout the cerebral cortex of the brain, causing nerve cells to degenerate. This type of dementia leads to problems with walking and balance, hallucinations, dizziness and other nervous system issues, and sleep disturbances.

Dendrites: These branched extensions of nerve cells carry impulses from one cell to another.

Diastolic blood pressure: The bottom number of a blood-pressure reading, diastolic pressure is the force inside your blood vessels as your heart relaxes between beats.

Endorphins: These brain and nervous system chemicals serve as natural pain-killers and mood elevators.

Executive control: This refers to your ability to connect past experiences with present actions so you can better plan, organize, and strategize.

Fasting blood glucose: A measure of the glucose (or sugar) present in your blood after you've gone without food or liquid (except water) for eight hours, a fasting glucose level less than 100 mg/dL is considered normal, 100 to 125 mg/dL is considered prediabetes, and more than 126 mg/dL, diabetes.

Frontotemporal dementia: Affecting the front and side of the brain, this type of dementia leads to changes in personality and behavior.

Glutamate: A brain chemical that is involved in the formation of memories.

HDL cholesterol: Cholesterol circulates in the bloodstream with the help of protein carriers, such as *high-density lipoprotein* (HDL). HDL is thought to be a healthy protein carrier (in contrast to LDL).

Hypothalamus: A part of the brain that controls automatic processes such as heartbeat and sweating.

Inflammation: A process of heightened immune response as white blood cells and other substances protect cells and tissues from infection.

LDL cholesterol: One of the proteins that carries cholesterol throughout the bloodstream. Low-density lipoprotein (LDL) is thought to be an unhealthy protein carrier.

Microglia: A type of an immune cell, *microglia* can interpret the formation of beta-amyloid plaques as an injury, leading to inflammation.

Neuron: Another word for a nerve cell or a brain cell.

Neurotransmitters: Chemicals that allow our brain cells to communicate.

Normal pressure hydrocephalus: Caused by the buildup of fluid in the brain, this rare form of dementia can bring on intense headaches and dizziness, changes in personality and behavior, trouble walking, and thinking and reasoning problems.

Oxidation: The interaction between cells and oxygen that causes cells to rust, eroding our health over time.

Oxytocin: The bonding hormone that is believed to be involved in trust.

Parkinson's disease: In this form of dementia, microscopic abnormal clumps of protein called Lewy bodies form deep in the brain, in an area called the *substantia nigra,* causing tremors and problems with movement.

Relational binding: When we meet new people, the memories of their names are stored with other memories of how we met them. This is called *relational binding.*

Sleep apnea: If you have this condition, your airways temporarily collapse as you sleep, causing you to stop breathing repeatedly for short periods of time.

Sundowning: The increase in arousal, irritability, and activity of someone with Alzheimer's disease that tends to start in late afternoon and progress into the evening.

Systolic blood pressure: The top number in the reading, your systolic pressure is a measure of the force inside your arteries as your heart beats.

Tau tangles: An otherwise normal protein called *tau* can twist into long, tangled threads (or tangles) that gradually strangle neurons.

Total cholesterol: A measure of the total amount of cholesterol in your blood, including your HDL and LDL cholesterol.

Vascular dementia: In this type of dementia, hardened, blocked, and leaking blood vessels stop blood from flowing to affected parts of the brain, causing brain cells to die.

Ventrolateral preoptic nucleus: A small cluster of brain cells involved in sleep.

Visuospatial attention: Placing your gaze on a particular object and selecting it to notice, or pay attention to.

White matter integrity: A measure of the pathways between neurons.

Endnotes

1. J.C. de la Torre, "A Turning Point for Alzheimer's Disease," *Biofactors* 38, no. 2 (March–April 2012):78–83.

2. J.C. Smith, K.A. Nielson, J.L. Woodard, M. Seidenberg, S. Durgerian, P. Antuono, A.M. Butts, N.C. Hantke, M.A. Lancaster, S.M. Rao, "Interactive Effects of Physical Activity and APOE-e4 on BOLD Semantic Memory Activation in Healthy Elders," *Neuroimage* 54, no. 1 (January 2011): 635–644, doi: 10.1016 j.neuroimage.2010.07.070.

3. A.N. Szaba, et al, "Cardiorespiratory Fitness, Hippocampal Volume and Frequency of Forgetting in Older Adults," *Neuropsychology* 5 (September 25, 2011): 545–553.

4. S. Norton, F. Matthews, D. Barnes, K. Yaffe, C. Brayne, "Potential for Primary Prevention of Alzheimer's Disease: An Analysis of Population-Based Data," *The Lancet Neurology* 13, no. 8 (August 2014): 788–794.

5. D.E. Barnes, K. Yaffe, "The Projected Effect of Risk Factor Reduction on Alzheimer's Disease Prevalence," *Lancet Neurology* 10, no. 9 (September 2011): 819–828.

6. M. Kivipelto, A. Solomon, S. Ahtiliuoto, et al, "A 2 Year Multidomain Intervention of Diet, Exercise, Cognitive Training, and Vascular Risk Monitoring Versus Control to Prevent Cognitive Decline in At-Risk Elderly People (FINGER): A Randomized Controlled Trial," *The Lancet* (March 12, 2015), *http: dx.doi.org 10.1016 S0140-6736(15)60461-5.*

7. Ibid.

8. M.C. Morris, C.C. Tangney, Y. Wang, L.L. Barnes, D. Bennett, N. Aggarwal, "MIND Diet Score More Predictive Than DASH or Mediterranean Diet Scores," *Alzheimer's & Dementia* 10, no 4 (July 2014): P166.

9. P. Vemuri, T. Lesnick, S.A. Przybelski, C.R. Jack, et al, "Association of Lifetime Intellectual Enrichment with Cognitive Decline in the Older Person," *JAMA Neurology* 71, no 8 (August 2014): 1017-1024 doi:10.1001 jamaneurol.2014.963.

10. Ibid.

11. F. Lopera et al, "Brain Imaging and Fluid Biomarker Analysis in Young Adults at Genetic Risk for Autosomal Dominant Alzheimer's Disease in the presenilin 1 E280A Kindred: A Case Control Study," *The Lancet Neurology* 11, no 12 (December 2012): 1048-1056.

12. M. Kivipelto, A. Solomon, S. Ahtiliuoto, et al, "A 2 Year Multidomain Intervention of Diet, Exercise, Cognitive Training, and Vascular Risk Monitoring Versus Control to Prevent Cognitive Decline in At-Risk Elderly People (FINGER): A Randomized Controlled Trial," *The Lancet* (March 12, 2015*), http: dx.doi.org 10.1016 S0140-6736(15)60461-5.*

13. M.C. Morris, C.C. Tangney, Y. Wang, L.L. Barnes, D. Bennett, N. Aggarwal, "MIND Diet Score More Predictive Than DASH or Mediterranean Diet Scores," *Alzheimer's & Dementia* 10, no. 4 (July 2014): 166.

14. P. Vemuri, T. Lesnick, S.A. Przybelski, C.R. Jack, et al, "Association of Lifetime Intellectual Enrichment with Cognitive Decline in the Older Person," *JAMA Neurology* 71, no. 8 (August 2014): 1017–1024, doi:10.1001 jamaneurol.2014.963.

15. W. F.A. den Dunnen, W.H. Brouwer, E. Bijlard, J. Kamphius, K. van Linschoten, E. Eggens-Meijer, G. Holstege, "No Disease in the Brain of a 115-Year-Old Woman," *Neurobiology of Aging* 29 (2008): 1127–1132, doi:10.1016 j.neurobiolaging.2008.04.010.

16. K. Ritchie, "Mental Status Examination of an Exceptional Case of Longevity J.C. Aged 118 Years," *British Journal of Psychiatry* 166 (1995): 229–235.

17. Alzheimer's Association, "Risk factors," accessed February 2015, *http: www.alz.org alzheimers_disease_causes_risk_factors.asp.*

18. J.C. Smith, K.A. Nielson, J.L. Woodard, M. Seidenberg, S. Durgerian, K.E. Hazlett, C.M. Figueroa, C.C. Kandah, C.D. Kay, M.A. Matthews, S.M. Rao, "Physical Activity Reduces Hippocampal Atrophy in Elders at Genetic Risk for Alzheimer's Disease," Frontiers in Aging Neuroscience 6, no 61 (April 2014): doi: 10.3389/fnagi.2014.00061.

19. Vemuri, T. Lesnick, S.A. Przybelski, C.R. Jack, et al, "Association of Lifetime Intellectual Enrichment with Cognitive Decline in the Older Person," *JAMA Neurology* 71, no. 8 (August 2014): 1017–1024, doi:10.1001 jamaneurol.2014.963.

20. K.S. Kosik, "The Fortune Teller," *The Sciences* 39, no. 4 (July-August 1999), 13–17.

21. National Institute on Aging, "Alzheimer's Disease Genetics Fact Sheet," accessed February 2015, *http: www.nia.nih.gov alzheimers publication alzheimers-disease-genetics-fact-sheet.*

22. Alzheimer's Association, "Risk factors", accessed February 2015, *http: www.alz.org alzheimers_disease_causes_risk_factors.asp.*

23. National Institute on Aging, "Alzheimer's Disease Genetics Fact Sheet," accessed February 2015: *http: www.nia.nih.gov alzheimers publication alzheimers-disease-genetics-fact-sheet.*

24. Alzheimer's Association, "2015 Alzheimer's Disease Facts and Figures" accessed June 18, 2015: *http://www.alz.org/facts/overview.asp.*

25. M Prince, R Bryce, et al, "The Global Prevalence of Dementia: A Systematic Review and Metaanalysis," *Alzheimer's & Dementia* 9, no 1 (January 2013) 63-75.e2.

26. Ibid.

27. K.A. Ertel, M. Glymour, L.F. Berkman, "Effects of Social Integration on Preserving Memory Function in a Nationally Representative U.S. Elderly Population," *American Journal of Public Health* 98, no. 7 (July, 2008): 1215–1220.

28. Lourida, et al, "Mediterranean Diet, Cognitive Function, and Dementia: a Systematic Review," *Epidemiology* 24, no. 4 (July, 2013):479–89.

29. F. Sofi, R. Abbate, G. F. Gensini, and A. Casini, "Accruing Evidence on Benefits of Adherence to the Mediterranean Diet on Health: an Updated Systematic Review and Meta-Analysis," *American Journal of Clinical Nutrition,* 92, no. 5 (November 2010): 1189–1196.

30. A. Bjørnebekk, A. Mathé, S. Brené, "The Antidepressant Effect of Running Is Associated with Increased Hippocampal Cell Proliferation," *The International Journal of Neuropsychopharmacology* 8, no. 3 (September 2005): 357–368.

31. L. Mah, M.A. Binns, D.C. Stevens, "Anxiety Symptoms in Amnestic Mild Cognitive Impairment are Associated with Medial Temporal Atrophy and Predict Conversion to Alzheimer's Disease," *The American Journal of Geriatric Psychiatry* (October 2014), DOI: http: dx.doi.org 10.1016 j.jagp.2014.10.005.

32. P. Vemuri, T. Lesnick, S.A. Przybelski, C.R. Jack, et al, "Association of Lifetime Intellectual Enrichment with Cognitive Decline in the Older Person," *JAMA Neurology* 71, no. 8 (August 2014): 1017–1024, doi:10.1001 jamaneurol.2014.963.

33. Christian Benedict, Liisa Byberg, Jonathan Cedernaes, Pleunie S. Hogenkamp, Vilmantas Giedratis, Lena Kilander, Lars Lind, Lars Lannfelt, and Helgi B. Schiöth, "Self-Reported Sleep Disturbance is Associated with Alzheimer's Disease Risk in Men," *Alzheimer's & Dementia* (October, 2014), DOI 10.1016 j.jalz.2014.08.104.

34. L.A. Profenno, A.P. Porsteinsson, S.V. Faraone, "Meta-Analysis of Alzheimer's Disease Risk with Obesity, Diabetes, and Related Disorders," *Biological Psychology* 67, no. 6 (March, 2010), 505-512 doi: 10.1016 j.biopsych.2009.02.013.

35. M. Kivipelto, A. Solomon, S. Ahtiliuoto, et al, "The Finnish Geriatric Intervention Study to Prevent Cognitive Impairment and Disability (FINGER): Study Design and Progress," *Alzheimer's & Dementia: The Journal of the Alzheimer's Association* 9, no. 6 (November 2013), 657-665 doi: 10.1016 j.jalz.2012.09.012.

36. AAIC 2014 Press Briefing 7 16.14 in Copenhagen Denmark, *https: www.youtube.com watch?v=mwNFRbfRVYk.*

37. N. Zilka, M. Novak, "The Tangled Story of Alois Alzheimer," *Bratislavské lekarske Listy* 107, no. 9-10 (2006), 343-345.

38. K. Maurer, S. Volk, H Gerbaldo, "Auguste D. and Alzheimer's Disease" *The Lancet* 349 (May 1997), 1546-1549.

39. Marist Poll, November 15, 2012, "Alzheimer's Most Feared Disease," MaristPoll.Marist.Edu, accessed December 2014, *http: maristpoll.marist.edu 1114-alzheimers-most-feared-disease*

40. Alzheimer's Association, "What is Dementia?" accessed June 18th, 2015: *http://www.alz.org/what-is-dementia.asp.*

41. K.M. Langa, D.A. Levine, "Diagnosis and Management of Mild Cognitive Impairment," *JAMA: The Journal of the American Medical Association* 312, no. 23 (December, 2014): 2551-2561.

42. J.D. Van Horn, A Irimia, C.M. Torgerson, M.C. Chambers, R. Kikinis, et al, "Mapping Connectivity Damage in the Case of Phineas Gage," *PLoS One* 7, no. 5 (May 2012): e37454 DOI: 10.1371 journal.pone.0037454.

43. K. O'Driscoll, J.P. Leach, "'No Longer Gage': An Iron Bar Through the Head," *BMJ* 317, no. 7174 (December 1998): 1673-1674.

44. Benedict Carey, "H.M., an Unforgettable Amnesiac, Dies at 82," *The New York Times*, December 4, 2008, accessed December 2014.

45. The Science Museum, "Transcript of Interview with Henry Molaison," *Who Am I? http: www.sciencemuseum.org.uk visitmuseum_old galleries who_am_i ~ media 8A897264B5064BC7BE1D5476CFCE50C5.ashx,* accessed December 2014.

46. J. Annese, et al, "Postmortem Examination of Patient H.M.'s Brain Based on Histological Sectioning and Digital 3D Reconstruction," *Nature Communications* 5, no. 3122 (January 2014): doi:10.1038 ncomms4122.

47. S. Banerjee, P. Neveu, K.S. Kosik, "A Coordinated Local Translational Control Point at the Synapse Involving Relief From Silencing and MOV10 Degradation," *Neuron* 64, no. 6 (December 2009): 871-874, doi: 10.1016 j.neuron.2009.11.023.

48. T. Wyss-Coray, J. Rogers, "Inflammation in Alzheimer's Disease–a Brief Review of the Basic Science and Clinical Literature," *Cold Spring Harbor Perspectives in Medicine* 2 no. 1 (January 2012): a006346.

49. A.M. Hedman, N.E. van Haren, H.G. Schnack, R.S. Kahn, H.E. Hulshoff Pol, "Human Brain Changes Across The Life Span: A Review Of 56 Longitudinal Magnetic Resonance Imaging Studies," *Human Brain Mapping,* 33, no. 8 (August, 2012): 1987-2002.

50. T.A. Salthouse, "The Processing-Speed Theory of Adult Age Differences in Cognition," *Psychological Review,* 103, no. 3 (1996): 403-428.

51. P. Rabbitt, C. Lowe, V. Shilling, "Frontal Tests and Models for Cognitive Aging," *European Journal of Cognitive Psychology,* 13, no. 1 2 (2001): 5-28.

52. L. Nyberg, M. Lovden, K. Riklund, U. Lindenberger, L. Backman, "Memory Aging and Brain Maintenance," *Trends in Cognitive Sciences,* 16, no. 5 (May 2012): 292-305.

53. D.C. Park, P. Reuter-Lorenz, "The Adaptive Brain: Aging and Neurocognitive Scaffolding," *Annual Review of Psychology* 60 (2006): 173-196 doi: 10.1146 annurev.psych.59.

54. A. Gutchess, "Plasticity of the Aging Brain: New Directions in Cognitive Neuroscience," *Science* 346, no. 6209 (October 2014): 579-582 ,DOI: 10.1126 science.1254604.

55. M. Ramscar, P. Hendrix, C. Shaoul, P. Milin, H. Baayen, "The Myth of Cognitive Decline: Non-Linear Dynamics of Lifelong Learning," *Topics in Cognitive Science* 6, no. 1 (January 2014): 5-42, DOI: 10.1111 tops.12078.

56. D.C. Park, P Reuter-Lorenz, "The Adaptive Brain: Aging and Neurocognitive Scaffolding," *Annual Review of Psychology* 60 (2009): 173–196, 10.1146 annurev.psych.59.103006.093656.

57. R.J. Kryscio, E.L. Abner, G.E. Cooper, D.W. Fardo, GA Jicha, P.T. Nelson, C.D. Smith, L.J. Van Eldik, L. Wan, F.A .Schmitt, "Self-reported memory complaints: Implications from a longitudinal cohort with autopsies," *Neurology* 83, no. 15 (October 7, 2014): DOI:10.1212 WNL.0000000000000856.

58. M.T. Weber, L.H. Rubin, P.M. Maki, "Cognition in Perimenopause: The Effect of the Transition Stage," *Menopause* 20 no. 5 (May 2013): 511–517.

59. Ellen Clegg, *ChemoBrain: How Cancer Therapies Can Affect Your Mind* (New York: Prometheus Books, 2008).

60. R.J. Caselli, J. Langbaum, G.E. Marchant, R.A. Lindor, K.S. Hunt, B.R. Henslin, A.C. Dueck, J.S. Robert, "Public Perceptions of Presymptomatic Testing for Alzheimer's Disease," *Mayo Clinic Proceedings* 89, no. 10 (Oct 2014): 1389–1396.

61. C. Kawas, S. Gray, R. Brookmeyer, J. Fozard, A. Zonderman, "Age-Specific Incidence Rates of Alzheimer's Disease: The Baltimore Longitudinal Study of Aging," *Neurology* 54, no. 11 (June 2000): 2072–2077.

62. E.J. Lampert, K.R. Choudhury, C.A. Hostage, J.R. Petrella, P. Murali Doraiswamy, "Prevalence of Alzheimer's Pathologic Endophenotypes in Asymptomatic and Mildly Impaired First-Degree Relatives," *PLoS ONE*, 8, no. 4 (April 2013): e60747 DOI: 10.1371 journal. pone.0060747.

63. L. Johansson, X. Gui, T. Hällström, M.C. Norton, M. Waern, S. Östling, C. Bengtsson, I Skoog, "Common Psychological Stressors in Middle-Aged Women Related to Longstanding Distress and Increased Risk of Alzheimer's Disease: A 38-year Longitudinal Population Study," *BMJ Open* 3, no. 9 (2013), e003142 *doi:10.1136 bmjopen-2013-003142.*

64. P. Washington, N. Morffy, M. Parsadanian, D.N. Zapple, M.P. Burns, " Experimental Traumatic Brain Injury Induces Rapid Aggregation and Oligomerization of Amyloid-Beta in an Alzheimer's Disease Mouse Model," *Journal of Neurotrauma* 30, no. 1 (January 2014): 125–134.

65. National Institute for Occupational Safety and Health, "Brain and Nervous System Disorders Among NFL Players," (January 2013): accessed December 2014, *http: www.cdc.gov niosh p.ms worknotify pdfs NFL_Notification_02.pdf.*

66. R.S. Wilson, Y Li, N.T. Aggarwal, L.L. Barnes, J.J. McCann, D.W. Gilley, D.A. Evans, "Education and the Course of Decline in Alzheimer's Disease," *Neurology* 63, no. 7 (Oct. 2004):1198–1202.

67. S. Edland, G. Peavy, D. Salmon, D. Galasko, "Elevated Blood Pressure and Risk of Incident Amnestic Mild Cognitive Impairment Alzheimer's Disease," *Neurology* 82, no. 10 (April 2014): S62.003.

68. K.J. Anstey, D.M. Lipnicki, L.F. Low, "Cholesterol as a Risk Factor for Dementia and Cognitive Decline: A Systematic Review of Prospective Studies with Meta-Analysis," *American Journal of Geriatric Psychiatry* 16, no. 5 (May 2008): 343–354, doi: 10.1097 JGP.0b013e31816b72d4.

69. C.J. Lavie, R.V. Milani, "Optimal Lipids, Statins, and Dementia," *Journal of the American College of Cardiology* 45, no. 6 (March 2005):963–964.

70. A. Ott, R.P. Stolk, A. Hofman, H.F. van Harskamp, D.E. Grobbee, M.M. Breteler, "Association of Diabetes Mellitus and Dementia: The Rotterdam Study," *Diabetologia* 39, no. 11 (1996):1392–1397.

71. W.L. Xu, A.R. Atti, M Gatz, N.L. Pedersen, B. Johansson, L. Fratigilioni, "Midlife Overweight and Obesity Increase Late-Life Dementia Risk," *Neurology* 76, no. 18 (May 2011):1568–1574, doi: 10.1212 WNL.0b013e3182190d09.

72. S. Norton, F.E. Matthews, D.E. Barnes, et al, "Potential for Primary Prevention of Alzheimer's Disease: An Analysis of Population-Based Data," *The Lancet Neurology*. Published online July 13, 2014, DOI: http: dx.doi.org 10.1016 S1474-4422(14)70136-X.

73. J.C.Smith, K.A. Nielson, S.M. Rao, "Physical Activity Reduces Hippocampal Atrophy in Elders at Genetic Risk for Alzheimer's Disease," *Frontiers in Aging Neuroscience* 6 (April 2014): 61.

74. M.C. Carlson, K.I. Erickson, A.F. Kramer, M.W. Voss, N. Bolea, M. Mielke, S. McGill, G.W. Rebok, T. Seeman, L.P. Fried, "Evidence for Neurocognitive Plasticity in At-Risk Older Adults: The Experience Corps Program," *The Journals of Gerontology, Series A Biological Sciences and Medical Sciences* 62, no. 12 (2009):1275–1282.

75. P. Vemuri, T.G. Lesnick, et al, "Association of Lifetie Intellectual Enrichment with Cognitive Decline in the Older Population," *JAMA Neurology* 71, no. 8 (August 2014): 1017–1024.

76. J.C. Lo, K.K. Loh, H. Zheng, S. Sim, M. Chee, "Sleep Duration and Age-Related Changes in Brain Structure and Cognitive Performance," *SLEEP* 37, no. 7 (2014): DOI: 10.5665 sleep.3832.

77. A.C. Trousier, C.M. Charley, J. Salleron, F. Richard, X. Delbueck, P. Derambure, F. Pasquier, S. Bombois, "Treatment of Sleep Apnea Syndrome Decreases Cognitive Decline in Patients with Alzheimer's Disease," *Journal of Neurology, Neurosurgery & Psychiatry* (May 2014): doi:10.1136 jnnp-2013-307544.

78. T.J. Holwerda, D.J. Deeg, A.T. Beekman, T.G. van Tilburg, M.L. Stek, C. Jonker, R.A. Schoevers, "Feelings of Loneliness, but Not Social Isolation, Predict Dementia Onset: Results From the American Study of the Elderly (AMSTEL)," *Journal of Neurology, Neurosurgery, and Psychiatry* 85, no. 2 (Feb. 2014): 135–142 doi: 10.1136 jnnp-2012-302755.

79. D.A. Bennett, J.A. Schneider, Y. Tang, S.E. Arnold, R.S. Wilson, "The Effect of Social Networks on the Relation Between Alzheimer's Disease Pathology and Level of Cognitive Function in Old People: A Longitudinal Cohort Study," *Lancet Neurology* 5 no. 5 (May 2006):406–412.

80. M. Rusanen, M. Kivipelto, C.P. Quesenberry, Jr, J. Zhou, R.A. Whitmer, "Heavy Smoking in Midlife and Long-term Risk of Alzheimer Disease and Vascular Dementia," *Archives of Internal Medicine* 171. No. 4 (February 28, 2011): 333–339, DOI: 10.1001 archinternmed.2010.393.

81. R. Boulay, M. Quagebeur, E.J. Godzinska, A. Lenoir, "Social Isolation in Ants: Evidence of Its Impact on Survivorship and Behavior in Camponotus Felluah," *Sociobiology* 33 no. 2 (1999): 111–124, *http: www.cataglyphis.fr Publis%20AL Boulay-etal-Sociobiol1999.pdf.*

82. L. Wang, Y. Xu, Z Di, B.M. Roehner, "How Does Group Interaction and Its Severance Affect Life Expectancy," Cornell University Library (April, 2013): arXiv:1304.2935 [q-bio.PE].

83. L.F. Berkman, S.L. Syme, "Social Networks, Host Resistance, and Mortality: A Nine-Year Follow-Up Study of Alameda County Residents," *American Journal of Epidemiology* 109, no. 2 (1979):186–204.

84. J. Holt-Lunstad, T.B. Smith, J.B. Layton, "Social Relationships and Mortality Risk: a Meta-Analytic Review," *PLOS Medicine* 7 no. 7 (July 27, 2010): e1000316 DOI: 10.1371 journal. pmed.1000316.

85. Sharon Shalev, "The Health Effects of Solitary Confinement," *Sourcebook on Solitary Confinement* (London: Mannheim Centre for Criminology, London School of Economics 2008): 1–24.

86. Woodburn Heron, "The Pathology of Boredom," *Scientific American* 196 (1956): 52–56.

87. R.I.M. Dunbar, "The Social Brain Hypothesis," *Evolutionary Anthropology* (1998): 178–190.

88. L.C. Aiello, R.I.M. Dunbar, "Neocortex Size, Group Size and the Evolution of Language," *Current Anthropology* 34, no. 2 (April 1993): 184–193.

89. M. McPherson, L. Smith-Lovin, M.E. Brashears, "Social Isolation in America: Changes in Core Discussion Networks over Two Decades," *American Sociological Review* 71, no 3 (June 2006): 353-375.

90. G.M. Walton, G.L. Cohen, A. Cwir, S.J. Spencer, "Mere Belonging: The Power of Social Connections," *Journal of Personality and Social Psychology* 102 no 3 (2012): 513-532.

91. B.D. James, R.S. Wilson, et al, "Late-Life Social Activity and Cognitive Decline in Old Age," *Journal of the International Neuropsychological Society* 17, no 6 (November 2011): 998-1005.

92. T.J. Holwerda, D.J. Deeg, A.T. Beekman, T.G. van Tilburg, M.L. Stek, C. Jonker, R.A. Schoevers, "Feelings of Loneliness, but Not Social Isolation, Predict Dementia Onset: results From the American Study of the Elderly (AMSTEL)," *Journal of Neurology, Neurosurgery, and Psychiatry* 85, no 2 (Feb. 2014): 135-142 doi: 10.1136 jnnp-2012-302755.

93. L.C. Hawkley, J.T. Cacioppo, "Loneliness Matters: A Theoretical and Empirical Review of Consequences and Mechanisms," *Annals of Behavioral Medicine* 40, No. 2 (October 2010): 1–14 10.1007 s12160-010-9210-8.

94. A. K. Barbey, R. Colom, E. J. Paul, A. Chau, J. Solomon, J. H. Grafman, "Lesion Mapping of Social Problem Solving," *Brain: A Journal of Neurology* (July 2014): DOI: 10.1093 brain awu207.

95. L.C. Hawkley, J.T. Cacioppo, "Loneliness Matters: A Theoretical and Empirical Review of Consequences and Mechanisms," *Annals of Behavioral Medicine* 40, No. 2 (October 2010): 1–14 10.1007 s12160-010-9210-8.

96. W.M. Troxel, D.J. Buysse, T.H. Monk, A. Begley, M. Hall, "Does Social Support Differentially Affect Sleep in Older Adults with Versus Without Insomnia?" *Journal of Psychosomatic Research* 69, no. 5 (Nov 2010): 459–466, doi: 10.1016 j.jpsychores.2010.04.003.

97. M.A. Aanes, J. Hetland, S. Pallesen, M.B. Mittelmark, "Does Loneliness Mediate the Stress-Sleep Quality Relation? The Hordaland Health Study," *International Psychogeriatrics* 23, no. 6 (August 2011): 994–1002.

98. M.L. Small, "Weak Ties and the Core Discussion Network: Why People Regularly Discuss Important Matters with Unimportant Alters," *Social Networks* 35, no. 3 (2011): 470–483.

99. L.C. Hawkley, J.T. Cacioppo, "Loneliness Matters: A Theoretical and Empirical Review of Consequences and Mechanisms," *Annals of Behavioral Medicine* 40, No. 2 (October 2010): 1–14, 10.1007 s12160-010-9210-8.

100. A. Karp, et al "Mental, Physical and Social Components in Leisure Activities Equally Contribute to Decrease Dementia Risk," *Dementia and Geriatric Cognitive Disorders* 21, no. 2 (2006): 65–73.

101. J.A. Anguera, J. Boccanfuso, J.L. Rintoul, O. Al-Hashimi, F. Faraji, J. Janowich, E. Kong, Y. Larraburo, C. Rolle, E. Johnston, A. Gazzaley, "Video Game Training Enhances Cognitive Control in Older Adults," *Nature* 501, no. 7465 (September 2013): 97–101.

102. S. Cooper, et al, "Prediction Protein Structures with a Multiplayer Online Game," *Nature* 477 no. 7307 (August 2010): 756–760, doi:10.1038 nature09304. *Nanocrafter*, beta, Accessed December 2014: http: nanocrafter.org .

103. Ibid.

104. S. Ofei Do-Doo, L.J. Medvene, K.M. Nilsen, R.A. Smith, A. DiLollo, "Exploring the Potential of Computers to Enrich Home and Community-Based Services Clients' Social Networks," *Educational Gerontology* 41 (2015): 216–225.

105. Nicholas Epley, Juliana Schroeder, "Mistakenly Seeking Solitude," *Journal of Experimental Psychology: General* 143, no. 5 (October, 2014): 1980–1999, doi: 10.1037 a0037323.

106. L. Wood, B. Giles-Corti, M. Bulsara, "The Pet Connection: Pets as a Conduit For Social Capital?" *Social Science & Medicine* 61, no. 6 (September, 2005): 1159–1173.

107. A.R. McConnell, CM Brown, "Friends With Benefits: On the Positive Consequences of Pet Ownership," *Journal of Personality and Social Psychology* 101, No. 6 (2011): 1239–1252.

108. PetsForTheElderly.org, "Help Support Pets for the Elderly," accessed December 2014.

109. S. Wesenberg, "Effects of an Animal-Assisted Intervention Program on Social Behavior and Emotional Expressions of Nursing Home Residents Suffering From Dementia," International Congress of the Royal College of Psychiatrists (RCPsych) 2014. Poster 40. Presented June 25, 2014: *http: www.rcpsych.ac.uk pdf Poster%20abstracts%2005%2006%2014%20(2).pdf.*

110. Israel21c, "Israel is first in the world to develop Alzheimer's guide dogs," Accessed December 2014: *http: www.israel21c.org health israel-first-in-the-world-to-develop-alzheimers-guide-dogs.*

111. C. R. Hooijmans, F. Rutters, P. J. Dederen et al., "Changes in Cerebral Blood Volume and Amyloid Pathology in Aged Alzheimer APP PS1 Mice on a Docosahexaenoic Acid (DHA) Diet or Cholesterol Enriched Typical Western Diet (TWD)," *Neurobiology of Disease* 28, no. 1 (October 2007): 16–29.

112. S. Singh Gill, N. Tuteja, "Reactive Oxygen Species and Antioxidant Machinery in Abiotic Stress Tolerance in Crop Plants," *Plant Physiology and Biochemistry* 48 (2010): 909–930.

113. N.W Milgram, E. Head, S.C. Zicker, C.I. Ikeda-Douglas, H. Murphey, B. Muggenburg, C. Siwak, D. Tapp, C.W. Cotman, "Learning Ability in Aged Beagle Dogs is Preserved by Behavioral Enrichment and Dietary Fortification: a Two-Year Longitudinal Study," *Neurobiology of Aging* 26, no. 1 (January 2005): 77–90.

114. M. Ozawa, T. Ninomiya, T. Ohara, et al., "Dietary Patterns and Risk of Dementia in an Elderly Japanese Population: the Hisayama Study," *The American Journal of Clinical Nutrition* 97, no. 5 (April 2013): 1076–1082.

115. H.H. Dodge, T.C. Buracchio, G. Fisher, Y. Kiyohara, K. Meguro, Y. Tanizaki, J.A. Kaye, "Trends in the Prevalence of Dementia in Japan," *International Journal of Alzheimer's Disease* (October 2012): 956354 doi: 10.1155 2012 956354 (PMC3469105).

116. I. Lourida, et al, "Mediterranean Diet, Cognitive Function, and Dementia: a Systematic Review," *Epidemiology* 24, no. 4 (July, 2013):479–89.

117. F. Sofi, R. Abbate, G. F. Gensini, and A. Casini, "Accruing Evidence on Benefits of Adherence to the Mediterranean Diet on Health: an Updated Systematic Review and Meta-Analysis," *American Journal of Clinical Nutrition* 92, no. 5 (November 2010): 1189–1196.

118. F. Sofi, C. Macchi, R. Abbate, G. F. Gensini, A. Casini, "Effectiveness of the Mediterranean Diet: Can It Help Delay or Prevent Alzheimer's Disease?" *Journal of Alzheimer's Disease* 20, no. 3 (2010): 795–801.

119. P. J. Smith, J. A. Blumenthal, M. A. Babyak et al., "Effects of the Dietary Approaches to Stop Hypertension Diet, Exercise, and Caloric Restriction on Neurocognition in Overweight Adults with High Blood Pressure," *Hypertension,* 55, no. 6 (June 2010): 1331–1338.

120. M.C. Morris, C.C. Tangney, Y. Wang, L.L. Barnes, D. Bennet, N. Aggarwal, "MIND Diet Score More Predictive Than DASH or Mediterranean Diet Scores," *Alzheimer's & Dementia* 10, no. 4 (July 2014): P166.

121. Y.Yokoyama, K. Nishimura, N.D. Barnard, M. Takegami, M. Watanabe, A. Sekikawa, T. Okamura, Y. Miyamoto, "Vegetarian Diets and Blood Pressure,"*JAMA Internal Medicine* 174, no. 4 (April 2014): doi: 10.1001 jamainternmed.2013.14547.

122. J.T. Sutliffe, L.D. Wilson, H.D. de Heer, R.L. Foster, M.J. Carnot, "C-Reactive Protein Response to a Vegan Lifestyle Intervention," *Complementary Therapies in Medicine* (December 2014): doi: http: dx.doi.org 10.1016 j.ctim.2014.11.001.

123. G.M. Turner-McGrievy, C.R. Davidson, E.E. Wingard, S. Wilcox, E.A. Frongillo, "Comparative Effectiveness of Plant-Based Diets for Weight Loss: A Randomized Controlled Trial of Five Different Diets," *Nutrition* (October 2014): doi: 10.1016 j.nut.2014.09.002.

124. S. Soret, A. Mejia, M. Batech, K. Jaceldo-Siegl, H. Harwatt, J. Sabate, "Climate Change Mitigation and Health Effects of Varied Dietary Patterns in Real-Life Settings throughout North America,"*American Journal of Clinical Nutrition* 100, Supplement 1 (2014): 490S doi: 10.3945 ajcn.113.071589.

125. P. Giem, W.L. Beeson, G.E. Fraser, "The Incidence of Dementia and Intake of Animal Products: Preliminary Findings from the Adventist Health Study," *Neuroepidemiology* 12, no. 1 (1993): 28–36.

126. D. Jenkins, et al, "Effect of a 6-Month Vegan Low-Carbohydrate ('Eco-Atkins') Diet on Cardiovascular Risk Factors and Body Weight in Hyperlipidaemic Adults: a Randomized Controlled Trial," *BMJ Open* 4 (2014): e003505doi:10.1136 bmjopen-2013-003505.

127. Y. Gu, J.W. Nieves, Y. Stern, J.A. Luchsinger, N. Scarmeas, "Food Combination and Alzheimer's Disease Risk: a Protective Diet," *Archives of Neurology* 67, no. 6 (June 2010): 699–706, doi: 10.1001 archneurol.2010.84.

128. G. Glazer, C. Greer, D. Barrios, C. Ochner, J. Galvin, R. Isaacson, "Evidence on Diet Modification for Alzheimer's Disease and Mild Cognitive Impairment," *Neurology* 82, no. 10 (April 2014): Supplement P5.224.

129. L. Olsén, L. Lind, M. Lind, "Associations Between Circulating Levels of Bisphenol A and Phthalate Metabolites and Coronary Risk in the Elderly," *Exotoxicology and Environmental Safety* 80 (June 2012): 179–183.

130. "Frequently Asked Questions," Saran Brands, accessed December 2014: *http: www. saranbrands.com faq.asp#1.*

131. "FAQs" Glad.com, accessed December 2014: *https: www.glad.com faq .*

132. C.Z. Yang, S.I. Yaniger, V.C. Jordan, D.J. Klein, G.D. Bittner, "Most Plastic Products Release Estrogenic Chemicals: A Potential Health Problem That Can Be Solved," *Environmental Health Perspectives* 119, no. 7 (July 2011): 989–996.

133. C.D. Kinch, K. Ibhazehiebo, J-H. Jeong, H.R. Habibi, DM Kurrasch, "Low-Dose Exposure to Bisphenol A and Replacement Bisphenol S Induces Precocious Hypothalamic Neurogenesis in Embryonic Zebrafish," *PNAS* 112, no. 5(January 12, 2015): 1475–1480 doi: 10.1073 pnas.1417731112.

134. C.Z. Yang, S.I. Yaniger, V.C. Jordan, D.J. Klein, G.D. Bittner, "Most Plastic Products Release Estrogenic Chemicals: A Potential Health Problem That Can Be Solved," *Environmental Health Perspectives* 119 no. 7 (July 2011): 989–996.

135. N. Hu, J-T. Yu, L. Tan, Y-L. Wang, L. Sun, L. Tan, "Nutrition and the Risk of Alzheimer's Disease," *BioMed Research International* 2013, no. 524820 (2013): 1–12, *http: dx.doi.org 10.1155 2013 524820.*

136. J.F. Fernandes, L.S. Araujo, M. de Lourdes, et al, "Restricting Calories May Improve Sleep Apnea, Blood Pressure in Obese People, *American Heart Association Meeting Report Abstract* #461" (paper presented at the American Heart Association's High Blood Pressure Research Scientific Sessions, San Francisco, California, September 9–12, 2014).

137. R. Gredilla, A. Sanz, M. Lopex-Torres, G. Barja, "Caloric Restriction Decreases Mitochondrial Free Radical Generation at Complex I and Lowers Oxidative Damage to Mitochondrial DNA in the Rat Heart," *FASEB J* 15, no. 9 (July 2001):1589–1591.

138. A.B. Crujeiras, D. Parra, I. Abete, J.Av Martinez, "A Hypocaloric Diet Enriched in Legumes Specifically Mitigates Lipid Peroxidation in Obese Subjects," *Free Radical Research* 41, no. 4 (April 2007): 498–506.

139. B. Wansink, K. van Ittersum, J.E. Painter, "Ice Cream Illusions: Bowl Size, Spoon Size, and Serving Size," *American Journal of Preventive Medicine*, 145, no 5 (September, 2006):240–243

140. Ibid.

141. I.N. Bezerra, C. Curioni, R. Sichieri, "Association Between Eating Out of Home and Body Weight," *Nutrition Reviews* 70, no. 2 (February 2012): 65–79,doi: 10.1111 j.1753-4887.2011.00459.x.

142. K.M. Purtell, E.T. Gershoff, "Fast Food Consumption and Academic Growth in Late Childhood," *Clinical Pediatrics* (December 2014): pii: 0009922814561742.

143. Suzanne Akterin, "From Cholesterol to Oxidative Stress in Alzheimer's Disease: a Wide Perspective on a Multifactorial Disease," (PhD diss., Karolinska Institutet, 2008).

144. J.R. Richardson, A. Roy, S.L. Shalat, RT von Stein, M.M. Hossain, B. Buckley, M. Gearing, A.Leavey, D.C. German, "Elevated Serum Pesticide Levels and Risk for Alzheimer's Disease," *JAMA Neurology* 71, no. 3 (March 2014): 284–290.

145. M. C. Morris, D. A. Evans, C. C. Tangney, J. L. Bienias, and R. S. Wilson, "Associations of Vegetable and Fruit Consumption with Age-Related Cognitive Change," *Neurology* 67, no. 8 (October, 2006): 1370–1376.

146. Ibid.

147. C. Gemma, J. Vila, A Bachstetter, P.C. Bickford, "Oxidative Stress and the Aging Brain: From Theory to Prevention," *Brain Aging: Models, Methods, and Mechanisms,* D.R. Riddle, ed. (Boca Raton, FL, CRC Press, 2007).

148. S. Subash, M.M. Essa, A. Al-Asmi, S. Al-Adawi, R. Vaishnav, "Chronic Dietary Supplementation of 4% Figs on the Modification of Oxidative Stress in Alzheimer's Disease Transgenic Mouse Model," *BioMed Research International* 2014, no. 546357 (June 2014): doi: 10.1155 2014 546357.

149. J.A. Vinson, L. Zubik, P. Bose, N. Samman, J. Proch, "Dried Fruits: Excellent in Vitro and in Vivo Antioxidants," *Journal of the American College of Nutrition* 24, no. 1 (February 2005): 44–50.

150. S. Subash, M.M. Essa, A. Al-Asmi, S. Al-Adawi, R. Vaishnav, N. Braidy, T. Manivasagam, G.J. Guillemin, "Pomegranate from Oman Alleviates the Brain Oxidative Damage in Transgenic Mouse Model of Alzheimer's Disease," *Journal of Traditional & Complementary Medicine* 4, no. 4 (October 2014): 232-238.

151. Ibid.

152. S. Subash, M.M. Essa, A. Al-Asmi, S. Al-Adawi, R. Vaishnav, G.J. Guillemin, "Effect of Dietary Supplementation of Dates in Alzheimer's Disease AAPsw 2576 Transgenic Mice on Oxidative Stress and Antioxidant Status," *Nutritional Neuroscience* (June 2014): doi: *http: dx.doi.org 10.1179 1476830514Y.0000000134.*

153. E. Fuentes, O. Forero-Doria, G. Carrasco, A. Maricán, L. Santos, M. Alarcón, I Palomo, " Effect of Tomato Industrial Processing on Phenolic Profile and Antiplatelet Activity," *Molecules* 18, no. 9 (2013): 11526–11536.

154. P.I. Moreira, "High-Sugar Diets, Type-2 Diabetes and Alzheimer's Disease," *Current Opinion in Clinical Nutrition and Metabolic Care* 16, no. 4 (July 2013): 440–445.

155. C. Carvalho, P.S. Katz, S. Dutta, P. V.g. Katakam, P.I. Moreira, D.W. Busija, "Increased Susceptibility to Amyloid-Ð Toxicity in Rat Brain Microvascular Endothelial Cells under Hyperglycemic Conditions," *Journal of Alzheimer's Disease* 38, no. 1 (October 2013): 74–83.

156. M. Tong, A. Neusner, L. Longato, M. Lawton, J.R. Wands, S. de la Monte, "Nitrosamine Exposure Causes Insulin Resistance Diseases: Relevance to Type 2 Diabetes Mellitus, Non-Alcoholic Steatohepatitis, and Alzheimer's," *Journal of Alzheimer's Disease* 17, no 4 (2009): 827-844

157. C. Mancuso, E. Barone, "Curcumin in Clinical Practice: Myth or Reality?" *Trends in Pharmacological Science* 30, no. 7 (July 2009): 333–334, doi:10.1016 j.tips.2009.04.004.

158. B. Qin, K.S. Panickar, R.A. Anderson, "Cinnamon: Potential Role in the Prevention of Insulin Resistance, Metabolic Syndrome, and Type 2 Diabetes," *Journal of Diabetes Science and Technology* 4, no. 3 (May 2010): 685–693.

159. A. Pengelly, J. Snow, S. Mills, A. Scholey, K. Wesnes, L. Butler, "Short-Term Study on the Effects of Rosemary on Cognitive Function in an Elderly Population," *Journal of Medicinal Food* 15, no. 1 (August, 2011): 10–17.

160. Ibid.

161. M. Moss, "Plasma 1,8-Cineole Correlates with Cognitive Performance Following Exposure to Rosemary Essential Oil Aroma," *Psychopharmacology* (February 24, 2012): doi: 10.1177 2045125312436573.

162. Food and Agriculture Organization of the United Nations, "World Health Organization. Summary Report of the Sixty-Fourth Meeting of the Joint FAO WHO Expert Committee on Food Additives (JECFA). Retrieved July 24, 2008, from: *http: www.who.int entity ipcs food jecfa summaries summary_ report_ 64_final.pdf.*

163. R.M. LoPachin, T. Gavin, D.S. Barber, "Type-2 Alkenes Mediate Synaptotoxicity in Neurodegenerative Diseases," *NeuroToxicity* 29, no 5 (September 2008): 871-882.

164. D.S. Mottram, B.L. Wedzicha, A.T. Dodson, "Acrylamide is Formed in the Maillard Reaction," *Nature* 2002; 419(6906):448–449.

165. "Acrylamide: Information on Diet, Food Storage, and Food Preparation," Food and Drug Administration, May 22, 2008, accessed December 2014: http: www.fda.gov Food FoodborneIllnessContaminants ChemicalContaminants ucm151000.htm.

166. L. Zhang, T. Gavin, R. LoPachin, et al, "Protective Properties of 2-Acetylcyclopentanone in a Mouse Model of Acetaminophen Hepatotoxicity," *The Journal of Pharmacology and Experimental Therapeutics* 346, no 2 (August 2013): 259-269.

167. R.M. LoPachin, T. Gavin, D.S. Barber, "Type-2 Alkenes Mediate Synaptotoxicity in Neurodegenerative Diseases," *NeuroToxicity* 29, no. 5 (September 2008): 871-882.

168. H. Vlassara, et al, "Oral Glycotoxins are a Modifiable Cause of Dementia and the Metabolic Syndrome in Mice and Humans," *PNAS* 11, no. 13 (April 2014): 4940-4945.

169. M. C. Morris, D. A. Evans, J. L. Bienias et al., "Consumption of Fish and n-3 Fatty Acids and Risk of Incident Alzheimer Disease," *Archives of Neurology*, 60, no. 7 (July 2003): 940-946.

170. R.A. Hites, J.A. Foran, D.O. Carpenter, M.C. Hamilton, B.A. Knuth, S.J. Schwager, "Global Assessment of Organic Contaminants in Farmed Salmon," *Science* 303, no. 5655 (January 2004): 226-229.

171. S.D. Shaw, D. Brenner, A. Bourakovsky, D.O. Carpenter, K. Kannan, C-S. Hong, "PCBs, Dioxin-like PCBs and Prganochlorine Pesticides in Farmed Salmon (Salmo salar) from Maine and Eastern Canada," Environmental *Science & Technology* 40, no. 17 (September 2006): 5347-5354.

172. University of Michigan Integrative Medicine, "Healing Foods Pyramid," Accessed December 2014: *http: www.med.umich.edu umim food-pyramid fish.htm.http: www.health.harvard.edu fhg updates update0404b.shtml.*

173. Ibid.

174. B. Muthaiyah, M.M. Essa, M. Leem V. Chauhan, K. Kaur, A. Chauhan, "Dietary Supplementation of Walnuts Improves Memory Deficits and Learning Skills in Transgenic Mouse Model of Alzheimer's Disease," *Journal of Alzheimer's Disease* 42, no. 4 ((2014): 1397-1405, doi: 10.3233 JAD-140675.

175. Ibid.

176. S.A. Mandel, et al, "Understanding the Broad-Spectrum Neuroprotective Action Profile of Green Tea Polyphenols in Aging and Neurodegenerative Diseases," *Journal of Alzheimer's Disease* 25, no. 2 (2011): 187-208, doi: 10.3233 JAD-2011-101803.

177. K. Rezai-Zadeh, G. W. Arendash, H. Hou et al., "Green Tea Epigallocatechin-3-Gallate (EGCG) Reduces Đ-amyloid Mediated Cognitive Impairment and Modulates Tau Pathology in Alzheimer Transgenic Mice," *Brain Research,* 1214 (June 2008): 177-187.

178. X. Peng, R.Z. Wang, X. Yu, X. Yang, K. Liu, M. Mi, "Effect of Green Tea Consumption on Blood Pressure: A Meta-Analysis of 13 Randomized Controlled Trials," *Nature Scientific Reports* 4, no. 6251 (September 2014): doi:10.1038 srep06251.

179. I. Onakpoya, E. Spencer, H. Heneghan, M. Thompson, "The Effect of Green Tea on Blood Pressure and Lipid Profile: A Systematic Review and Meta-Analysis of Randomized Clinical Trials," *Nutrition, Metabolism and Cardiovascular Disease* 24, no. 8 (August 2014): 823-836.

180. D.L. McKay, C-Y. Chen, E. Saltzman, J.B. Blumberg, "Hibiscus Sabdariffa L. Tea (tisane) Lowers Blood Pressure in Prehypertensive and Mildly Hypertensive Adults," *The Journal of Nutrition* 140, no. 2 (February, 2010): 298-303.

181. "Product Review: Green Tea Supplements, Drinks, and Brewable Teas Review," ConsumerLab. com, posted October 26, 2014, accessed December 2014: *https: www.consumerlab.com reviews Green_Tea_Review_Supplements_and_Bottled Green_Tea .*

182. G. Basurto-Islas, J. Blanchard, Y.C. Tung, J.R. Fernandez, M. Voronkov, M. Stock, S. Zhang, J.B. Stock, K. Iqbal," Therapeutic Benefits of a Component of Coffee in a Rat Model of Alzheimer's Disease," *Neurobiology of Aging* 35, no. 12 (December 2014): 2701-2712.

183. C. Laurent, S. Eddarkaoui, M. Derisbourg, et al, "Beneficial Effects of Caffeine in a Transgenic Model of Alzheimer's Disease-Like Tau Pathology," *Neurobiology of Aging* 35, no. 9 (September 2014): 2079-2090.

184. D. Borota, E. Murray, G. Keceli, A. Chang, J.M.Watabe, M. Ly, J.P. Toscano, M.A. Yassa, "Post-Study Caffeine Administration Enhances Memory Consolidation in Humans,"*Nature Neuroscience* 17 (2014): 201-203, doi: 10.1038 nn.3623.

185. N. Yamada-Fowler, M. Fredrikson, P. Söderkvist, "Caffeine Interaction with Glutamate Receptor Gene GRIN2A: Parkinson's Disease in Swedish Population," *PLoS ONE*, 9 no. 6 (June 2014): e99294 doi: 10.1371 journal.pone.0099294.

186. Y. Ma, M. Gao, D. Liu, "Chlorogenic Acid Improves High Fat Diet-Induced Hepatic Steatosis and Insulin Resistance in Mice," *Pharmaceutical Research* (September 2014): doi: 10.1007 s11095-014-1526-9.

187. George Boon-Bee Goh, Wan-Cheng Chow, Renwei Wang, Jian-Min Yuan, Woon-Puay Koh, "Coffee, Alcohol and Other Beverages in Relation to Cirrhosis Mortality: the Singapore Chinese Health Study,"*Hepatology* 60 no. 2 (August 2014):661–669, doi: 10.1002 hep.27054.

188. H. Jang, H. Ryul Ahn, H. Jo, K.A. Kim, E.H. Lee, K.W. Lee, S.H. Jung, C.Y. Lee, "Chlorogenic Acid and Coffee Prevent Hypoxia-Induced Retinal Degeneration,"*Journal of Agricultural and Food Chemistry*, 62, no. 1 (2014): 182 doi: 10.1021 jf404285v.

189. Q. Xiao, R. Sinha, B.I. Graubard, N.D. Freedman, "Inverse Associations of Total and Decaffeinated Coffee with Liver Enzyme Levels in NHANES 1999–2010,"*Hepatology*, 60, no. 6 (December 2014): 2091–2098, doi: 10.1002 hep.27367.

190. "Caramel Brulee Frappuccino Blended Coffee," Starbucks corporate website, accessed December 2014: *http: www.starbucks.com menu drinks frappuccino-blended-beverages caramel-brul%C3%A9e-frappuccino#size=11005501&milk=67&whip=125.*

191. C.Carvalho, P.S. Katz, S. Dutta, P.Vg. Katakam, P.I. Moreira, D.W. Busija, "Increased Susceptibility to Amyloid-Ð Toxicity in Rat Brain Microvascular Endothelial Cells Under Hyperglycemic Conditions," *Journal of Alzheimer's Disease* 38, no. 1 (October 2013): 75–83.

192. A.M. Brickman, U.A. Khan, F.A. Provenzano, et al, "Enhancing Dentate Gyrus Function with Dietary Flavanols Improves Cognition in Older Adults," *Nature Neuroscience* 17 (November 2014): 1798–1803, doi:10.1038 nn.3850.

193. Ibid.

194. X. Feng, N. Liang, D. Zhu, L. Peng, H. Dong, et al, "Resveratrol Inhibits B-Amyloid-Induced Neuronal Apoptosis through Regulation of S1RT1-ROCK1 Signaling Pathway," *PLOS ONE* (March 2013): doi: 10.1371 journal.pone.0059888.

195. D.R. Zamzow, V. Elias, L.L. Legette, J. Choi, J.F. Stevens, K.R. Magnusson, "Xanthohumol Improved Cognitive Flexibility in Young Mice," *Behavioural Brain Research* 275, no. 15 (December 2014): 1-10 doi: 10.1016 j.bbr.2014.08.045.

196. D. G. Harwood, A. Kalechstein, W. W. Barker et al., "The Effect of Alcohol and Tobacco Consumption, and Apolipoprotein E Genotype, on the Age of Onset in Alzheimer's Disease," *International Journal of Geriatric Psychiatry* 25, no. 5 (May 2010): 511–518.

197. D Walker, L Smarandescu, B Wansink "Half Full or Empty: Cues That Lead Wine Drinkers to Unintentionally Overpour," *Substance Abuse & Misuse* 49, no 3 (2014): 295-302.

198. "Air Popped Popcorn," Calorie King, accessed December 2014: *http: www.calorieking.com foods calories-in-popcorn-air-popped_f-ZmlkPTYxNzI5.html.*

199. J. Vinson, "Popcorn: The Snack with Even Higher Antioxidants Levels than Fruits and Vegetables," (presented at the 243rd National Meeting & Exposition of the American Chemical Society (ACS) March 23–28, San Diego, California).

200. "Teflon and Perfluorooctanoic Acid," American Cancer Society website, accessed December 2014: *http: www.cancer.org cancer cancercauses othercarcinogens athome teflon-and-perfluorooctanoic-acid--pfoa.*

201. K.D. Brownell, J.L. Pomeranz, "The Trans-Fat Ban Food Regulation and Long-Term Health," *The New England Journal of Medicine* 370 (May 8, 2014): 1773–1775.

202. "News About Microwave Popcorn,' Orville Redenbacher's website, accessed December 2014: *http: www.orville.com news-and-offers latest-news.*

203. "Recent Consumer Lab.com Reviews," *ConsumerLab.com*, accessed December 2014: *https: www.consumerlab.com .*

204. B. Vellas, N. Coley, P.J. Ousset, et al, "Long-Term Use of Standardised Ginkgo Biloba Extract for the Prevention of Alzheimer's Disease (GuidAge): A Randomized Placebo-Controlled Trial," *Lancet Neurology* 11, no. 10 (October 2012): 851–859.

205. A.M. Canevelli, E. Kelaiditi, C. Cantet, P.J. Ousset, M. Cesari, "Effects of Gingko Biloba Supplementation in Alzheimer's Disease Patients Receiving Cholinesterase Inhibitors: Data From the ICTUS Study," *Phytomedicine* 21, no. 6 (May 2014): 888–892.

206. G.C. Shearer, O.V. Savinova, W.S. Harris, "Fish Oil—How Does It Reduce Plasma Triglycerides?" *BBA Molecular and Cell Biology of Lipids* 1821, no. 5 (May 2012): 843–851.

207. K.A. Kennel, M.T. Drake, D.L. Hurley, "Vitamin D Deficiency in Adults: When to Test and How to Treat," *Mayo Clinic Proceedings* 85, no. 8 (August 2010): 752–758.

208. A.F. Kramer, K.I. Erikson, S.J. Colcombe, "Exercise, Cognition and the Aging Brain," *Journal of Applied Physiology* 101, no. 4 (October 2006): 1237–1242.

209. A.F. Kramer, K.I. Erikson, S.J. Colcombe, "Exercise, Cognition, and the Aging Brain," *Journal of Applied Physiology* 101 (June 2006): 1237–1242 ,doi:10.1152 japplphysiol.00500.2006.

210. S.B. Chapman, S. Aslan, J.S. Spence, L.F. DeFina, M.W. Keebler, N. Didehbani, H. Lu, "Shorter Term Aerobic Exercise Improves Brain, Cognition, and Cardiovascular Fitness in Aging," *Frontiers in Aging Neuroscience* (November 2013): doi: 10.3389 fnagi.2013.00075.

211. Centers for Disease Control and Prevention, "Injury Prevention & Control: Motor Vehicle Safety," Accessed December 2014: *http: www.cdc.gov motorvehiclesafety Pedestrian_Safety index.html.*

212. L. Chaddock, M.B. Neider, M.W. Voss, J.G. Gaspar, A.F. Kramer, "Do Athletes Excel at Everyday Tasks," *Medicine in Science & Sports and Exercise* 43 no. 10 (October 2011): 1920-1926, doi: 10.1249 MSS.0b013e318218ca74.

213. N.C. Berchtold, N. Castello, C.W. Cotman, "Exercise and Time-Dependent Benefits to Learning and Memory," *Neuroscience* 16, no. 3 (May 19, 2010): 588–597.

214. James Michael Monti, "Aerobic Fitness Enhances Relational Memory in Preadolescent Children," (PhD diss., University of Illinois, 2011).

215. M. Voss, C. Vivar, A.F. Kramer, H. van Praag, "Bridging Animal and Human Models of Exercise-Induced Brain Plasticity," *Trends in Cognitive Sciences* 17, no. 10 (October 2013): 525–544.

216. L.S. Nagamatsu, A. Chenm T Liu-Ambrose, et al, "Physical Activity Improves Verbal and Spacial Memory in Older Adults with Probably Mild Cognitive Impairment: A 6-Month Randomized Controlled Trial," *Journal of Aging Research* 2014 (2013): 861893.

217. The Centers for Disease Control,"Falls Among Older Adults: An Overview,", Accessed December 2014: *http: www.cdc.gov homeandrecreationalsafety falls adultfalls.html.*

218. M.D. Newman, J.H. Silber, J.S. Magaziner, M.A. Oassarella, S. Mehta, R.M. Werner, "Survival and Functional Outcomes After Hip Fracture Among Nursing Home Residents," *JAMA Internal Medicine* 174, no. 8 (August 2014): 1273–1280.

219. Dave Morgan, "Water Maze Tasks in Mice: Special Reference to Alzheimer's Transgenic Mice," in *Methods of Behavior Analysis in Neuroscience, 2nd Edition,* Jerry J. Buccafusco, ed. (Boca Raton, FL: CRC Press, 2009).

220. A. Pinto, D. Di Raimondo, A. Tuttolomondo, C. Butta, G. Millo, G. Licata, "Effects of Physical Exercise on Inflammatory Markers of Atherosclerosis," *Current Pharmaceutical Design* 18, no. 28 (2012): 4326–4349.

221. M.W. Voss, C. Vivar, A.F. Kramer, H. van Praag, "Bridging Animal and Human Models of Exercise Induced Plasticity," *Trends in Cognitive Sciences* 17, no. 10 (October 2013): 525–544

222. R.R. Pate, G.W. Heath, M. Dowda, S.G. Trost, "Associations Between Physical Activity and Other Health Behaviors in a Representative Sample of US Adolescents," *American Journal of Public Health* 86, no. 11 (November 1996): 1577–1581.

223. P.D. Loprinzi, E. Smit, S. Mahoney, "Physical Activity and Dietary Behavior in US Adults and Their Combined Influence on Health," *Mayo Clinic Proceedings* 89, no. 2 (February 2014): 190–198.

224. S. Taddei, F. Galetta, A. Virdis, L. Ghiadoni, Salvetti, F. Franzoni, C. Giusti, A. Salvetti, "Physical Activity Prevents Age-Related Impairments in Nitric Oxide Availability in Elderly Athletes," *Circulation* 101, no. 25 (June 2000): 2896–2901.

225. C.W. Cotman, N.C. Berchtold, "Exercise: A Behavioral Intervention to Enhance Brain Heath and Plasticity," *Trends in Neuroscience* 25, no. 6 (June 2002): 295–301.

226. J.C. Smith, K.A. Nielson, J.L. Woodard, M. Seidenberg, S. Durgerian, K.E. Hazlett, C.M. Figueroa, C.C. Kandah, C.D. Kay, M.A. Matthews, S.M. Rao, "Physical Activity Reduces Hippocampal Atrophy in Elders at Genetic Risk for Alzheimer's Disease," Frontiers in Aging Neuroscience 6, no 61 (April 2014): doi: 10.3389/fnagi.2014.00061.

227. A.N. Szaba, et al "Cardiorespiratory Fitness, Hippocampal Volume and Frequency of Forgetting in Older Adults," *Neuropsychology* 5 (September 25, 2011): 545–553.

228. T. Brinke, N. Bolandzadeh, L.S. Nagamatsu, C.L. Hsu, J.C. Davis, K. Miran-Khan, T. Liu-Ambrose, "Aerobic Exercise Increases Hippocampal Volume in Older Women and Probable Mild Cognitive Impairment: A 6-Month Randomised Controlled Trial," *British Journal of Sports Medicine* 49, no. 4 (February 2015): 248–254.

229. A.Z. Burzynska, L. Chaddock-Heyman, et al, "Physical Activity and Cardiorespiratory Fitness are Beneficial for White Matter in Low-Fit Adults," *PLOS One* 17, no. 9 (September 2014): e107413 doi: 10.1371 journal.pone.0107413.

230. P.A. Adlard, V.M. Perreau, V. Pop, C.W. Cotman, "Voluntary Exercise Decreases Amyloid Load in Transgenic Model of Alzheimer's Disease," *The Journal of Neuroscience* 27, no. 17 (April 2005): 4217–4221 doi: 10.1523 JNEUROSCI.0496-05.2005.

231. R.C. Cassilhas, K.S. Lee, J. Fernandes, M.G. Oliveira, S. Tufik, R. Meeusen, M.T. de Mello, "Spatial Memory is Improved by Aerobic and Resistance Exercise Through Divergent Molecular Mechanisms," *Neuroscience* 202 (January 2012): 309–317.

232. J.M. Tucker et al, "Physical Activity in the US: Adults Compliance with the Physical Activity Guidelines for Americans," *American Journal of Preventative Medicine* 40 no, 4 (2011): 454–461.

233. E.B. Larson, L Wang, J.D. Brown, W. McCormick, L. Teri, "Exercise Is Associated with Reduced Risk for Incident Dementia Among Persons 65 Years of Age and Older," *Annals of Internal Medicine* 44 no. 2 (January 2006): 73–81.

234. M.J. Biondolillo, D.B. Pillemer, "Using Memories to Motivate Future Behaviour: An Experimental Exercise Intervention," *Memory* (February, 2014): 1 doi: 10.1080 09658211.2014.889709.

235. A. Pesola, A. Laukkanen, P. Haakana, M. Havu, A. Saakslahti, S. Sipila, T. Finnni, "Muscle Inactivity and Activity Patterns after Sedentary Time-Targeted Randomized Controlled Trial," *Medicine & Science in Sports and Exercise* 46, no. 11 (November 2014): 2122–2131.

236. T. Noice, H. Noice, A. Kramer, "Participatory Arts for Older Adults: A Review of Benefits and Challenges," *The Gerontologist* 54, no. 5 (2014): 741–753, 10.1093 geront gnt138.

237. J. Verghese, et al, "Leisure Time Activities and the Risk of Dementia in the Elderly," *The New England Journal of Medicine* 348 (June 2003): 2508–2516, doi: 10.1056 NEJMoa022252.

238. H. Alves, M.W. Voss, W.R. Boot, A. Deslandes, V. Cossich, J.I. Salles, A.F. Kramer, "Perceptual Cognitive Expertise in Elite Volleyball Players," *Frontiers in Psychology* 4, no. 36 (March 2013): doi: 10.3389 fpsyg.2013.00036. eCollection 2013.

239. M.E. Francois, J.C. Baldi, P.J. Manning, S.J.E. Lucas, J.A. Hawley, M.J.A. Williams, J.D. Cotter, "'Exercise snacks' before meals: a novel strategy to improve glycaemic control in individuals with insulin resistance,"*Diabetologia* 57, no. 7 (May 2014): 1437–1445 doi: 10.1007 s00125-014-3244-6.

240. B. Kilka, C. Jordan, "High-Intensity Circuit Training Using Body Weight: Maximum Results with Minimum Investment," *ACSM's Health and Fitness Journal* 17, no. 3 (June 2013): 8–13.

241. E. Graessel, R. Stemmer, B. Eichenseer, S. Pickel, C. Donath, J. Kornhuber, K. Luttenberger, "Non-Pharmacological, Multicomponent Group Therapy in Patients with Degenerative Dementia: a 12-Month Randomized, Controlled Trial," *BMC Medicine* 9 no. 129 (2011): 1–11.

242. N.P. Gothe, A.F. Kramer, E. McAuley, "The Effects of an 8-Week Hatha Yoga Intervention on Executive Function in Older Adults," *The Journals of Gerontology Series A: Biological Sciences and Medical Sciences* 69, no. 9 (Sept 2014):1109–1116. XX

243. L. Ching, C. Ssu-Y.uan, W. May-Kuen, L. Jin Shin, "Tai Chi Chuan Exercise for Patients with Cardiovascular Disease," *Evidence Based Complementary and AlternativeMedicine* 2013 (2013): Article ID 983208.

244. R. Jahnke, L. Larkey, C. Rogers, J. Etnier, F. Lin, "A Comprehensive Review of Health Benefits of QiGong and Tau Chi," *American Journal of Health Promotion* 26, no 6 (July 2011): e1-e25.

245. A.A. Thorp, A.B. Kingwell, P. Sethi, L. Hammond, O. Neville, D. Dunstan, "Alternating Bouts of Sitting and Standing Attenuate Postprandial Glucose Responses," *Medicine & Science in Sports and Exercise* 46, no. 11 (November 2014): 2053–2061.

246. K.H. Pitkala, et al "Effects of the Finnish Alzheimer Disease Exercise Trial," *JAMA Internal Medicine* 173 no. 10 (May 2013): 901–902 doi:10.1001 jamainternmed.2013.1215.

247. L. Teri, et al, "Exercise and Activity Level in Alzheimer's Disease: A Potential Treatment Focus," *Journal of Rehabilitation Research and Development* 35 no. 4 (October 1998): 411–419: *http: www.rehab.research.va.gov JOUR 98 35 4 teri.pdf.*

248. H. Mairer, et al, "Jeanne Calment and Her Successors. Biographical Notes on the Longest Living Humans," in *Supercentenarians* (Berlin Heidelberg: Springer-Verlag, 2010).

249. "Jean Calment, World's Elder, Dies at 122," *The New York Times Archives*, accessed December 2014: *http: www.nytimes.com 1997 08 05 world jeanne-calment-world-s-elder-dies-at-122. html.*

250. E.D. Kirby, S.E. Muroy, W.G. Sun, D. Covarrubias, M.J. Leong, L.A. Barchas, D. Kaufer, "Acute Stress Enhances Adult Rat Hippocampal Neurogenesis and Activation of Newborn Neurons Via Secreted Astrocytic FGF2," *eLife* 2 (April 2013): e00362 *http: dx.doi.org 10.7554 eLife.00362.*

251. R.S. Wilson, G.M. Hoganson, K.B. Rajan, L.L. Barnes, C.F. Mendes de Leon, and D.A. Evans, "Temporal course of depressive symptoms during the development of Alzheimer disease," 75, no. 1 *Neurology* (July 2010): 21–22.

252. K.N. Green, L.M. Billings, B. Roozendaal, J.L. McGaugh, F.M. LaFerla, "Glucocorticoids Increase Amyloid-B and Tau pathology in a Mouse Model of Alzheimer's Disease," *The Journal of Neuroscience* 26, no. 35 (August 2006): 9047–9056.

253. R.A. Rissmann, M.A. Staup, A.R. Lee, N.J. Justice, K.C. Rice, W. Vale, and P.E. Sawchenko "Corticotropin-releasing factor receptor-dependent effects of repeated stress on tau phosphorylation, solubility, and aggregation," *PNAS* 109, no. 16 (April 2012): 6277–6282.

254. J. L. Hanson, et al, "Behavioral Problems After Early Life Stress: Contributions of the Hippocampus and Amygdala," *Biological Psychiatry* (May 2014): pii: S0006-3223(14)00351- 5. doi: 10.1016 j.biopsych.2014.04.020.

255. L. Mah, M.A. Binns, D.C. Stevens, "Anxiety Symptoms in Amnestic Mild Cognitive Impairment are Associated with Medial Temporal Atrophy and Predict Conversion to Alzheimer's Disease," *The American Journal of Geriatric Psychiatry* (October 2014): doi: http: dx.doi.org 10.1016 j.jagp.2014.10.005.

256. A. Keller, K. Litzelman, L.E. Wisk, T. Maddox, E.R. Cheng, P.D. Creswell, W.P. Witt, "Does the Perception That Stress Affects Health Matter? The Association with Health and Mortality," *Health Psychology* 31 no. 5 (September 2012): 677–684.

257. D. Head, T. Singh, J.M. Bugg, "The Moderating Role of Exercise on Stress-Related Effects on the Hippocampus and Memory in Later Adulthood," *Neuropsychology* 26, no. 2 (March 2012): 133–143.

258. A.S. Moss, H. Roggenkamp, A.B. Newberg, D. Monti, M.R. Waldman, N. Wintering, D.S. Khalsa, "Effects of an 8-Week Meditation Program on Mood and Anxiety in Patients with Memory Loss," *Journal of Alternative and Complementary Medicine* 18, no. 1 (Jan 2012): 48–53 doi: 10.1089 acm.2011.0051.

259. A.B. Newberg, N. Wintering, D.S. Khalsa, H. Roggenkamp, M.R. Waldman, "Meditation Effects on Cognitive Function and Cerebral Blood Flow in Subjects with Memory Loss: A Preliminary Study," *Journal of Alzheimer's Disease* 20, no. 2 (2010): 517–526 doi: 10.3233 JAD-2010-1391.

260. H. Lavretsky, E.S. Epel, P. Siddarth, N. Nazarian, N.S. Cyr, D.S. Khalsa, E. Blackburn, M.R. Irwin, "A Pilot Study of Yogic Meditation for Family Dementia Caregivers with Depressive Symptoms: Effects on Mental Health, Cognition, and Telomerase Activity," *International Journal of Geriatric Psychiatry* 28, no. 1 (Jan 2013): 57–65.

261. E.M. Seppala, J.B. Nitschke, D.L. Tudorascu, A. Hayes, M.R. Goldstein, D.T. Nguyen, D. Perlman, R.J. Davidson, "Breathing-Based Meditation Decreases Posttraumatic Stress Disorder Symptoms in US Military Veterans: A Randomized Controlled Longitudinal Study," *Journal of Traumatic Stress* 27, no. 4 (August 2014): 397–405 doi: 10.1002 jts.21936.

262. S. Subramaian, T. Elango, H. Malligarjunan, V. Kochupillai, H. Dayalan, "Rolse of Sudarshan Kriya and Pranayam on Lipid Profile and Blood Cell Parameters During Exam Stress: A Randomized Controlled Trial," *International Journal of Yoga* 5, no. 1 (January 2012): 21–27.

263. H. Lavretsky, E.S. Epel, P. Siddarth, N. Nazarian, N.S. Cyr, D.S. Khalsa, E. Blackburn, M.R. Irwin, "A Pilot Study of Yogic Meditation for Family Dementia Caregivers with Depressive Symptoms: Effects on Mental Health, Cognition, and Telomerase Activity," *International Journal of Geriatric Psychiatry* 28, no. 1 (Jan 2013): 57–65.

264. T. Gard, B.K. Holzel, S.W. Lazer, "The Potential Effects of Meditation on Age-Related Cognitive Decline: A Systematic Review," *Annals of the NY Academy of Sciences* 1307 (Jan 2004): 89–103 doi: 10.1111 nyas.12348.

265. I. Amihai, M. Kozhevnikov, "Arousal vs. Relaxation: A Comparison of the Neurophysiological and Cognitive Correlates of Vajrayana and Theravada Meditative Practices," *PLoS ONE* 9, no. 7 (July 2014): e102990 doi: 10.1371 journal.pone.0102990.

266. L.S. Colzato, A. Szapora, D. Lippelt, B. Hommel, "Prior Meditation Practice Modulates Performance and Strategy Use in Convergent- and Divergent-Thinking Problems," *Mindfulness* (October 2014): doi: 10.1007 s12671-014-0352-9.

267. J.T. Ramsburg, R.J. Youmans, "Meditation in the Higher-Education Classroom: Meditation Training Improves Student Knowledge Retention during Lectures," *Mindfulness* 5 no. 4 (March 2013): 431–441 doi: 10.1007 s12671-013-0199-5.

268. M. Maslar et al, "Benefits of Mindfulness Training for Patients With Progressive Cognitive Decline and Their Caregivers," *American Journal of Alzheimer's Disease and Other Dementias* (August 25 2014): doi: 10.1177 1533317514545377 Springer-Verlag Berlin Heidelberg *http: www.demogr.mp..de books drm 007 3-4.pdf.*

269. H. Eastman-Mueller, T. Wilson, A.K. Jung, J. Tarrant, "iRest Yoga-Nidra on the College Campus: Changes in Stress, Depression, Worry and Mindfulness," *International Journal of Yoga Therapy* 23 (2013): 15–24.

270. N. Markil, M. Whitehurst, P.L. Jacobs, R.F. Zoeller, "Yoga Nidra Relaxation Increases Heart Rate Variability and is Unaffected by a Prior Bout of Hatha Yoga," *Journal of Alternative and Complementary Medicine* 10 (October 2012): 953–958 doi: 10.1089 acm.2011.0331.

271. S. Amita, S. Prabhakar, I. Manoj, S. Harminder, T. Pavan, "Effect of Yoga-Nidra on Blood Glucose Level in Diabetic Patients," *Indian Journal of Physiology and Pharmacology* 53, no. 1 (Jan-March 2009): 97–101.

272. M. Kosfeld, M. Heinrichs, P.J. Zak, U. Fischbacher, E. Fehr, "Oxytocin Increases Trust in Humans," *Nature* 435 (June 2005): 673–676 doi:10.1038 nature03701.

273. S. Jourard, M. Sidney, J. Rubin, "Self Disclosure and Touching: A Study of Two Modes of Interpersonal Encounter and Their Inter-Relation," *Journal of Humanistic Psychology* 8, no. 1 (1968): 39–48 *http: psycnet.apa.org psycinfo 1968-13772-001.*

274. M.J. Herenstein, R. Holmes, M. McCullough, D. Keltner, "The Communication of Emotion Through Touch," *Emotion* 9, no. 4 (August 2009): 566–573.

275. J.A. Coan, H.S. Schaefer, R.J. Davidson, "Lending a Hand," *Psychological Science* 17 no. 12 (December 2006): 1032–1039.

276. T. Field, M. Hernandez-Reif, M. Diego, S. Schanberg, C. Kuhn, "Cortisol Decreases and Serotonin and Dopamine Increase Following Massage Therapy," *International Journal of Neuroscience* 115, no. 10 (2005): 1397–1413.

277. R. Inzelberg, A.E. Afgin, et al, "Prayer at Midlife is Associated with Reduced Risk of Cognitive Decline in Arabic Women," *Current Alzheimer Research* 10, no. 3 (March 2013): 340–346.

278. J. Tartaro, L.J. Luecken, H.E. Gunn, "Exploring Heart and Soul: Effects of Religiosity Spirituality and Gender on Blood Pressure and Cortisol Stress Responses," *Journal of Health Psychology* 10, no. 6 (December 2005): 753–766.

279. J.E. Rubenstein et al "Executive Control of Thought Processes in Task Switching," *Journal of Experimental Psychology* 27, no. 4 (August 2001): 763–797.

280. M.B. Neider, J.G. Gasper, J.S. McCarley, J.A. Crowell, H. Kaczmarski, A.F. Kramer, "Walking and Talking: Diel-Task Effects on Street Crossing Behavior in Older Adults," *Psychology and Aging* 26, no. 2 (June 2011): 260–268.

281. B. Jeune, J.M. Robine, R. Young, B. Desjardins, A. Skytthe, J.W. Vaupel, "Jeanne Calment and Her Successors. Biographical Notes on the Longest Living Humans," *Supercentenarians* Demographic Research Monographs (2010): doi 10.1007 978-3-642-11520-2_16.

282. L.F. Low, et al, "The Effects of Humor Therapy on Nursing Home Residents Measured Using Observational Methods: The SMILE Cluster Randomized Trial," *Journal of the American Medical Directors Association* 15, no 8 (August 2014): 564–569.

283. M. Poulin, S.L. Brown, A.J. Dillard, D.M. Smith, "Giving to Others and the Association Between Stress and Mortality," *American Journal of Public Health* 103, no. 9 (September 2013): 1649–1655 doi: 10.2105 AJPH.2012.300876.

284. S. Post, "It's Good to Be Good: 2011 5th Annual Scientific Report on Health, Happiness, and Helping Others," *The International Journal of Person Centered Medicine* 1 no. 4 (September 2011): 814–829.

285. Ibid.

286. M. Van Willigen, "Differential Benefits of Volunteering Across the Life Course," *The Journals of Gerontology. Series B, Psychological Sciences and Social Sciences* 55, no. 5 (September 2000): S308–S318.

287. M.A. Musick, A.R. Herzog, J.S. House, "Volunteering and Mortality Among Older Adults: Findings From a National Sample," *Journal of Gerontology*, Social Sciences 54B, no. 3 (1999): S173–S180.

288. A. Guinote, I. Cotzia, S. Sandhu, P. Siwa, "Social Status Modulates Prosocial Behavior and Egalitarianism in Preschool Children and Adults," *PNAS* 112, no. 3 (January 20, 2015) 731–736.

289. J.J. Froh, G. Bono, and R.A. Emmons, "Being Grateful is Beyond Good Manners: Gratitude and Motivation to Contribute to Society Among Early Adolescents," *Motivation and Emotion*, 34, no. 2 (June 2010) 144–157.

290. J.G. Serpa, S.L. Taylor, K. Tillisch, "Mindfulness-based Stress Reduction (MBSR) Reduces Anxiety, Depression and Suicidal Ideation in Veterans," *Medical Care* 52, Supp 5 (December 2014): S19–24 doi: 10.1097 MLR.0000000000000202.

291. E.J. Lenze, S. Hickman, T. Hershey, L. Wendleton, K. Ly, D. Dixon, P. Dore, J.L. Wetherell, "Mindfulness-Based Stress Reduction for Older Adults with Worry Symptoms and Co-Occurring Cognitive Dysfunction," *International Journal of Geriatric Psychiatry* 29, no. 10 (October 2014): 991–1000 doi: 10.1002 gps.4086.

292. N. Wu-Chainani-Wu, G. Weidner, D.M. Purnell, S. Frenda, T. Merritt-Worden, C. Pischke, R. Campo, C. Kemo, E.S. Kersh, D. Ornish, "Changes in Emerging Cardiac Biomarkers After an Intensive Lifestyle Intervention," *American Journal of Cardiology* 108, no 4 (August 2011): 498–507 doi: 10.1016 j.amjcard.2011.03.077.

293. M. Suzuki et al, "Physical and Psychological Effects of 6-Week Tactile Massage on Elderly Patients with Severe Dementia," *American Journal of Alzheimer's Disease and Other Dementias* 25, no. 8 (December 2010): 680–686 doi: 10.1177 1533317510386215.

294. M. Rowe, D. Alfred, "The Effectiveness of Slow-Stroke Massage in Diffusing Agitated Behaviors in Individuals with Alzheimer's Disease," *Journal of Gerontological Nursing* 25, no. 6 (June 1999): 22–34.

295. D. Jimbo, Y. Kimura, M. Tanguchi, M. Inoule, K. Urakami, "Effect of Aromatherapy on Patients with Alzheimer's Disease," *Psychogeriatrics* 9, no. 4 (December 2009): 173–179 *http: www.ncbi.nlm.nih.gov pubmed 20377818.*

296. S.Y. Lee, "The Effect of Lavender Aromatherapy on Cognitive Function, Emotion, and Aggressive Behavior of Elderly with Dementia," *Taehan Kanho Hakhoe Chi* 35, no. 2 (April 205): 303–312.

297. L.A. Gerdner, "Effects of Individualized Versus Classical "Relaxation" Music on the Frequency of Agitation in Elderly Persons with Alzheimer's Disease and Related Disorders," *International Psychogeriatrics* 12, no. 1 (March 200):49–65.

298. J. Verghese, R.B. Lipton, M.J. Katz, C.B. Hall, C.A. Derby, G. Kuslansky, A.F. Ambrose, M. Sliwinski, H. Buschke, "Leisure Activities and the Risk of Dementia in the Elderly," *The New England Journal of Medicine,*" 348 (June 19, 2003): 2508–2516.

299. T.N. Akbaraly, F. Portet, S. Fustioni, et al, "Leisure Activities and the Risk of Dementia in the Elderly," *Neurology* 73, no. 11 (September 15, 2009): 854–861.

300. R.S. Wilson, D.A. Bennett, J.L. Bienias, C.F. Mendes de Leon, M.C. Morris, D.A. Evans, "Cognitive Activity and Cognitive Decline in a Biracial Community Population," *Neurology* 61, no 6 (September 23, 2003):812-816.

301. R.S. Wilson, P.A. Scherr, J.A. Schneider, Y. Tang, D.A. Bennett, "Relation of Cognitive Activity to Risk of Developing Alzheimer's Disease," *Neurology* 69, no. 20 (November 2007): 1911–1920.

302. P. Vemuri, T. Lesnick, S.A. Przybelski, C.R. Jack, et al, "Association of Lifetime Intellectual Enrichment with Cognitive Decline in the Older Person," *JAMA Neurology* 71, no. 8 (August 2014): 1017–1024 doi:10.1001 jamaneurol.2014.963.

303. S.L. Willis, S.L. Tennstedt, M. Marsiske, K. Ball, J. Elias, K.M. Koepke, J.N. Morris, G.W. Rebok, F.W. Unverzagt, A.M. Stoddard, E. Wright, "Long-term Effects of Cognitive Training on Everyday Functional Outcomes in Older Adults," *JAMA* 296, no. 23 (December 2006): 2805–2814.

304. LondonCouncils.gov, "London Facts and Statistics," accessed June 24, 2015: http://www. londoncouncils.gov.uk/who-runs-london/london-facts- and-statistics.

305. E.A. Maguire, D.G. Gadian, I.S. Johnsrude, C.D. Good, J. Ashburner, R. Frackowiak, C.D. Frith, "Navigation-Related Structural Change in the Hippocampi of Taxi Drivers," *PNAS* 97, no. 8 (April, 2000): 4398–4403.

306. E.A. Maguire, K. Wollett, H.J. Spiers, "London Taxi and Bus Drivers: A Structural MRI and Neuropsychological Analysis," *Hippocampus* 16, no. 2 (2006): 1091-1101.

307. Sharp Brains, "New Neurons: Good News, Bad News," Accessed June 24, 2015: http:// sharpbrains.com/blog/2008/04/25/new-neuronsgood- news-bad-news/.

308. Sharp Brains, "Can brain training work? Yes, if it meets these 5 conditions," accessed June 24, 2015: http://sharpbrains.com/blog/2013/05/22/does-brain-training-work-yes-if-it-meets-these-5-conditions.

309. B. Hanna-Pladdy, A. MacKay, "The Relation Between Instrumental Musical Activity and Cognitive Aging," Neuropsychology 25, no. 3 (2011): 378–386 *http: www.apa.org pubs journals releases neu-25-3-378.pdf.*

310. T. Särkämö, M. Tervaniemi, S. Laitinen, A. Numminen, M. Kurki, J.K. Johnson, P. Rantanen, "Cognitive, Emotional, and Social Benefits of Regular Musical Activities in Early Dementia: Randomized Controlled Study," *Gerontologist* 54, no. 4 (August 2014):634–50.

311. J.A. Bugos, W.M. Perlstein, C.S. McCrae, T.S. Brophy, P.H. Bedenbaugh, "Individualized Piano Instruction Enhances Executive Functioning and Working Memory in Older Adults," *Aging and Mental Health* 11, no. 4 (July 2007): 464–471.

312. Ibid.

313. S. Schultz, O.C. Okonkwo, et al, "Participation in Cognitively-Stimulating Activities is Associated with Brain Structure and Cognitive Function in Preclinical Alzheimer's Disease," *Brain Imaging and Behavior (October 2014): ePub http: www.ncbi.nlm.nih.gov pubmed 25358750.*

314. S. Schultz, D. Hartley, Alzheimer's Association International Conference, Copenhagen, DE (July 2014): *http: www.med.wisc.edu news-events cognitive-activities-may-help-protect-the-brain-from-alzheimers 43886.*

315. E. Woumans, P. Santens, A. Sieben, J. Versijpt, M. Stevens, W. Duyck, "Bilingualism Delays Clinical Manifestation of Alzheimer's Disease," *Bilingualism: Language and Cognition* (December 2014): doi: http: dx.doi.org 10.1017 S136672891400087X.

316. P. Li, J. Legault, K.A. Litcofsky, "Neuroplasticity as a Function of Second Language Learning: Anatomical Changes in the Human Brain," *Cortex* 58, (September 2014): 301-324 doi: 10.1016 j.cortex.2014.05.001.

317. T. Bak, J.J. Nissan, M.M. Allerhand, I.J. Deary, "Does Bilingualism Influence Cognitive Aging?" *Annals of Neurology* 75, no. 6 (June 2014): 959–963.

318. J. Mårtensson, J. Eriksson, N.C. Bodammer, M. Lindgren, M. Johansson, L. Nyberg, M. Lövdén, "Growth of Language-Related Brain Areas After Foreign Language Learning," *NeuroImage,* 63, no. 1 (October 2012): 240–244 doi: 10.1016 j.neuroimage.2012.06.043.

319. R.O. Roberts, R.H. Cham M.M. Mielke, Y.E. Geda, B.F. Boeve, M.M. Machulda, D.S. Knopman, R.C. Peterson, "Risk and Protective Factors for Cognitive Impairment in Persons Aged 85 Years and Older," *Neurology* 8, no. 4 (2015): 1–7.

320. A. Bolwerk, J. Mack-Andrick, F.R. Lang, A. Dörfler, C. Maihöfner, "How Art Changes Your Brain: Differential Effects of Visual Art Production and Cognitive Art Evaluation on Functional Brain Connectivity," *PLOS One* 9, no. 7 (July 1, 2014): e101035.

321. H. Noice, T. Noice, "An Arts Intervention for Older Adults Living in Subsidized Retirement Homes," Neuropsychology, Development and Cognition. Section B, Aging, Neuropsychology and Cognition 16, no. 1 (2009): 56–79.

322. H. Noice, T. Noice, "Extending the Reach of an Evidence-Based Theatrical Intervention," *Experimental Aging Research* 39, no. 4 (2013): 398–418.

323. M.C. Carlso, K.I. Erickson, A.F. Kramer, M.W. Voss, N. Bolea, M. Mielke, S. McGill, G.W. Rebok, T. Seeman, L.P. Fried, "Evidence for Neurocognitive Plasticity in At-Risk Older Adults: The Experience Corps Program," *The Journals of Gerontology. Series A, Biological Sciences and Medical Sciences* 62, no. 12 (December 2009):1275–1282.

324. S. Belleville, S. Mellah, C. de Boysson, J-F. Demonet, B. Bier, "The Pattern and Loci of Training-Induced Brain Changes in Healthy Older Adults Are Predicted by the Nature of the Intervention," *PLoS ONE* 9, no. 8 (August 2014): e102710 doi: 10.1371 journal.pone.0102710.

325. J.A. Anguerra, J. Boccanfuso, J.L. Rintoul, O. Al-Hashimi, F. Faraji, J. Janowich, E. Kong, Y. Larraburo, C. Rolle, E. Johnson, A. Gazzaley, "Video Game Training Enhances Cognitive Control in Older Adults," *Nature* 501 (September 2013): 97–101 doi:10.1038 nature12486.

326. Ibid.

327. Ibid.

328. J.G. Gasper, M.B. Neider, J.A. Crowell, A. Lutz, H. Kaczmarski, A.F. Kramer, "Are Gamers Better Crossers? An Examination of Action Video Game Experience and Dial Task Effects in a Simulated Street Crossing Task," *Human Factors* 56, no. 3 (May 2014): 443–452.

329. A. Nikolaidis, M.W. Voss, H. Lee, L.T. Vo, A.F. Kramer, "Parietal Plasticity After Training with a Complex Video Game is Associated with Individual Differences in Improvements in an Untrained Working Memory Task," *Frontiers in Human Neuroscience* 8, no. 169 (March 2014): doi: 10.3389 fnhum.2014.00169. eCollection 2014.

330. B.P. Lucey, R.J. Bateman, "Amyloid-B Diurnal Pattern: Possible Role of Sleep in Alzheimer's Disease Pathogenesis," *Neurobiology of Aging* 35, no. 2 (September 2014): S29–S34 *http: www.neurobiologyofaging.org article S0197-4580%2814%2900350-9 abstrac.*

331. J.J. Iliff, M. Nedergaard, "Is there a cerebral lymphatic system," *Stroke* 44, no. 601 (June 2013): S93S95.

332. L. Yang, B.T. Kress, H.J. Weber, M. Thiyagarajan, B. Wang, R. Deane, H. Benveniste, J.J. Iliff, M. Nedergaard, "Evaluating glymphatic pathway function utilizing clinically relevant intrathecal infusion of CSF tracer," *Journal of Translational Medicine* 11 no. 107 (May 2013): doi: 10.1186 1479-5876-11-107.

333. G. Tononi, C. Cirelli, "Sleep and the Price of Plasticity: From Synaptic and Cellular Homeostasis to Memory Consolidation and Integration," *Neuron*, 81, no. 1 (January 2014): 12–34 doi: 10.1016 j.neuron.2013.12.025.

334. A.P. Spira et al, "Self-reported Sleep and Ð-Amyloid Deposition in Community-Dwelling Older Adults," *JAMA Neurology* 70 no. 12 (December, 2013): 1537–1543 doi: 10.1001 jamaneurol.2013.4258.

335. J.C. Lo, K.K. Loh, H. Zheng, S. Sim, M. Chee, "Sleep Duration and Age-Related Changes in Brain Structure and Cognitive Performance," *SLEEP* 37, no. 7 (2014) doi: 10.5665 sleep.3832.

336. WebMD, "Sleep Disorders Health Center," accessed December 2014: *http: www.webmd.com sleep-disorders guide sleep-101.*

337. National Sleep Foundation, "What Happens When You Sleep," accessed December 2014 *http: sleepfoundation.org how-sleep-works what-happens-when-you-sleep.*

338. A.W. Varga, A. Kishi, J. Mantua, J. Lim, et al, "Apnea-Induced Rapid Eye Movement Sleep Disruption Impairs Human Spatial Navigational Memory," *The Journal of Neuroscience* 34, no. 44 (October 2014): 14571-14577.

339. R. Leproult, E.F. Colecchia, M. L.'Hermite-Baleriaux, E. Van Cauter, "Transition from Dim to Bright Light in the morning Induces an Immediate Elevation of Cortisol Levels," *The Journal of Clinical Endocrinology & Metabolism* 86 no. 1 (July 2013): doi: *http: dx.doi.org 10.1210 jcem.86.1.7102.*

340. M.G. Figueriro, "24-hr Lighting Scheme for Older Adults," *http: www.aia.org aiaucmp groups aia documents pdf aiab092627.pdf.*

341. Medline Plus, "Aging Changes in Sleep," accessed December 2014: *http: www.nlm.nih.gov medlineplus ency article 004018.htm.*

342. A.S.P. Lim, B.A. Ellison, J.L. Wang, L. Yu, J.A. Schneider, A.S. Buchman, D.A. Bennett, C.B. Saper, "Sleep Is Related to Neuron Numbers in the Ventrolateral Preoptic Intermediate Nucleus in Older Adults with and Without Alzheimer's Disease," *Brain* (August 2014): doi: *http: dx.doi.org 10.1093 brain awu222.*

343. P. A. Parmelee, C. A. Tighe, N. D. Dautovich, "Sleep disturbance in Osteoarthritis: Linkages with pain, disability and depressive symptoms," *Arthritis Care & Research*, (October, 2014): doi: 10.1002 acr.22459.

344. C.E. Sexton, A.B. Storsve, K.B. Walhovd, H. Johansen-Berg, A.M. Fjell, "Poor Sleep Quality is Associated with Increased Cortical Atrophy in Community-Dwelling Adults," *Neurology* 83, no. 11 (September 2014): 967–973.

345. S. J. Frenda, L. Patihis, E. F. Loftus, H. C. Lewis, K. M. Fenn, "Sleep Deprivation and False Memories," *Psychological Science* (July 2014): doi: 10.1177 0956797614534694.

346. C. Benedict, L. Byberg, J. Cedernaes, P.S. Hogenkamp, V. Giedratis, L. Kilander, L. Lind, L. Lannfelt, H. B. Schiöth, "Self-reported sleep disturbance is associated with Alzheimer's disease risk in men," *Alzheimer's & Dementia* (October, 2014): doi 10.1016 j.jalz.2014.08.104.

347. E. E. Devore, F. Grodstein, J.F. Duffy, M.J. Stampfer, C.A. Czeisler, E.S. Schernhammer, "Sleep Duration in Midlife and Later Life in Relation to Cognition," *Journal of the American Geriatrics Society* 62, no. 6 (June 2014): doi: 10.1111 jgs.12790.

348. M.A. Miller, H. Wright, C. Ji, F.P. Cappuccio, "Cross-Sectional Study of Sleep Quantity and Quality and Amnestic and Non-Amnestic Cognitive Function in an Ageing Population: The English Longitudinal Study of Ageing (ELSA)," *PLoS ONE*, 9, no. 6 (June 2014): e100991 doi: 10.1371 journal.pone.0100991.

349. J. Martinson, "So Marissa Mayer will be Skipping Maternity Leave—How Very American," *The Guardian* (July 2012), Accessed December 2014: *http: www.theguardian.com lifeandstyle the-womens-blog-with-jane-martinson 2012 jul 17 marissa-mayer-yahoo-working-childbirth.*

350. M. Lewis, "Obama's Way," *Vanity Fair* (October 2012) Accessed December, 2014: *http: www. vanityfair.com politics 2012 10 michael-lewis-profile-barack-obama.*

351. E. Rasskazova, I. Zavalko, A. Tkhostov, V. Dorohov, "High Intention to Fall Asleep Causes Sleep Fragmentation," *Journal of Sleep Research* 23 no. 3 (June 2014): 295–301 doi: 10.1111 jsr.12120.

352. M.G. Figueriro, "24-hr Lighting Scheme for Older Adults," *http: www.aia.org aiaucmp groups aia documents pdf aiab092627.pdf.*

353. N. Hanford, M. Figueiro, "Light Therapy and Alzheimer's Disease and Related Dementia: Past, Present and Future," *Journal of Alzheimer's Disease* 33, no. 4 (January 2013): 913–922.

354. Mariana Figuerio, "24-HR Lighting Scheme for Older Adults," Rensselaer Polytechnic Institute Lighting Research Center report: *http: www.aia.org aiaucmp groups aia documents pdf aiab092627.pdf.*

355. N. Hanford, M. Figueiro, "Light Therapy and Alzheimer's Disease and Related Dementia: Past, Present and Future," *Journal of Alzheimer's Disease* 33, no. 4 (January 2013): 913–922.

356. M. Figuerio, "24-HR Lighting Scheme for Older Adults," Rensselaer Polytechnic Institute Lighting Research Center report: *http: www.aia.org aiaucmp groups aia documents pdf aiab092627.pdf.*

357. K. Lanaj, R.E. Johnson, C.M. Barnes, "Beginning the workday yet already depleted? Consequences of late-night smartphone use and sleep," *Organizational Behavior and Human Decision Processes* 124, no. 1 (May 2014): 11–23 doi:10.1016 j.obhdp.2014.01.001.

358. A.S. Rahman, E.E. Flynn-Evans, D. Aeschbach, G.C. Brainard, et al, "Diurnal Spectral Sensitivity of the Acute Alerting Effects of Light," *SLEEP* 37, no. 2 (February 2014): 271–281.

359. J.J. Gooley, K. Chamberlain, K.A. Smith, et al, "Exposure to Room Light Before Bedtime Suppresses Melatonin Onset and Shortens Melatonin Duration in Humans," *The Journal of Clinical Endocrinology & Metabolism* 96, no. 3 (December 2010): doi: *http: dx.doi.org 10.1210 jc.2010-2098.*

360. J.A. Horne, A.J. Reid, "Night-time sleep EEG changes following body heating in a warm bath," *Electroencephalography and Clinical Neurophysiology* 62, no. 2 (February 1985): 154–157.

361. P.J. Murphy, S.S. Campbell, "Nighttime drop in body temperature: a physiological trigger for sleep onset?" *Sleep* 10, no. 7 (July 1997): 505–511.

362. P.D. Loprinzi, B.J. Cardinal, "Association Between Objectively-Measured Physical Activity and Sleep, NHANES 2005-2006," *Mental Health and Physical Activity* 4, no. 2 (December 2011): 65–69.

363. L.A. Irish, C.E. Kline, H.E. Gunn, D.J. Buysse, M.H. Hall, "The Role of Sleep Hygiene in Promoting Public Health," *Sleep Medicine Reviews* (October, 2014): doi: *http: dx.doi.org 10.1016 j.smrv.2014.10.001.*

364. S.S. Campbell, M.D. Stanchina, J.R. Schlang, P.J. Murphy, "Effects of a Month-Long Napping Regimen in Older Adults," *Journal of American Geriatric Society* 59, no. 2 (Feb. 2011): 224–232 doi: 10.1111 j.1532-5415.2010.03264.x.

365. B. Faraut, K.Z. Boudjeltia, M. Dyzma, A. Rousseau, E. David, P. Stenuit, T. Franck, P. Van Antwerpen, M. Vanhaeverbeek, M. Kekhors, "Benefits of Napping and an Extended Duration of Recovery Sleep on Alertness and Immune Cells After Acute Sleep Restriction," *Brain Behavior and Immunity* 25, no. 1 (Jan 2011): 16–24 doi: 10.1016 j.bbi.2010.08.001.

366. N. Novanto, L. Lack, "The effects of napping on cognitive functioning," *Progress in Brain Research* 185 (2010): 155–166 doi: 10.1016 B978-0-444-53702-7.00009-9.

367. Ibid.

368. Ibid.

369. C. Drake, T. Roehrs, J. Shambroom, T. Roth, "Caffeine Effects on Sleep Taken 0, 3, or 6 Hours Before Going to Bed," *Journal of Clinical Sleep Medicine* 11, no. 3 (2013): *http: dx.doi.org 10.5664 jcsm.3170.*

370. Y. Sagawa, H. Kondo, N. Matsubucci, T. Takemura, H. Kanayama, Y. Kaneko, T. Kanbayashi, Y. Hishikawa, Y. Shimizu, "Alcohol Has a Dose-Related Effect on Parasympathetic Nerve Activity During Sleep," *Alcoholism Clinical & Experimental Research* 35, no. 11 (November 2011): 2093–2100.

371. DrinkAware.co.uk "Alcohol and Sleep," Accessed December 2014: *https: www.drinkaware. co.uk check-the-facts health-effects-of-alcohol effects-on-the-body alcohol-and-sleep .*

372. L.A. Irish, C.E. Kline, H.E. Gunn, D.J. Buysse, M.H. Hall, "The Role of Sleep Hygiene in Promoting Public Health," *Sleep Medicine Reviews* (October, 2014): doi: *http: dx.doi.org 10.1016 j.smrv.2014.10.001.*

373. A.G. Harvey, S. Payne, "The management of unwanted pre-sleep thoughts in insomnia: Distraction with imagery versus general distraction," *Behaviour Research and Therapy*, 40, no 3 (March 2002): 267–277.

374. C.M. Portas, K. Krakow, P.A. Allen, O. Josephs, J.L. Armony, C.D. Frith," Auditory Processing Across the Sleep-Wake Cycle," *Neuron* 28. no 3 (December 2000): 991-999.

375. A. Rechtschaffen, P. Hauri, M. Zeitlin, "Auditory Waking Thresholds in REM and NREM Sleep Stages," *Perceptual and Motor Skills* 22 (1966): 927–942.

376. M.L. Stanchina, M. Abu-Hijeh, B.K. Chaudhry, V.V. Carlisle, R.P. Millman, "The Influence of White Noise on Sleep in Subjects Exposed to Noise," *Sleep Medicine* 6, no. 5 (September 2004): 423–428.

377. L. Krahn, B. Miller, "Where Do Companion Animals Sleep?" Presented at the 29th Annual Meeting of the Associated Professional Sleep Societies, June 2014.

378. W.R. Pigeon, M. Carr, C. Gorman, M.L. Perlis, "Effects of a tart cherry juice beverage on the sleep of older adults with insomnia: a pilot study," *Journal of Medicinal Food* 13, no. 3 (June, 2010):579–83.

379. H.H. Lin, P.S. Tsai, S.C. Fang, J.F. Liu, "Effect of kiwifruit consumption on sleep quality in adults with sleep problems," *Asia Pacific Journal of Clinical Nutrition* 20, no. 2 (2011): 169–174.

380. P. Montgomery, et al, "Fatty Acids and Sleep in UK Children: Subjective and Pilot Objective Sleep Results from the DOLAB Study—a Randomized Controlled Trial," *Journal of Sleep Research* 23, no. 4 (March 2014): 364–388 doi: 10.1111 jsr.12135.

381. A.L. Hansen, L. Dahl, G. Olson, D. Thornton, I.E. Graff, L. Froyland, J.F. Thayer, S. Paliesen, "Fish Consumption, Sleep, Daily Functioning and Heart Rate Variability," *Journal of Clinical Sleep Medicine* 10, no. 5 (2010): 567–575 10.5664 jcsm.3714.

382. N. Goel, H. Kim, R. Lao, "An Olfactory Stimulus Modifies Nighttime Sleep in Young Men and Women," *Chronobiology International* 22 no. 5 (2005): 889–904.

383. W. Sayorwan, V. Siripornpanich, T. Piriyapunyaporn, N. Kotachabhakdi, N. Ruangrungsi, "The Effects of Lavender Oil Inhalation on Emotional States, Autonomic Nervous System, and Brain Electrical Activity," *Journal of Medical Association of Thailand* 95, no. 4 (April 2012): 598–606.

384. M.J. Cordi, A.A. Schlarb, B. Rasch, "Deepening Sleep by Hypnotic Suggestion," *SLEEP* 37, no. 6 (2014): doi: 10.5665 sleep.3778.

385. H. Kadotani, T. Kadotani, T. Young, P.E. Peppard, L. Finn, I.M. Colrain, G.M. Murphy, E. Mignot, "Association Between Alipoprotein E epsilon4 and sleep-disordered breathing in adults," *JAMA* 285, no. 22 (June 2001): 2888–2890.

386. N. Canessa, L. Ferini-Strambi, "Sleep-Disordered Breathing and Cognitive Decline in Older Adults," *JAMA* 306, no. 6 (August 2011):654–655.

387. K. Yaffe, A.M. Laffan, S.L. Harrison, S. Redline, A.P. Spira, K.E. Ensrud, S. Ancoli-Israel, K.L. Stone, "Sleep-Disordered Breathing, Hypoxia, and Risk of Mild Cognitive Impairment and Dementia in Older Women," *JAMA* 306, no. 6 (August 20111): 613–619.

388. S. Ancoli-Israel, B. Palmer, J.R. Cooke, J. Corey-Bloom, L. Florentino, L. Liu, L. Ayalon, F. He, J. Loredo, "Cognitive Effects of Treating Obstructive Sleep Apnea in Alzheimer's Disease: a Randomized Controlled Study," *Journal of the American Geriatrics Society* 56, no. 11 (November 2008): 2076–2081.

389. H. Bao, X. Pan, et al, "Acupuncture for Treatment of Insomnia: A Systematic Review of Randomized Controlled Trials," *Journal of Alternative and Complementary Medicine* 15, no. 11 (November 2011): 1171–1186.

390. A.O. Freire, G.C. Sugai, F.S. Chrispin, S.M. Togeiro, Y. Yamamura, L.E. Mello, S. Tufik, "Treatment of Moderate Obstructive Sleep Apnea Syndrome with Acupuncture: A Randomized, Placebo-Controlled Pilot Trial," *Sleep Medicine* 8, no 1 (January 2007): 43–50.

391. T. Kwok, P.C. Leung, Y.K. Wing, I. Ip, B. Wong, D.W. Ho, W.M. Wong, F. Ho, "The Effectiveness of Acupuncture on the Sleep Quality of Elderly with Dementia," *Journal of Clinical Interventions in Aging* 8 (2013): 923–929 doi: 10.2147 CIA.S45611.

392. B.P. Kolla, J.K. Lovely, M.P. Mansukhani, T.I. Morgenthaler, "Zolpidem is Independently Associated with Increased Risk of Inpatient Falls," *Journal of Hospital Medicine* 8, no. 1 (Jan 2013): 1–6.

393. D.J. Frey, J.D. Ortega, C. Wiseman, C.T. Farley, K.P. Wright, "Influence of Aolpididem and Sleep Inertia on Balance and Cognition During Nighttime Awakening: a Randomized Placebo-Controlled Trial," *Journal of the American Geriatric Society* 59, no. 1 (Jan 2011): 73–81 doi: 10.1111 j.1532-5415.2010.03229.x.

394. The Centers for Disease Control and Prevention "Falls Among Older Adults: An Overview," accessed December 2014: *http: www.cdc.gov homeandrecreationalsafety falls adultfalls.html.*

395. E.S. LeBlanc, T.A. Hillier, K.L. Pedula, et al, "Hip Fracture and Increased Short-Term but not Long-Term Mortality in Healthy Older Women," *Archives of Internal Medicine* 171, no. 20 (November 2011): 1831–1837.

396. N. Hanford, M. Figueiro, "Light Therapy and Alzheimer's Disease and Related Dementia: Past, Present and Future," *Journal of Alzheimer's Disease* 33, no. 4 (January 2013): 913–922 *http: www.ncbi.nlm.nih.gov pmc articles PMC3553247* .

397. M.G. Figueiro, "24-hr Lighting Scheme for Older Adults," http: www.aia.org aiaucmp groups aia documents pdf aiab092627.pdf.

398. N. Hanford, M. Figueiro, "Light Therapy and Alzheimer's Disease and Related Dementia: Past, Present and Future," *Journal of Alzheimer's Disease* 33, no. 4 (January 2013): 913–922.

399. P. Ranasignhe, S. Pigera, G.A. Premakumara, P. Galappaththy, G.R. Constantine, P. Katulanda, "Medicinal Properties of 'Tue' Cinnamon (CinnamomumZeylanicum): a Systematic Review," *BMC Complementary Alternative Medicine* 13 (October 2013): 275.

400. A.W. Allen, E. Schwartzman, W.L. Baker, C.I. Coleman, O.J. Phung, "Cinnamon Use in Type 2 Diabetes: An Updated Systematic Review and Meta Analysis," *Annals of Family Medicine* 11, no. 5 (September-October 2013): 452–459.

401. M. Peppa, J. Uribarri, H. Vlassara, "Glucose, Advanced Glycation End Products and Diabetes Complications: What Is New and What Works," *Clinical Diabetes* 21, no. 4 (October 2003): 186–187.

402. American Diabetes Association, "How Stress Affects Diabetes," accessed December 2014: *http: www.diabetes.org living-with-diabetes complications mental-health stress.html.*

403. J.W. Hughes, D.M. Fresco, R. Myerscough, M.H.M. van Dulmen, L.E. Carlson, R. Josephson, "Randomized Controlled Trial of Mindfulness-Based Stress Reduction for Prehypertension," *Psychosomatic Medicine* 75, no. 8 (October, 2013): 721–728 doi: 10.1097 %u200BPSY.0b013e3182a3e4e5.

404. S. G. Sheps, "Does Drinking Alcohol Affect Your Blood Pressure?" of the Mayo Clinic, accessed December 2014: *http: www.mayoclinic.org diseases-conditions high-blood-pressure expert-answers blood-pressure faq-20058254.*

405. E.B. Rimm, et al, "Prospective Study of Moderate Alcohol Consumption and Risk of Hypertension in Young Women," *JAMA Internal Medicine* 162, no. 5 (March 2002): 569–574.

406. M. Duncan, N. Clarke, S. Birch, J. Tallis, J. Hankey, E. Bryant, E. Eyre, "The Effect of Green Exercise on Blood Pressure, Heart Rate and Mood State in Primary School Children," *International Journal of Environmental Research and Public Health* 11, no. 4 (2014): 3678–3688 doi: 10.3390 ijerph110403678.

407. D. Liu, B. Fernandez, A. Hamilton, N.N. Lang, J.M.C. Gallagher, D. Newby, M. Feelisch, R.B. Weller, "UVA Irradiation of Human Skin Vasodilates Arterial Vasculature and Lowers Blood Pressure Independently of Nitric Oxide Synthase," *Journal of Investigative Dermatology* 134, no. 7 (January 2014): 1–38.

408. F. Zeidan, N.S. Gordon, J. Merchant, P. Goolkasian, "The Effects of Brief Mindfulness Meditation Training on Experimentally Induced Pain," *The Journal of Pain* 11, no. 3 (March 2010):1–11.

409. J.C. Norcross, D.J. Vangarelli, "The Resolution Solution: Longitudinal Examination of New Year's Resolutions," *Journal of Substance Abuse* 1, no. 2 (1988–1999): 127–134.

410. A.M. Graybiel, "Habits, Rituals and the Evaluative Brain," *Annual Review of Neuroscience* 31 (2008): 359–387.

411. D.T. Neal, W. Wood, M. Wu, D. Kuriander, "The Pull of the Past: When Do Habits Persist Despite Conflict with Motives," *Personality and Social Psychology Bulletin* 37, no. 11 (November 2011): 1428–1437.

412. M. Muraven, R.E. Baumeister, "Self-Regulation and Depletion of Limited Resources: Does Self-Control Resemble a Muscle?" *Psychological Bulletin* 126 no. 2 (2000): 247–259.

413. R.F. Baumeister, E. Bratslavsky, M. Muraven, D.M. Tice, "Ego Depletion: Is the Active Self a Limited Resource?" *Journal of Personality and Social Psychology* 74, no. 5 (May 1998): 1252–1265.

414. A. R. Silva, S. Pinho, L.M. M. Macedo, and C. J. Moulin, "Benefits of SenseCam Review on Neuropsychological Test Performance," *American Journal of Preventative Medicine* 44, no. 3 (March 2013): 302–307 doi: 10.1016 j.amepre.2012.11.005.

415. K. Van Ittersum, B Wansink, "Plate Size and Suggestibiliy: The Deboeuf Illusion's Bias and Eating Behavior," *The Journal of Consumer Research* 39, no. 2 (August 2012): http: www.jstor.org stable 10.1086 662615.

416. L. Lipsitz, M. Lough, J. Niemi, T. Travison, H. Howlett, B. Manor, "A Shoe Insole Delivering Subsensory Vibratory Noise Improves Balance and Gait in Healthy Elderly People," *Archives of Physical Medicine* 96, no. 3 (March 2015): 432–439.

417. B. Borah, P. Sacco, V. Zarotsky, "Predictors of Adherence Among Alzheimer's Disease Receiving Oral Therapy," *Current Medicine Research and Opinion* 26, no. 8 (August 2010): 1957–1965.

418. M.T. Brown, J.K. Bussell, "Medication Adherence: WHO Cares?" *Mayo Clinic Proceedings* 86, no. 4 (April 2011): 304–314.

419. J.L. Molinuevo, F.J. Arranz, "Impact of Transdermal Drug Delivery on Treatment Adherence in Patients with Alzheimer's Disease," *Expert Reviews of Neurotherapeutics* 12, no. 1 (January 2012):31–37.

Index

About the Author

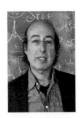

Since 2004, **Kenneth S. Kosik, MD,** has been the Harriman Professor of Neuroscience Research and Co-Director of the Neuroscience Research Institute at the University of California, Santa Barbara. Previously, he was a professor of neurology and neuroscience at Harvard Medical School, and a senior neurologist at Brigham and Women's Hospital, where he was one of the founding physicians of the Memory Disorders Clinic. His lifelong work is research into the cause and treatment of neurodegeneration, particularly Alzheimer's disease. His study of a group of interrelated families in rural Colombia who suffer from early onset Alzheimer's has been the subject of several documentaries. Dr. Kosik also founded and served as Medical Director of the non-profit Cognitive Fitness and Innovative Therapies (CFIT), a model "brain shop" that helped clients maintain and improve their cognitive function. Dr. Kosik, who received his medical degree from the Medical College of Pennsylvania and served as chief resident at Tufts New England Medical Center, has been featured in the *New York Times, Wall Street Journal,* and on CNN as an expert on brain health. He lives and works in Santa Barbara, California. Visit his website at KennethSKosikMD.com.

Alisa Bowman is a journalist, book collaborator, and author and co-author of several books, including *Project: Happily Ever After* and *Pitch Perfect.* She also has family members who have suffered from Alzheimer's. She lives and works in Pennsylvania.

Photograph by Jen Messecar